Principles of X-Ray Diagnosis of the Skull

Second Edition

G. H. du Boulay
FRCR, FRCP
Professor and Head of Lysholm Radiological Department,
National Hospital for Nervous Diseases, Queen Square
London; formerly Consultant Radiologist,
St. Bartholomew's Hospital, London

BUTTERWORTHS
LONDON – BOSTON
Sydney–Wellington–Durban–Toronto

THE BUTTERWORTH GROUP

ENGLAND

Butterworth & Co (Publishers) Ltd
London: 88 Kingsway, WC2B 6AB

AUSTRALIA

Butterworths Pty Ltd
Sydney: 586 Pacific Highway, Chatswood, NSW 2067
Also at Melbourne, Brisbane, Adelaide and Perth

SOUTH AFRICA

Butterworth & Co (South Africa) (Pty) Ltd
Durban: 152–154 Gale Street

NEW ZEALAND

Butterworths of New Zealand Ltd
Wellington: T & W Young Building,
77–85 Customhouse Quay 1, CPO Box 472

CANADA

Butterworth & Co (Canada) Ltd
Toronto: 2265 Midland Avenue, Scarborough, Ontario M1P 4S1

USA

Butterworths (Publishers) Inc
Boston: 10 Tower Office Park, Woburn, Mass. 01801

First published 1965
Second edition 1980
© Butterworth & Co (Publishers) Ltd, 1980

ISBN 0 407 001174

British Library Cataloguing in Publication Data

Du Boulay, George Houssemayne
    Principles of X-ray diagnosis of the skull. –
2nd ed.
    1. Skull – Radiography
    I. Title
    617'.514'07572   RC936   78-40364

ISBN 0-407-00117-4

Typeset by Butterworths Litho Preparation Department
Printed and bound by Wm. Clowes & Sons Ltd, Beccles and London

PREFACE TO THE SECOND EDITION

Most medical teaching changes radically in 14 years, but skull radiology is a mature subject; advances in basic knowledge have been less than those concerned with the use to be made of that knowledge. Two important determinants of practice have been the need to economize and the introduction of CT scanning. It has been shown by Bull and his co-workers that in skilled hands a single lateral view together with a reliable neurological examination are enough to indicate whether further views are necessary, but skill is as valuable as ever it was. So, too, is neurological training. As for the impact of CT scanning, neuroradiologists are making fools of themselves every week and delaying diagnoses by interpreting scans without looking at the plain radiographs, at the same time it has to be admitted that there are some neurological conditions in which plain x-rays are less important than they used to be.

The literature of the late 1960's and early 1970's was full of work on developmental deformity. This is a highly specialized field and a problem to integrate into a book designed like this one to teach basic principles. It is hoped that the new chapter and additions to other chapters will be adequate without overweighting the text. I am especially grateful to my friends Dr Dick Hoare and Dr Alan Chrispin for providing illustrations of developmental abnormalities.

The reproduction of x-ray pictures requires great attention. No less should be given to the way they are looked at. These are designed to be used in ordinary domestic illumination and not, for instance, in bright sunshine. Examined under the appropriate illumination they nearly all show what they are intended to.

The bibliography is not exhaustive but is nevertheless large enough to be useful to the established neuroradiologist. A simple method has been sought to help those who are looking up the literature of specific subjects by adding an index letter while keeping the arrangement alphabetical.

Finally, I wish to thank my secretary, Miss Johns, for an enormous amount of work in typing, checking the text and the not inconsiderable records of 14 years, reading.

G.H. du Boulay

ACKNOWLEDGEMENTS

A textbook such as this is written around a collection of cases and could not be begun without the radiographs. They have nearly all been made over a long period of time by a comparatively few radiographers. The care and skill that radiographers exercise is the basis of radiology, and although I do not thank them all by name here, I would like them to know how grateful I am.

My radiological and clinical colleagues at St. Bartholomew's Hospital and the National Hospitals for Nervous Diseases, Queen Square and, Maida Vale, may recognize the pictures I have borrowed. These colleagues are the sources of a great deal of the knowledge I have tried here to organize and I am in their debt. Dr David Sutton, in particular, investigated many of the Maida Vale patients, and Dr R. A. Kemp Harper, Dr George Simon and Dr W. D. Nichol collected a number of the earlier radiographs of the neurological and neurosurgical patients at St Bartholomew's Hospital.

I have used cases seen by Dr Hugh Davies, Dr James Bull, Dr Brian Kendall and Dr Ivan Moseley at Queen Square, and I owe a particular debt to my secretary at Queen Square, Miss Johns, for her help in finding the new illustrations for the Second Edition. I have previously acknowledged much help with the First Edition. Here I must repeat my thanks to the staff of Butterworths for their editorial work and encouragement.

G.H. du Boulay

CONTENTS

INTRODUCTION

This book is intended for students of radiology, before and after their diploma examination, and for those clinicians to whom the head is of special concern. There are already a number of text-books in which the skull is mentioned incidentally as part of a description of general skeletal pathology. The principal aim here is to explain more fully the effects of disease of the nervous system, and although generalized non-neurological conditions are included, both for their own sake and as differential diagnoses, much more space and fundamental thought is given to subjects such as raised intracranial pressure than to the local effects of general bone disease.

The author believes that in the process of examining a set of skull radiographs, the system of thought is something of the nature suggested in the central eight chapters—that the eye being directed in turn to different regions of the head, the memory ruminates upon possible causes of any translucencies, sclerotic areas or malformations that may be seen. For this reason the arrangement of chapters is a hybrid of many possible (and on the surface more logical) classifications.

The particular regional subdivision which has been adopted reflects the traditional method of neuroradiology which is to describe in turn the vault, the sella and the base, and then any intracranial calcification which may be present.

There are two main disadvantages of this method. In the first place, a good deal of repetition is unavoidable and will irritate the more knowledgeable (but will perhaps help the beginner). In the second place, it is very difficult to write a text-book of this style in such a way that it is easy to read, for the attention is broken by a multitude of subheadings.

The reader's best approach is to use the subheadings for a preliminary reconnaissance of each main section

and not to attempt more until the general scheme has been appreciated.

It is hoped that by cross-references tedious duplication has been avoided; and that the quantity of illustrations, including the new and improved ones in this second edition, will enliven a pictorial memory. There are 390 of them.

The radiology of ears, nose, throat and eyes has much common ground with neuroradiology, and in a fairly simple form these subjects are also dealt with. The radiology of the ear falls into its place in the chapters devoted to the skull base, but the nose, the nasopharynx, the sinuses and the orbits have a chapter on their own. The mandible and teeth have little connection with neuroradiology and are not dealt with.

Four subjects merit individual discussion because of their practical importance. These are Raised Intracranial Pressure, Head Injuries, Developmental Abnormalities (an entirely new chapter) and Radiography (in the last-named chapter a number of normal radiographs may be found, their features are numbered and the key is facing page 372. In order to give the reader an overall view at an early stage, Raised Intracranial Pressure appears first in the book.

The reader should be warned that the description of changes in the sella due to raised intracranial pressure goes somewhat beyond the usual teaching, particularly in asserting that these changes may be recognized and are significant in the old as well as in the young. A further warning is necessary (it is repeated in the text)—much skull radiography is done without high definition screens, with inexact technique and with film and processing which so interfere with definition that the fine structure of the vault and early erosions or loss of clear-cut shadows of the walls of the sella are counterfeited. As noted in the introduction to the first edition, radiology continues to head in the direction of histology where there is a place for both high and low power lenses—high and low definition techniques; high definition where radiation dose is of less importance and immobility makes it possible, lower definition where radiation must be cut or speed is essential. With further technical developments these two forms of examination will become more obviously distinct and may require quite different apparatus.

A few more references have been addded to the text, but these have in general been kept to a minimum in order to make the book less cumbersome for the beginner and not because of a lack of indebtedness to the works of others. To those whose published works seem to have been incorporated into the pages, but who find no acknowledgement, apologies are offered.

This is, in a special sense, a personal book and as the illustrations will show, a real attempt has been made to write nothing that has not come within the author's experience. Where this has proved impossible, an indication is usually given.

The reader should be aware of the division between generally accepted fact and statements of the author's original opinion. His ideas about the sella are already sufficiently hedged, and work on the effect of raised intracranial pressure in childhood has been published previously. At the time of the first edition there was no other mention in the literature of the nature of the thickening which takes place in the vault when pressure is relieved but this is now probably accepted by all. One perhaps original observation about osteoporosis circumscripta added in the first edition has been left in the second although it still awaits confirmation. With these exceptions the book contains nothing which has not already been accepted by most radiologists, and any differences which may be discovered are only those of emphasis or omission.

The book may be read in a variety of ways. The text is short enough to manage from cover to cover in a few hours. Any chapter may be taken separately, but the cross-references should always be followed if such a method is used. For those who need to refer to a few specific diseases, for example meningioma, an index is given on page 395. Lastly, since the captions to the illustrations are lengthy, a considerable amount may be learned simply by turning over the pages and looking at the pictures.

G.H. du Boulay

1 RAISED INTRACRANIAL PRESSURE

The intracranial pressure may be raised as a result of a number of different conditions.

(1) A large intracranial mass, such as new growth, abscess or haematoma, raises pressure by displacement and if it appears quickly will have a greater effect than if the brain and blood vessels have time for accommodation.

(2) Obstructive hydrocephalus may follow a partial or complete block of the cerebrospinal fluid pathways by an intracranial mass or congenital anatomical abnormalities or may be post-infective or post-haemorrhagic. Hydrocephalus may be associated with a choroid plexus papilloma. Raised intracranial pressure has been described in severe chronic enphysema with cough.

(3) Cerebral oedema may occur around a neoplasm or abscess. It may also be present as a result of encephalitis, cerebral infarction or vascular hypertension.

(4) Craniostenosis (in those severe cases where skull growth falls short of the requirements of the growing brain).

The manifestations of raised intracranial pressure in radiographs of the skull are few in number and, in the main, not peculiar to particular causes. The changes to be described are acute and chronic with variations in infancy, childhood and adult life. In certain cases of chronic obstructive hydrocephalus, the radiographs show some features which are an aid in the localization of the obstruction. The most chronic changes are more likely to be seen with slow-growing frontal tumours.

In the systematic description which follows, it may not be easy for those unfamiliar with neuroradiology to understand which observations are of most frequent clinical importance. They are, in the adult, the changes in the sella turcica, and in the child, the changes in the vault.

About one-third of all patients whose raised intracranial pressure persists for more than 5 or 6 weeks eventually show evidence of its effect upon the routine skull radiographs. Headache and papilloedema are found in many of them but not in all.

INFANCY

VAULT

In the ante-natal period and in the first few weeks of life the head is able to enlarge very rapidly, due to spreading of the unformed sutures. The bones of the vault may be thinner than normal, and sometimes if the cause of the rise in intracranial pressure has begun early enough there will be defects in ossification in the parietal or frontal bones — one form of craniolacunia (*Figures 1, 2, 3a* and *80*).

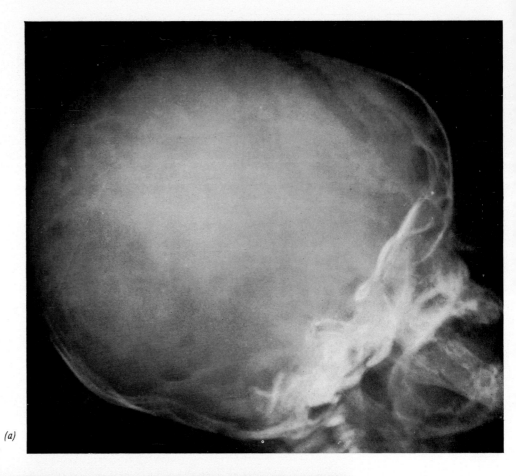

(a)

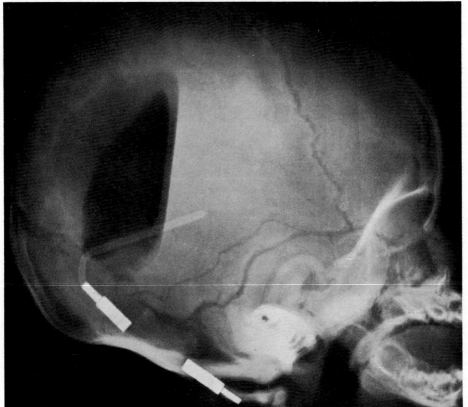

Figure 1. An example of the type of craniolacunia associated with congenital hydrocephalus. (a) Aged 1 week. (b) At 3 months after operation for the meningomyelocoele and for hydrocephalus. The skull is much more normal though still very thin posteriorly

(b)

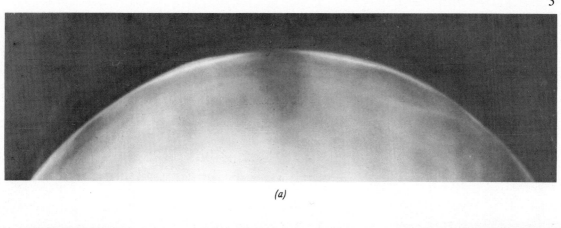

(a)

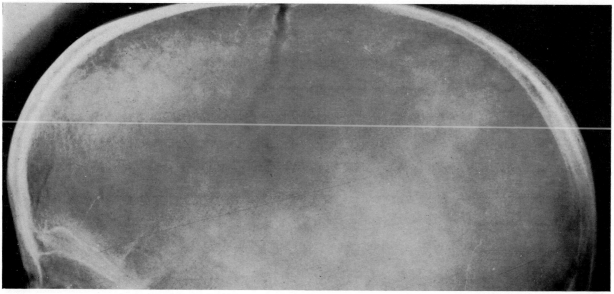

(b)

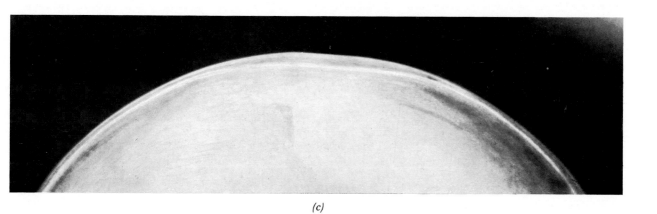

(c)

Figure 2. Progress of hydrocephalus. (a) Half-axial view. A boy aged 5 months with communicating hydrocephalus. The head is large, the sutures are spread and the bones thin. A theca-peritoneal anastomosis was performed. (b) The fontanelle became indrawn and the anastomosis appeared to function well for 3 months, but drainage of cerebrospinal fluid into the peritoneum then ceased and the operation was repeated on the opposite side, producing a further improvement for another 9 months. The intracranial pressure then again increased. The lateral and half axial views show how much thicker the bones have become. The sagittal suture has closed but suture diastasis is present elsewhere. There is little attempt at interdigitation, and it may be that this is because closure had almost occurred before this fresh episode of spreading (cont.)

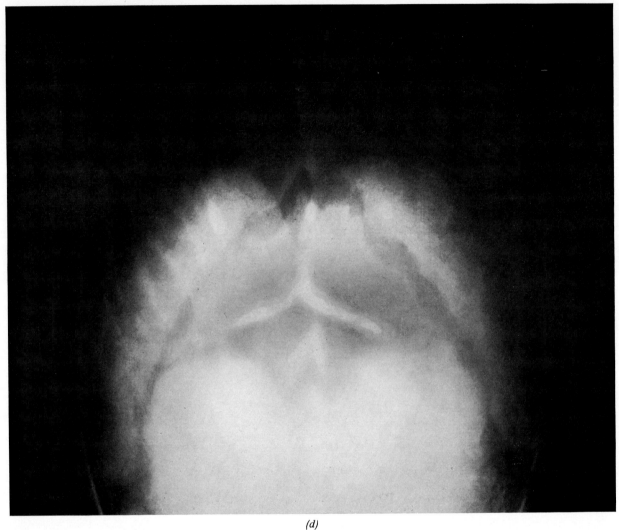

(d)

Figure 2 (cont.). (d) One month later there has been a great increase in diastasis; but a further operation reduced the intracranial pressure and the child subsequently improved

However, only very few faint convolutional impressions are usually visible on the vault bones either in the normal or in infants with hydrocephalus.

SELLA

After a few weeks of raised intracranial pressure, a loss of the crisp outline of the lamina dura of the sella turcica may be observed even in infancy but is always less obvious than suture diastasis.

Evidence of the cause

The commonest cause of raised intracranial pressure in infancy is hydrocephalus, due to a defect of absorption, or to a congenital block at some point in the posterior ventricular pathways. There is frequently an associated meningocoele of the spine.

The skull radiographs may provide some evidence of the position of the obstruction.

In aqueduct stenosis the supratentorial part of the skull may enlarge out of proportion to the posterior fossa which remains shallow. In the author's experience this is most difficult to assess, and in general is a sign of limited value.

In the Dandy–Walker syndrome of atresia of the exits from the fourth ventricle (*Figure 3*), the great dilatation of the fourth ventricle may cause a visible ballooning of the posterior fossa, particularly the squamous occipital bone as well as upward displacement of the attachment of the tentorium (transverse sinus).

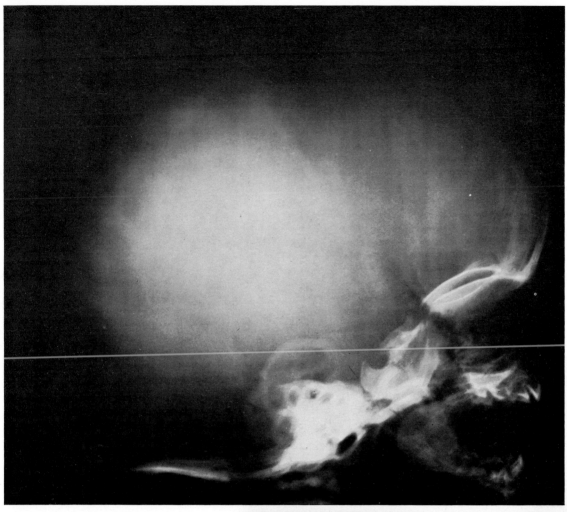

(a)

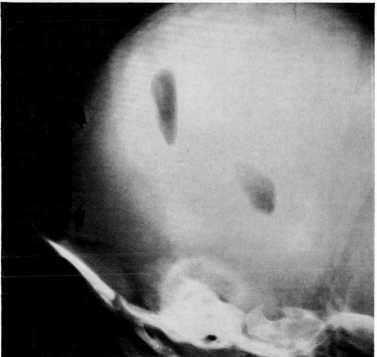

Figure 3. (a) A lateral radiograph showing great enlargement of the posterior fossa with elevation of the grooves for the transverse sinuses due either to developmental atresia of the exits from the fourth ventricle or to enlargement of the cisterna magna. (b) Atresia of the fourth ventricle foramina (Dandy–Walker syndrome). A baby aged 5 weeks who was well for the first 4 weeks of life and then rapidly developed progressive signs of hydrocephalus. At the age of 8 weeks, when bulging of the occiput had become more obvious, ventriculography showed air outlining a small part of the enormously expanded fourth ventricle (arrows). A very similar appearance, with or without signs of hydrocephalus, is found in both conditions. The cisterna magna may even protrude upwards through an opening in the tentorium near the torcula. Not all cases of atresia of the fourth ventricle exits show bony deformity

(b)

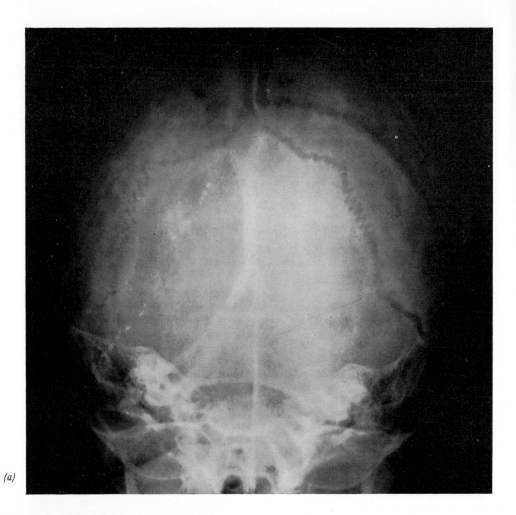

(a)

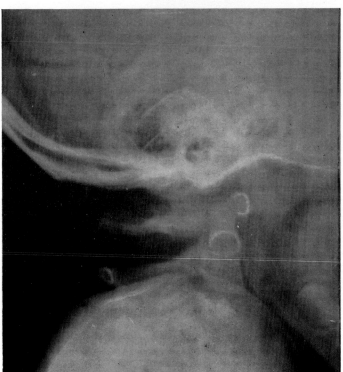

Figure 4a and b. Arnold–Chiari malformation in a child aged 2 years who had had a myelomeningocoele operated on in infancy and later developed hydrocephalus. There is suture diastasis, asymmetrical because the right half of the coronal suture fused during a period of relief from raised intracranial pressure. The foramen magnum is very large and the upper cervical canal is wide. (There is also an unfused posterior arch of atlas.) A large Arnold–Chiari malformation occupied the canal down to C 3

(b)

Meningocoele is commonly associated with an Arnold—Chiari malformation (*Figure 4*). In such cases it may be possible to see that the upper cervical spinal canal is unusually wide.

In the management of infants with hydrocephalus, treated by surgical methods, radiological assessment of progress may be very valuable. Repeated examinations may show changes which are bewildering unless the alterations which may occur following relief of raised pressure are also understood. These are dealt with at the end of this chapter and are illustrated particularly in *Figures 25* and *26*.

It is interesting, as yet unexplained but of clinical importance, that neonates with spinal meningocoeles may show increased convolutional impressions (craniolacunia) on their skull radiographs *before* there is any obvious enlargement of the head. In such cases, in the author's experience, hydrocephalus soon declares itself.

There is still confusion and doubt about the relationship of craniolacunia (Lückenschödel) and increased convolutional impressions. It is said that in craniolacunia the strands of bone between the defects do not correspond to cerebral sulci (Harwood Nash, personal communication). In the beaten silver skull of older children the thicker bone does certainly lie over some of the sulci (look at the Sylvian fissure in *Figure 11a*). It was because the question is unresolved that in the first paragraph of this section on page 1 the phrase 'one form of craniolacunia' was used. In neonates with meningomyelocoele or related defects the association with subsequent rapid development of hydrocephalus is so strong (McRae, 1966) that it is reasonable to believe the interaction of intracranial and intrauterine pressures determine the abnormal form of vault ossification. McRae has denied that raised intracranial pressure is necessary for the formation of craniolacunia on the grounds that it may be found in babies with meningoencephalocoeles and small heads, but perhaps one should not presuppose that the intracranial pressure of these babies was normal *in utero*.

After birth craniolacunia defects gradually disappear. In many children they are replaced by the signs of rapidly developing hydrocephalus. By 4—8 months, if the child survives, the vault generally shows no sign of this specific abnormality, though exceptions may be found (*Figure 80*).

CHILDHOOD

In childhood, raised intracranial pressure may be of recent onset or long-standing; each has its own radiographic signs.

Raised intracranial pressure of recent onset (acute) (*Figures 5* and *6*)

VAULT

Up to the age of 8 or 9 years, diastasis of the sutures of the vault occurs easily and may sometimes take place in a few days. After the age of 10 years, suture diastasis becomes uncommon except in very chronic conditions which may have had their origin before the age at which the sutures knit firmly. Very rarely, suture diastasis begins in late childhood or even in adult life, but it is not then evidence of a recent rise in intracranial pressure.

Severe degrees of suture diastasis are easy to diagnose, except when the vault bones are so thin that their edges are difficult to make out, but small degress of suture diastasis can be difficult to recognize unless the observer is familiar with the normal. Erasmie and Ringertz (1976) have published normal measurements which may be helpful. The sutures which spread most easily are the coronal and sagittal, and the ideal radiograph on which to observe these is taken in the full axial (submento-vertical) position in which the sutures, free of optical enlargement may be observed clearly through the structures of the middle fossa. This is one of the reasons for the importance of the full axial view in childhood.

SELLA

In childhood, as well as in the adult, raised intracranial pressure due to any cause may be associated with alterations in the bones of the sella turcica. Microscopically, the change in the bones consists of small confluent erosions in the thin cortical layer and loss of trabeculae in the cancellous structure. The erosions are most commonly seen on the anterior surface of the dorsum sellae near its base and in the floor of the pituitary fossa. The earliest radiographic evidence may sometimes be observed after 5 weeks of raised intracranial pressure in both child and adult, the affected cortex becoming interrupted or disappearing altogether. In many cases, however, the abnormality will be much slower to appear and in as many as two-thirds of all cases of raised intracranial pressure is not seen at all. If the disease continues and the rise in intracranial pressure becomes chronic, these alterations from the normal become more severe. It should be emphasized that the smaller, early (and therefore more important) erosions may only be visible on very good radiographs made with a high definition technique by modern apparatus.

The diagnosis of raised intracranial pressure must not be made from such evidence on indifferent pictures.

Long-standing raised intracranial pressure (*Figures 7—13*)

VAULT

Sutures

Up to the age of 8 or 9 years, suture diastasis is likely to be present and it may be found after this if the cause for the raised intracranial pressure is sufficiently long-standing. Although growth may tend to close the widened sutures, this closure is rarely complete until the raised intracranial pressure has been relieved. In children with long-standing raised intracranial pressure, the sutures often show very deep interdigitations, having a spiky appearance and a still translucent, irregular gap persisting between the bones. A somewhat similar appearance may be found in disseminated neuroblastoma or in the reticuloses where extradural and subpericranial metastatic deposits cause erosion and interference with ossification as well as an increase in the intracranial pressure. In these cases there may also be some spicular subpericranial new bone formation. Other bones may also be involved.

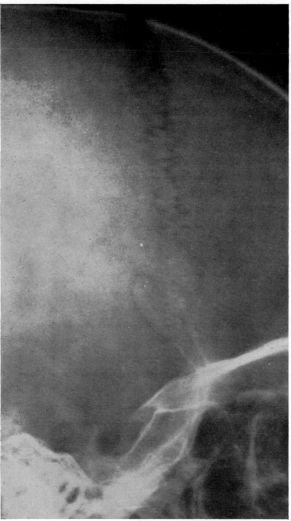

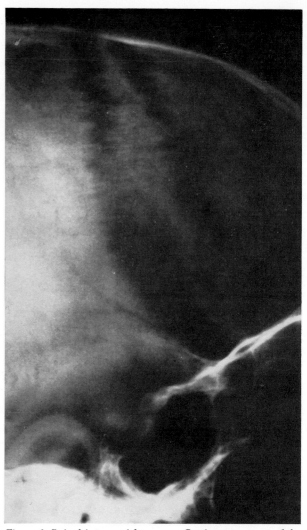

Figure 5. Raised intracranial pressure. A child aged 5 years with a history of raised intracranial pressure of 8 week's duration. The lamina dura of the posterior part of the sella turcica has disappeared (there is possibly also early suture diastasis)

Figure 6. Raised intracranial pressure. Cystic astrocytoma of the cerebellum in a child. The sella shows complete loss of bone detail of its whole floor, in spite of a well-developed sphenoid sinus, and of the front of the dorsum. There is diastasis of sutures, particularly the coronal suture

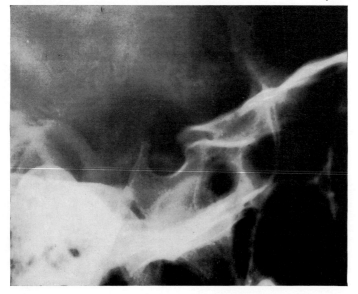

Figure 7. A patient aged 8 years with papilloedema in one half of one retina and cerebellar signs of 5 weeks' duration. The anterior surface of the dorsum sellae has lost its cortex. The tip of the dorsum sellae is more affected than the base

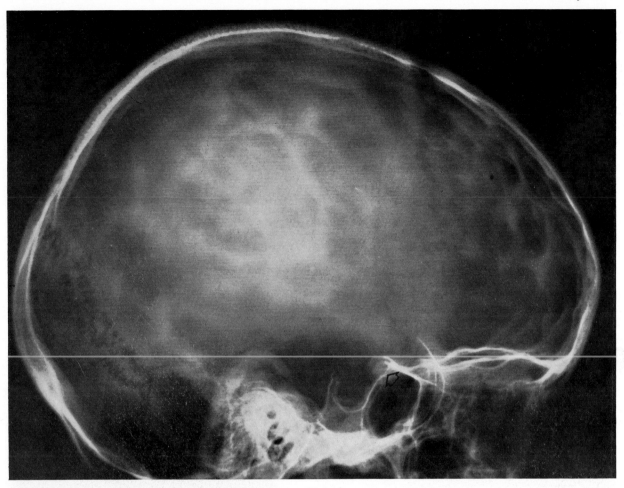

(a)

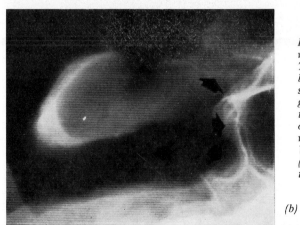

(b)

Figure 8. A child suffering from a posterior fossa tumour. (a) Lateral view. The sella appears deep because of a sloping sulcus chiasmaticus. The tip of the dorsum sellae or the posterior clinoids, or both, may be slightly eroded. It is possible that the large and steeply sloping sulcus chiasmaticus may be due to hydrocephalus during active skull growth. This is the appearance which probably gave rise originally to the term 'J sella'. It is a definite indication of a very long-standing obstruction beginning in childhood or infancy (or before). The convolutional impressions are very prominent, even over the vertex. (b) Ventriculogram showing the front end of the ballooned third ventricle (closed arrows) lying against the sulcus chiasmaticus and the top of the dorsum. (c) Diastasis of the coronal suture (open arrows)

(c)

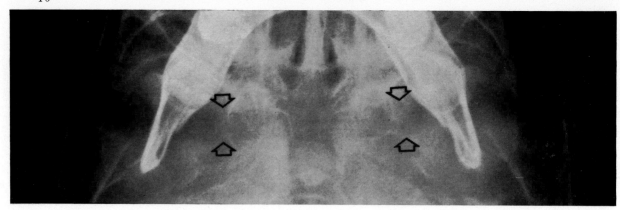

Figure 9. Suture diastasis in a girl aged 1½ years with hydrocephalus controlled by a ventriculo-caval shunt. There is severe diastasis of the coronal suture

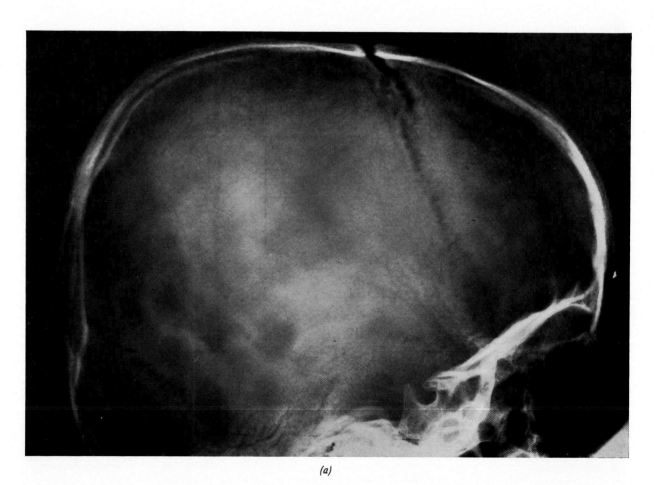

(a)

Figure 10. The progress of suture diastasis in a child aged 2 years who had had a theca-peritoneal anastomosis for hydrocephalus soon after birth. He had remained well until 2 weeks before these radiographs were made. He then vomited several times and became listless. (a) The coronal suture in lateral view (cont.)

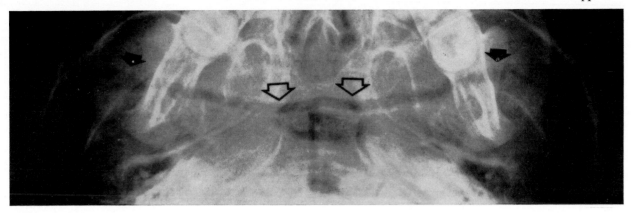

(b)

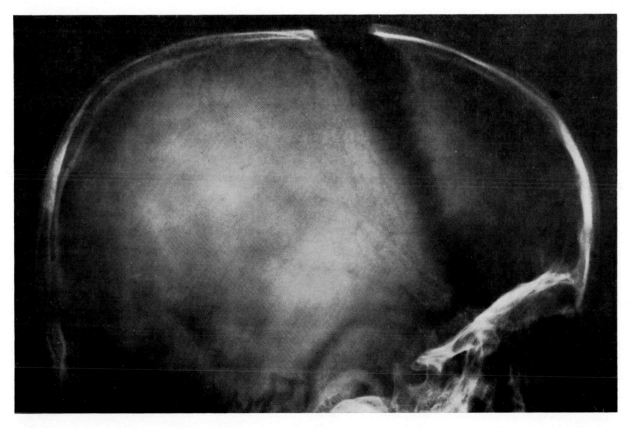

(c)

Figure 10 (cont.). (b) Full axial view. The central part of the coronal suture has never interdigitated (open arrows), but the interdigitations of the more peripheral part are apparent (closed arrow). It was found that the anastomosis tube had fractured, and the shunt was then replaced by one into the epidural space. The patient's head continued to enlarge but his condition improved greatly, and he now (at the age of 9 years) leads an active life. (c) Two months after the previous radiograph the sutures are much wider. Note how 'spikey' the digitations have become as the growing edge of bone attempts to fill the sutural gap

12

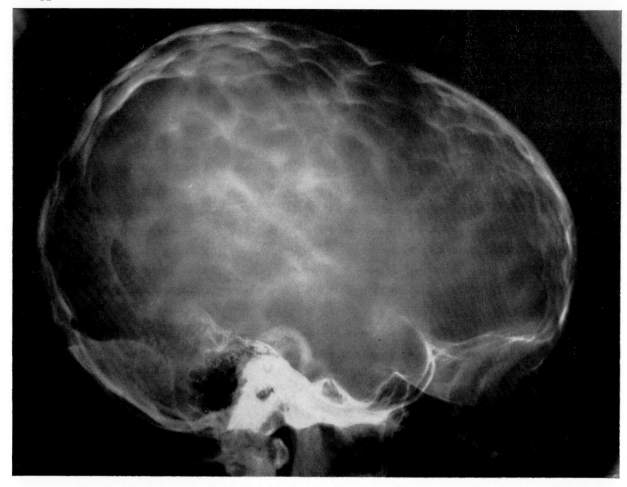

(a)

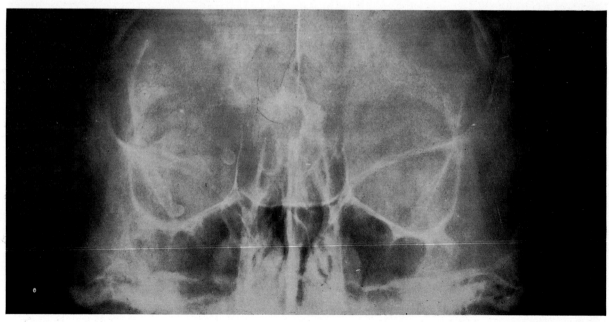

(b)

Figure 11. Legend on facing page

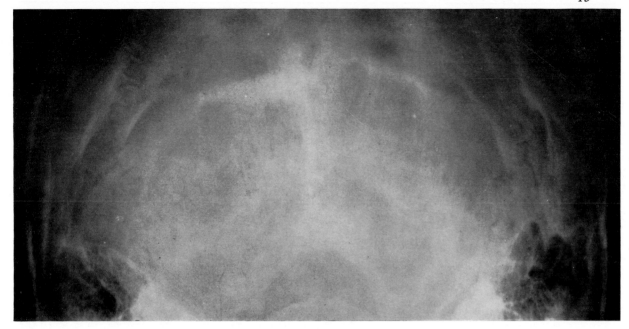

(c)

Figure 11. Chronic raised intracranial pressure and hydrocephalus due to aqueduct stenosis in a child aged 12 years with a 3-year history of headaches and recent deterioration in intelligence. There was some evidence of hypopituitarism and bitemporal hemianopia. On examination the patient had bilateral optic atrophy; but 3 years before when her eyes were examined they were thought to be normal. Ventriculography showed aqueduct stenosis. She made a very good recovery after a Torkildsen operation. (a) The lateral radiograph shows a large head with depression of the middle of the floor of the anterior fossa. The skull is very thin and convolutional impressions are extreme. The slightly enlarged sella has an indistinct floor, and the dorsum has disappeared. (b) The orbits are wide apart, the sphenoid fissures enormously expanded. (c) The sutures are not spread, but many of them show excessive interdigitation. The diagnosis from such films must be chronic hydrocephalus due to an obstruction at or behind the posterior part of the third ventricle

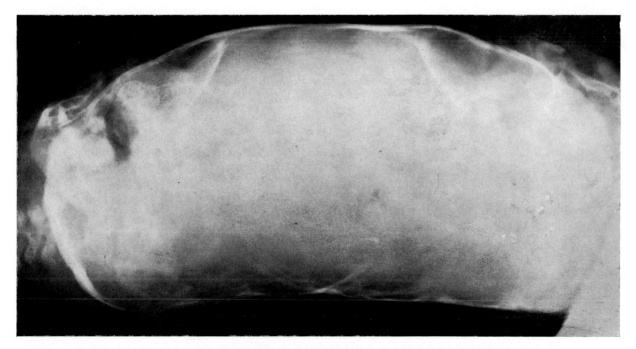

Figure 12. Craniopagus twins. Convolutional impressions are confined to the side upon which they habitually lie. This is a normal feature. There was no evidence of raised intracranial pressure and the finding has been present in other pairs seen by the author

An appearance similar to suture diastasis may be found for a few months in some children who, after a prolonged period of nutritional deficiency, are put on an adequate diet and rapidly gain brain weight. The history is sufficient to avoid confusion with raised intracranial pressure due to a pathological process (Sondheimer, 1970).

Other causes of widened sutures are discussed in Chapter 2.

Size

Sometimes along with general enlargement of the head there is an increase in the depth of the anterior fossa between the orbits, which tend to be displaced laterally. Raised intracranial pressure of long enough standing to affect the shape of the skull in this way gives evidence of itself in the vault as well; a distinction can thus be made from Soto's syndrome which does not cause increased convolutional markings or suture diastasis (Poznanski and Stephenson, 1967).

Cronqvist (1968) devised an index of cranial size such that

$$C \text{ index} = \frac{L + H + W}{M} \times 10$$

where the measurements are made between the inner tables and are = L, the greatest length; H, the greatest perpendicular distance from a line drawn from the nasion to the posterior margin of the foramen magnum; W, the greatest width; M, is the maximum distance between the inner margin of the two necks of the mandible in the antero-posterior film. The mean is $53.5 \pm 2 \times 1.21$. These are useful basic data but in the clinical field it is rarely necessary to make measurements.

Convolutional impressions

Long-standing raised intracranial pressure may result in an increase in the convolutional impressions over the upper parts of the frontal and parietal bones. Such changes, when gross, are almost always accompanied by widening of the sutures and commonly by abnormalities of the sella, and then they are an indication of a rise in intracranial pressure of several months' duration.

By themselves the convolutional impressions are of no diagnostic importance.

A more severe manifestation of the same process is generalized thinning of the bones of the vault.

Convolutional impressions are caused by moulding of the inner table of the skull in response to growth of the underlying brain: pulsation is probably an important factor in their development. They are seen throughout life on those parts of the skull which are least protected from the brain by a layer of cerebrospinal fluid. They are, for instance, always present on the orbital plates of the frontal bones and in the floor of the middle fossa. In childhood, particularly during the ages from 4 to 8 years, these convolutional impressions are often very prominent in skull radiographs, but even during these years, they tend to be confined to the base and the lower two-thirds of the vault. A clear indication of the importance of gravity on the situation of the most prominent convolutional impressions is provided by radiographs of children who for different reasons have remained for long periods in recumbency.

In the past, long-term nursing in the Trendelenburg position for Pott's disease of the cervical spine resulted in deep convolutional impressions, particularly noticeable over the occiput and posterior parietal regions.

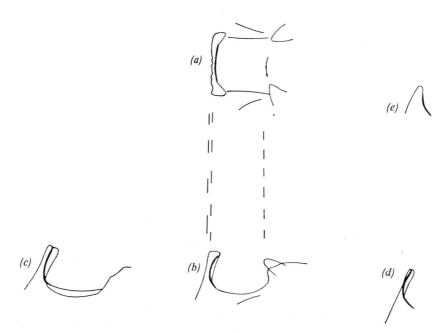

Figure 13. The cortex of the dorsum sellae. This part of the lamina dura often shows the earliest evidence of erosion. Because of the shape of the dorsum the cortex of the central part may lie behind the apparent anterior edge in lateral view. (a) Plan of the sella. (b) Lateral. (c) Another shape which may be seen when the floor of the sella is uneven. (d) A thin dorsum. (e) A thick dorsum, common in childhood

In three pairs of craniopagus twins, the convolutional impressions were only present on the side on which the children habitually lay.

SELLA

Usually, after weeks or months, severe destruction of the cortical layers of bone interferes with visualization of the sella turcica. Furthermore, there are many cases in which hydrocephalus is added to the picture (*see* below). Occasionally, however, alterations from the normal may be slight, and it is important to bear in mind the anatomy of the region (*Figure 13*).

Evidence of the cause

In infants and children before the age of 8 years, suture diastasis nearly always accompanies or precedes severe changes in the sella turcica. Apart from the characteristic appearances accompanying chronic obstruction of the ventricular pathway, erosion of the sella may come about as a result of a variety of intracranial tumours; but if in young children the sella shows erosion while the sutures remain normal, the cause is almost certainly a local process such as a craniopharyngioma.

If, due to a chronic obstruction in the distal cerebro-spinal pathways, there is marked dilatation of the anterior end of the third ventricle, additional changes may take place in the sella turcica. These are due to the front of the third ventricle impinging on the dorsum sellae, on the diaphragma and on the bone anterior to the attachment of the diaphragma. The changes are most commonly seen in developmental aqueduct stenosis, with long-standing mid-brain tumours and with slow-growing tumours within the fourth ventricle. The sella in these patients may appear to be enlarged unless its shape is more closely analysed. In addition, the dorsum sellae may be shortened by erosion from above or it may have the appearance of being slightly tipped forwards as well as being shortened.

Although it may appear at first to be enlarged, the sella is often actually flattened and the upper part of what is thought to be its long anterior wall is not part of the sella at all, but is formed by the elongated and vertically disposed sulcus chiasmaticus. Due perhaps to coincident growth and the downward pressure of the enlarged lateral ventricles upon the tentorium, the axis of the sulcus chiasmaticus has been changed, the anterior clinoid processes have become large and the vertically directed sulcus chiasmaticus has been enlarged by the direct pressure of the expanded front of the third ventricle. In its fully developed shape this deformity closely resembles the capital letter 'J', the sella itself, with its shortened dorsum, constituting the little bowl at the bottom. The sulcus chiasmaticus is responsible for the upper part of the long stem and anterior clinoids provide the cross piece at the top.

The shape is quite clearly distinguished from that due to a pituitary tumour and there can be little doubt that it originally gave rise to the description 'J' sella (*q.v.*).

Although nearly 90 per cent of children and infants with choroid plexus papillomas have hydrocephalus (Thompson, Harwood-Nash and Fitz, 1973), evidence of it was not detected in one-third and only a few showed the localizing features of an expansion of the vault over the affected trigone which may also be found with other trigonal masses.

In general, abnormalities of some kind are to be seen in the skull radiographs of half the children who have brain tumours, and abnormalities are more common in younger than in older children (Grossman *et al.*, 1971).

THE ADULT

Raised intracranial pressure of recent onset (*Figure 14*)

VAULT

It will be many months before a rise in intracranial pressure affects any change in the radiographic appearance of the bones of the vault or the sutures.

SELLA

The changes are the same as those described in childhood. They occur in about one-third of patients with raised intracranial pressure and the erosions are more likely to be found early in cases in which the sphenoid air sinuses do not reach the floor of the pituitary fossa. The erosions may be seen after 5 or 6 weeks illness, but the change becomes more obvious and is found more commonly after several months.

It should be noted that the author believes erosion of the lamina dura is recognizable at any age, and in the absence of a generalized bone disease the loss of this cortex is good evidence of raised intracranial pressure even in the old. Many neuroradiologists tend to discount 'osteoporosis' of the sella after middle age, but make no distinction between the cortex and the cancellous bone.

As time progresses, confluence of the erosions may result in more extensive destruction of the dorsum sellae which may virtually disappear, only a ghost shadow remaining to mark its position. The histological changes which are taking place have been beautifully illustrated by Mahmoud (1958).

Long-standing raised intracranial pressure (*Figures 15–24, 137, 148–151, 167–170*)

VAULT

Very long-standing raised intracranial pressure may affect the vault of the adult skull in a variety of ways.

Size

If the cause for the high intracranial pressure was present in childhood during the active phase of growth, the whole head may be enlarged or (for example, in cases of aqueduct stenosis) there may be enlargement of the supratentorial part of the vault with sparing of the squamous occipital.

16

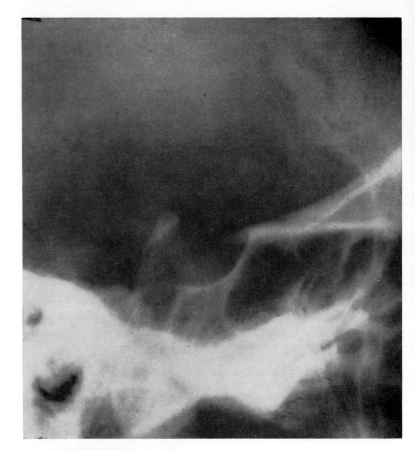

Figure 14. Raised intracranial pressure. Cerebral (parietal) metastasis from carcinoma of the breast. Three month's diplopia. Two months' headache. The anterior surface of the dorsum sellae has lost its cortex. The tip of the dorsum and the posterior clinoids are better preserved than the rest. A similar change may be found in rare cases of vascular hypertension. Perhaps the mechanism is the same

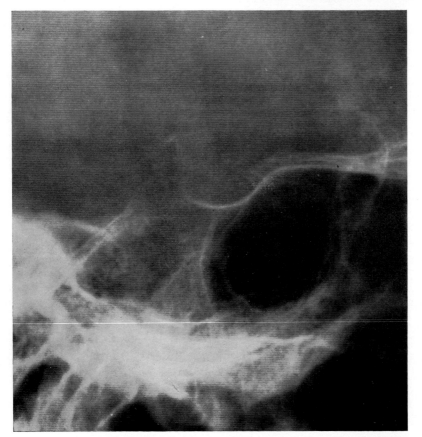

Figure 15. Osteoporosis and erosion of the sella. A patient aged 52 years with several months' history of fits and the recent appearance of papilloedema. Not only is the anterior surface of the dorsum sellae destroyed, but there are erosions through its cancellous structure and of the posterior surface

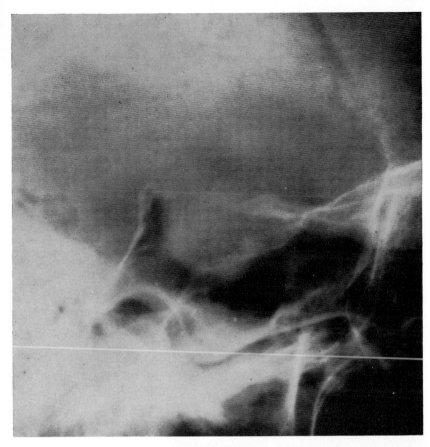

Figure 16. An adult with a 14-year history of Jacksonian epilepsy, recent status epilepticus and gross bilateral papilloedema. He had a frontal oligo-dendroglioma. The sella shows complete destruction of its lining lamina dura in spite of full pneumatization of the sphenoid. Such a change as this is unlikely to be seen except with long-standing intracranial pressure. When erosion reaches this degree, the floor of the sella may suddenly give way so that in rare cases expansion into the sphenoid sinus may be observed to progress over a few weeks. It is beginning in the middle of the floor of this sella

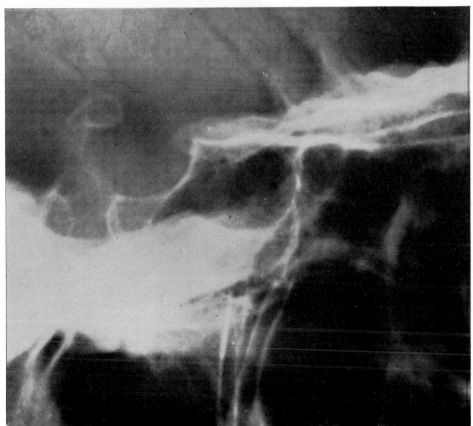

Figure 17. A patient aged 52 years with raised intracranial pressure of many months' duration, due to cerebral metastases. Papilloedema is present. The base of the dorsum sellae has lost its cortex and the cancellous bone is ill-defined

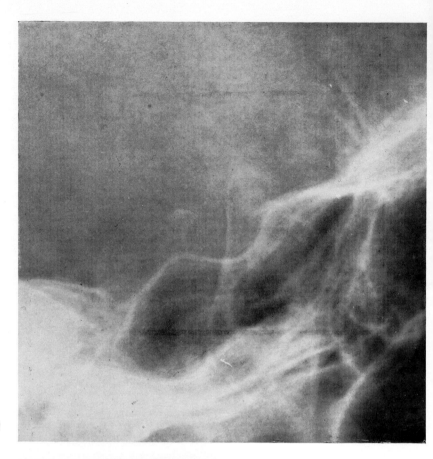

(a)

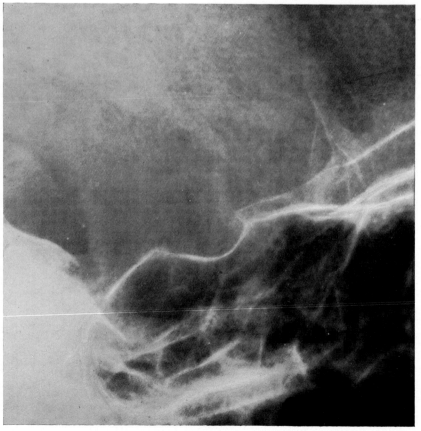

(b)

Figure 18. A woman aged 54 years with a 15-month history of cerebellar disturbance of gradual onset, but recent rapid deterioration. There was doubt about the presence of papilloedema. At ventriculography the pressure was slightly raised, and at operation after ventriculography a membranous occlusion of the aqueduct and of the exits from the fourth ventricle was found, with gross dilatation of the fourth ventricle. (a) The dorsum sellae was probably intact when this rather indifferent radiograph was made on 24.2.62, but (b) had disappeared by 25.11.62. The anterior end of the third ventricle lay in contact with the clivus and posterior part of the floor of the sella

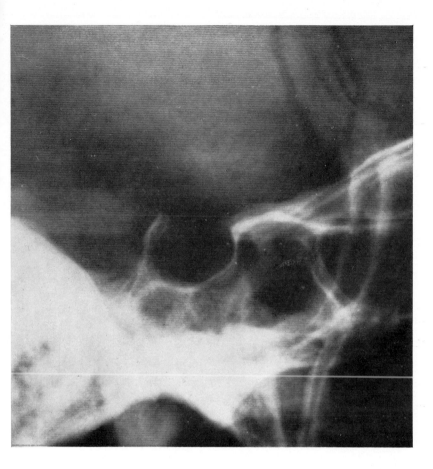

Figure 19. Raised intracranial pressure, sella. A woman aged 34 years with a 6-month history of headache, vomiting and unsteadiness. She had bilateral chronic papilloedema. At ventriculography the pressure was grossly raised and at operation a cerebellar haemangioblastoma was removed. The anterior surface of the dorsum and perhaps the floor of the sella show pin-point erosions

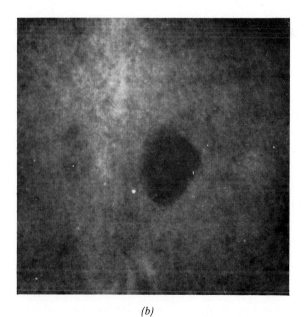

(a)   *(b)*

Figure 20. Enlargement of a depression for Pacchionian granulations. The patient had a proven brain-stem glioma. (a) A posterior fossa Pacchionian granulation depression is shown near the midline in a plain radiograph prior to encephalography. (b) Six months later. Plain radiograph prior to ventriculography. ((a) and (b) are for comparison and have been reproduced as near to the same size as possible)

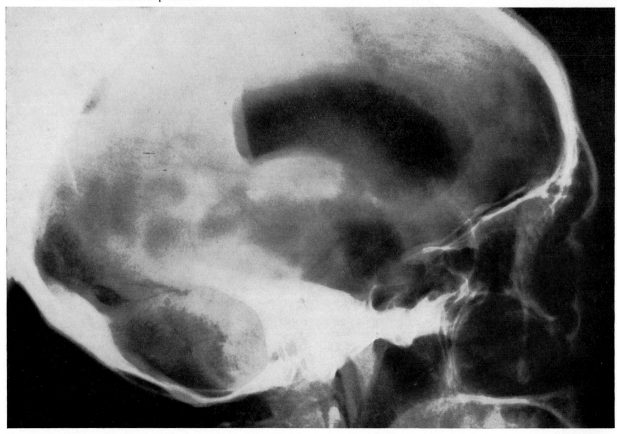

Figure 21. Raised intracranial pressure. Hydrocephalus. Tentorial meningioma. A patient with a 5-year history including 2 years of headache. Brow-up lateral ventriculogram shows the dorsum sellae eroded to a thin-pointed spike which is probably tipped slightly forwards. The appearance of the dorsum sellae was strongly in favour of pressure from above, due either to the third ventricle or a tumour such as a craniopharyngioma. The pineal is elevated rather than depressed which, together with the appearance of the sella, indicates a posterior fossa tumour

If the cause of the rise in intracranial pressure did not begin until normal skull growth had ceased, the head is unlikely to have enlarged to any noticeable degree.

Thickness

Chronic raised intracranial pressure, even in the adult, will sometimes result in a general thinning of the calvaria. When, however, there has been a long period of remission from the intracranial hypertension, the vault may sometimes be found unusually thick (*see* the section on 'Relief of raised intracranial pressure').

Shape

Local bulging due to some very long-standing expanding process may be observed. Sufficiently long-standing hydrocephalus, even if it does not enlarge the whole head, may cause a rounding and even a suggestion of ballooning of its contours which, together with other abnormalities observed on the radiograph, will give a clue to the presence of hydrocephalus. This rounding is observed most easily in the anterior fossa and the frontal bones.

Convolutional impressions

These are not normally visible over the upper part of the skull of an adult, although they are regularly present in the lower part of the vault and over the base. If well-marked convolutional impressions are observed over the vertex, this is a strong indication of the presence, probably for many years, of an intracranial condition which has resulted in prolonged (perhaps intermittent) raised intracranial pressure usually with internal hydrocephalus.

Sutures

Diastasis of sutures is very rarely seen in an adult but it may sometimes be observed when the increased intracranial pressure has persisted since before the normal time of their closure. Its rare onset in later life is presumably due to an unusual anatomical formation of the sutures which are poorly interlocked.

Foramina, venous channels and Pacchionian depressions

It has been pointed out that long-standing raised intracranial pressure may increase the size of the emissary

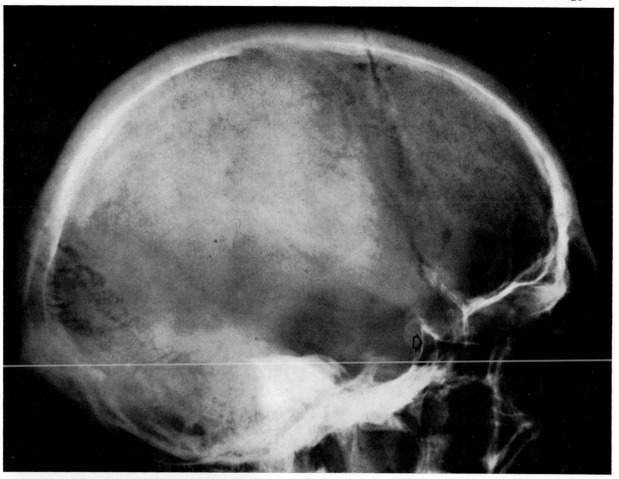

(a)

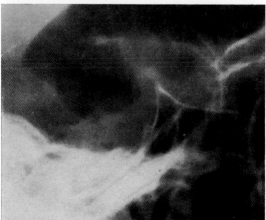

Figure 22. Hydrocephalus in a patient aged 42 years with a history of epilepsy since childhood. He had had severe headaches for 6 months and the fundi showed some pallor. Angiography and ventriculography demonstrated aqueduct stenosis with gross dilatation of the lateral and third ventricles. (a) Lateral view. The anterior margin of the sella remains. The sulcus chiasmaticus (arrow) shows up clearly through the short wide anterior clinoids. The posterior part of the sella floor is so deeply depressed that it cannot be seen distinct from the lateral part of the middle fossa. The dorsum sellae, although severely eroded, is still visible and is seen to be tipped forwards. All this is the result of long-continued pressure from the front of the third ventricle. (b) The relationship of the third ventricle. (c) Full axial view. Slight suture diastasis (arrowed) is seen although the patient is aged 42 years

(b)

(c)

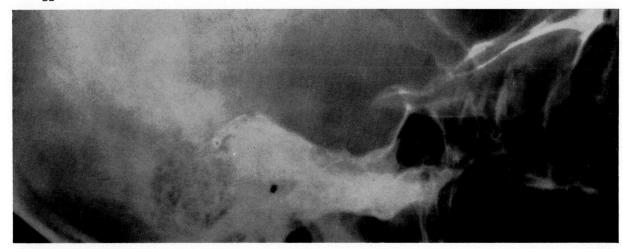

(a)

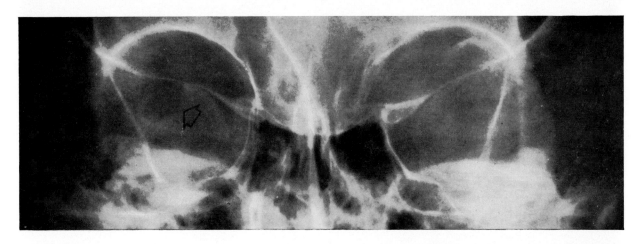

(b)

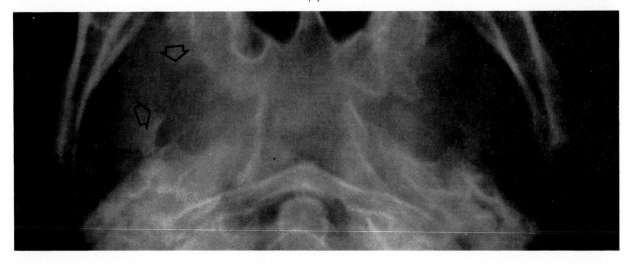

(c)

Figure 23. Long-standing raised intracranial pressure with hydrocephalus due to obstruction of the aqueduct from a quadrigeminal-plate tumour. No headache. No papilloedema. (a) Lateral view. The sella is elongated and the dorsum has disappeared. (b) Postero-anterior view. The lesser wings of the sphenoid are very thin. There is a defect, partial or complete, in the right greater wing. (c) Full axial view. The floor of the middle fossa is very thin, particularly on the right where the foramina ovale and spinosum are lost in the translucency (cont.)

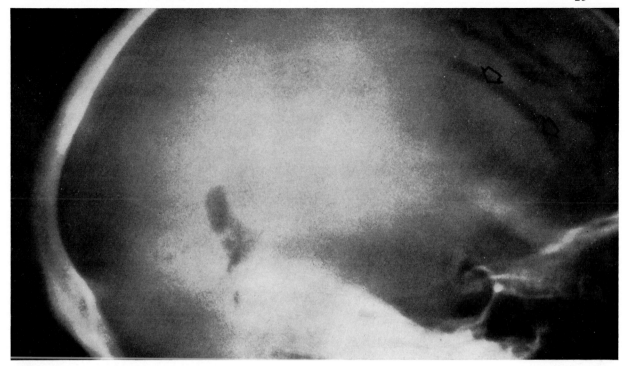

(d)

Figure 23 (cont.). (d) Tomography at pneumoencephalography demonstrates the chiasmatic cistern lying deep in the expanded sella. It also shows the wide-swept corpus callosum

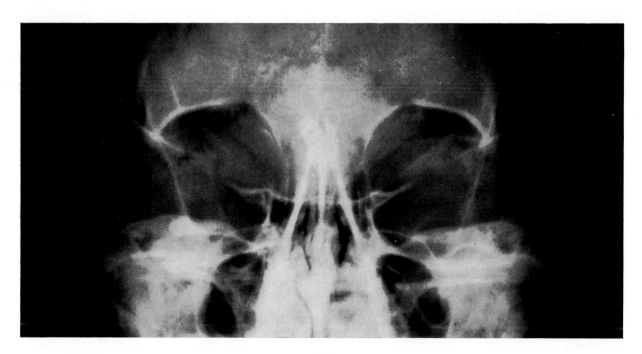

(a)

Figure 24. Chronic raised intracranial pressure. Expansion of the anterior fossa. There was an Arnold–Chiari malformation in this girl, aged 22 years, as well as aqueduct stenosis giving rise to severe tentorial herniation and expansion of the suprapineal recess of the third ventricle (she also had congenital pulmonary stenosis and an A.S.D.). (a) Postero-anterior view. There is expansion of the anterior fossa showing as a depression of its floor in the midline and thinning of the lesser wings of the sphenoid. The eyes are wide apart (cont.)

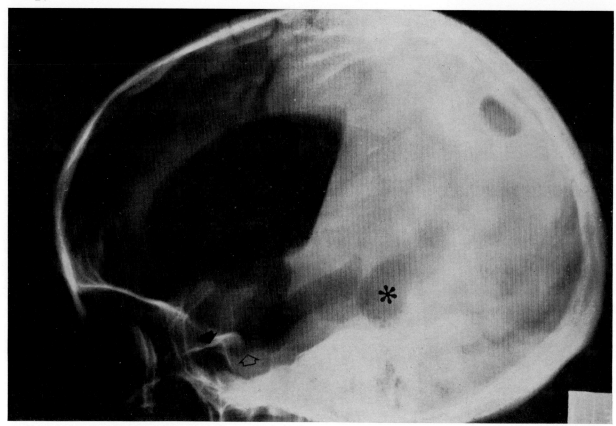

(b)

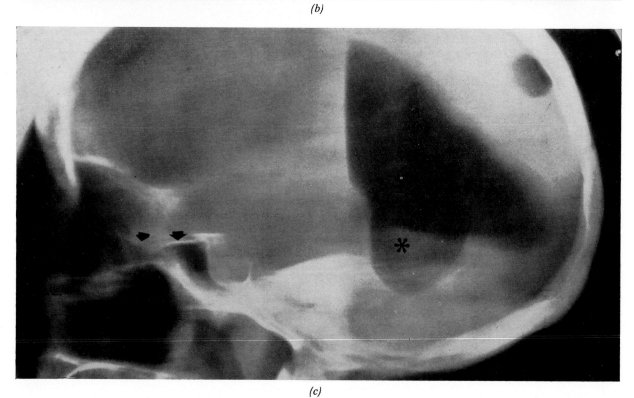

(c)

Figure 24 (cont.). (b) and (c) The laterals (brow-up ventriculogram and brow-down air tomogram) also show ballooning of the anterior fossa (closed arrows). There is slight erosion of the tip of the dorsum sellae and the dilated third ventricle (open arrow) is seen protruding into the pituitary fossa. Marked convolutional impressions are present over the vertex (Note: Infratentorial cystic dilatation of the herniated suprapineal recess (asterisk). A rare occurrence)

foramina and perhaps of the venous channels of the vault, but it is so difficult to judge the normal from the abnormal that this is not a sign of great clinical significance. Yuhl and Schmitz (1969) have recorded normal channels of 2 mm and more in diameter.

SELLA

Raised intracranial pressure causes progressive changes in the sella turcica in some patients. The proportion who show an abnormality must depend upon the number of chronic cases in the material as well as on some unknown factor which makes one patient's sella more susceptible to damage than another. Overall, in the author's material between one-fifth and one-third of patients with tumours have shown sellar erosion in their pre-operative films. Although sellar changes are somewhat uncommon it is important to remember that of patients who present with tumours but without papilloedema or headache, 20 per cent show abnormalities of the sella due to pressure. The changes may be severe. Many of these cases have benign or slow-growing tumours and plain radiographs of the skull fulfil a very useful function in pointing to the necessity for further investigation.

du Boulay and El Gammal (1966) demonstrated that the erosions and deformations of the sella pass through certain stages and reflect, to some degree, their causes. In bringing out this point they divided erosions of the region into categories.

Category I, destruction of the lamina dura as described above, when unaccompanied by other changes in the region gives no help in the localization or the determination of the cause of raised intracranal pressure. The most that can be said definitely and dogmatically is that it does not seem to occur in pure communicating hydrocephalus.

Category II was defined as destruction of the top and/or back of the dorsum sellae. This includes the posterior clinoid processes. When unaccompanied by Category I erosion it is often due either to a local expanding process, usually a craniopharyngioma, or to hydrocephalus causing the front of the third ventricle to impinge on the dorsum. In such cases (without Category I erosion) the C.S.F. obstruction lies along the aqueduct or in the fourth ventricle and is usually very long-standing. Category II erosion forms part of the characteristic change seen in the sella in aqueduct stenosis (*q.v.*).

Category II erosion is, however, not infrequently accompanied by Category I. Most of these patients have more rapidly growing tumours, either in the posterior fossa, causing hydrocephalus, or so placed that they thrust the base of the brain directly down upon the sella without actually dilating the third ventricle. Thus, many have tumours in the posterior frontal region.

If such a case goes clinically unrecognized (and the great majority of such tumours will be posterior frontal slow-growing gliomas, or meningiomas in several situations), destruction advances to include the planum sphenoidale which becomes difficult to see. This is the Category III change. Finally, the whole of the bony roof of the sphenoid sinus, including the floor of the sella, the sulcus chiasmaticus and the planum sphenoidale may be so weakened that they bulge downwards, herniating into the cavity of the sphenoid sinus and giving an appearance which superficially resembles sellar enlargement due to pituitary tumour. A close scrutiny should always show the difference, for pituitary tumours do not push the planum sphenoidale directly downwards and do not tilt the dorsum sellae forwards as may sometimes happen in Category III erosion.

du Boulay and El Gammal (1966) have added to these recognizably different categories of sellar abnormality a Category IV, an unwontedly deep pituitary fossa which may be associated with what has come to be called the 'empty sella' syndrome. In some cases slowly progressive enlargement of the intrasellar subarachnoid space may accompany a long period of moderately raised intracranial pressure. In other cases the reason for enlargement of the intrasellar subarachnoid space is not clear. In still other cases the 'emptiness' of a large part of the pituitary fossa may be a normal feature. At pneumoencephalography, after fairly vigorous manipulation, air can be made to replace the C.S.F. in the cavity if the pituitary fossa and this will show that the pituitary gland is confined to the bottom of it. In extreme cases the pituitary may suffer from pressure atrophy.

Pituitary tumours are responsible for a further two groups of 'empty sellas', either when the tumour undergoes spontaneous regression or when it shrinks following radiotherapy.

An 'empty sella' is recognizable at CT scanning which therefore provides a useful adjunct to plain x-ray when the sella is enlarged.

SKULL BASE

In addition to the changes in the sella, long-standing raised intracranial pressure may affect the skull base in three different ways. All of them are difficult to assess and none is a reliable sign in the absence of obvious changes elsewhere.

Thinning of the bones of the base

In the submento-vertical view, it may seem that the structures of the base are abnormally translucent, giving rise in some parts to difficulty in recognition of the margins of foramina because of thinning and even erosions and in other parts to an increase in clarity of definition of the overlying structures. In the postero-anterior view this thinning of the skull base may sometimes be seen affecting the lesser wing of the sphenoid whose upper surface may become invisible.

Thinning may occasionally be extreme and cause actual defects in the bony structure of the greater wing of the sphenoid so that a hole with a more or less obvious margin may be shown in the postero-anterior view.

It has been said that the upper surface of the petrous bones may be flattened or hollowed out by sufficiently chronic pressure.

Abnormality of shape

The effect of long-standing raised intracranial pressure beginning in infancy or childhood upon the general direction of axis of the pituitary fossa has already been described. Sometimes hydrocephalus also affects the floor of the anterior fossa, the central portion of which

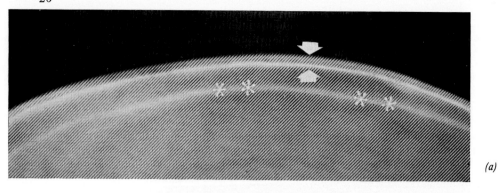

(a)

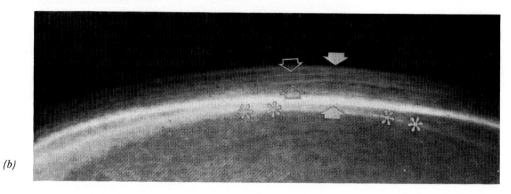

(b)

Figure 25. The relief of raised intracranial pressure. (a) Tangential view of the vault. A child aged 1 year suffering from hydrocephalus associated with a cervical meningocoele and Arnold–Chiari malformation. The vault is thin but normal in structure (arrows). The inner-most white line is the shadow of the inner table of the opposite frontal bone (asterisks). A ventriculo-caval shunt operation was performed. (b) One year later: the vault (closed arrows) has greatly increased in thickness by deposition on both surfaces (particularly the inner table). The relic of the original inner table (open arrows) is visible within the new diploë. The laminated appearance produced by this 'ghost' shadow does not persist indefinitely. The dynamic processes of bone remoulding remove it after a few months. A very similar change to the one described here occurs after the sudden onset of cerebral atrophy in young children

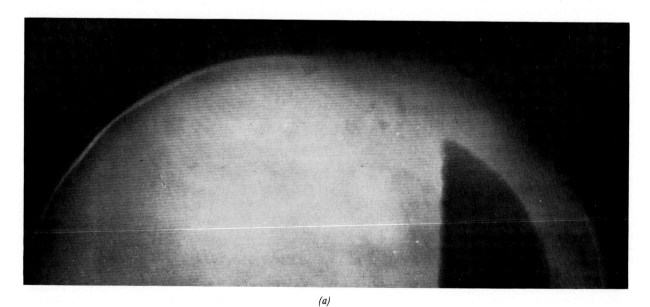

(a)

Figure 26. Effects of the relief of raised intracranial pressure in a child aged 3 months with a non-communicating hydrocephalus following meningitis. (a) The vault is very thin. The anterior fontanelle bulges (cont.)

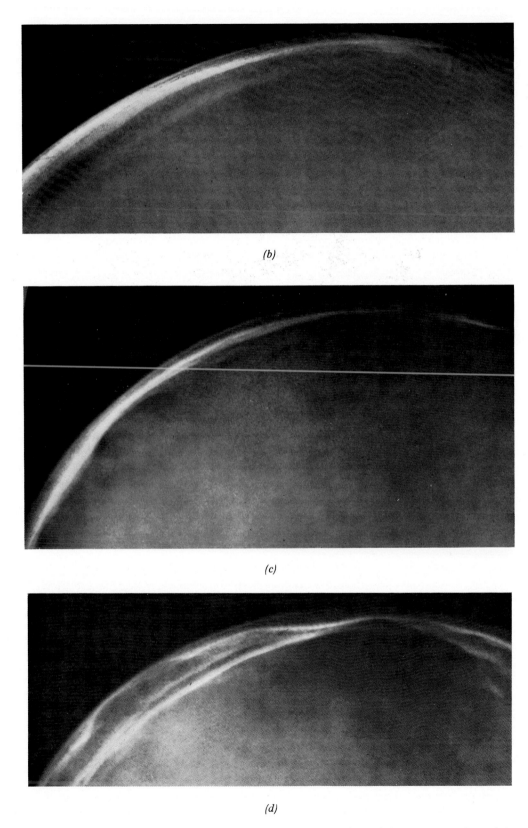

(b)

(c)

(d)

Figure 26 (cont.). (b) Eight months after the successful performance of a ventriculo-caval shunt operation the vault has increased in thickness, but a ghost of the previous inner table persists. The coronal suture is closing. (c) Eight months later this ghost has disappeared, the vault is thicker, the coronal suture has fused, as sometimes happens when pressure is relieved. (d) Two years later because of premature closure of the suture, the vault has begun to show exaggerated convolutional impressions, so that in places the vault is again becoming thinned

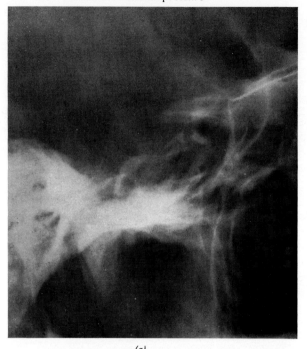

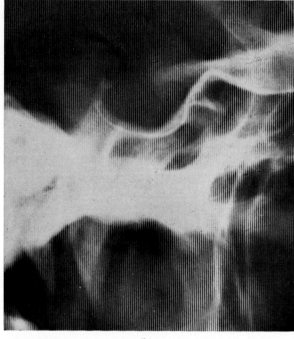

(a)   (b)

Figure 27. The relief of raised intracranial pressure. (a) Frontal cystic glioma. A frontal lobectomy was performed. The floor of the sella and the dorsum have lost their cortex. There is also erosion which has thinned the dorsum; but it is not displaced. (b) The same patient 3 years later. In the interval she had been free of clinical evidence of raised intracranial pressure until shortly before this radiological examination. An unusual amount of re-ossification has occurred. (Note: The scale of these two reproductions is slightly different)

may be deepened and widened. The cribriform plate and the roofs of the ethmoid sinuses then lie unusually far below the level of the lateral parts of the orbital plates of the frontal bones. This abnormality will be apparent in both lateral and postero-anterior views and is usually accompanied by thinning of the upper surfaces of the lesser wings of the sphenoid.

Enlargement of foramina

This enlargement of foramina may be part of a general thinning of the base of the skull, but it is always difficult to assess and usually of a mild degree.

ALTERATIONS FOLLOWING THE RELIEF OF RAISED INTRACRANIAL PRESSURE (*Figures 2, 4, 25–27, 102, 167, 170*)

VAULT

Particularly during the period of most active skull growth in childhood, the bones of the vault may be thinned by long-standing raised intracranial pressure, the head may be large and suture diastasis is likely to be present. The relief of pressure in such cases may then produce a recognizable appearance, the skull bones increasing in thickness by deposition of bone on the inner as well as the outer table. This deposition causes a double inner table shadow consisting of concentric lines which persist for a few months leaving, as it were, a ghost of the original vault buried in the new one. The thickening of

the bones takes place at the expense of convolutional markings which may recently have been prominent. These observations, first recorded in 1965 and 1966, have been confirmed by other writers.

The sutures may revert to normal or sometimes show very deep interdigitation. If only slight enlargement of the intracranial cavity had occurred, the disparity between head and body may disappear with further growth of the body.

In infants and young children the sudden relief of raised intracranial pressure is sometimes followed by premature closure of the sutures. This premature synostosis may be of little significance if the head is already much enlarged, or if it affects only part of the skull; but in other patients, subsequent pictures show the beginning of the typical secondary deformities of craniostenosis.

If raised intracranial pressure recurs, diastasis can only take place where the sutures have remained unfused, and bizarre and asymmetrical expansion of the head may follow.

SELLA

Re-ossification may be seen to convert osteoporotic areas to normal density and will sometimes cause the disappearance of small erosions, but when there has been a severe degree of destruction some abnormality of shape tends to remain permanently after the removal of raised intracranial pressure. One has the impression that once the lamina dura has formed again following the relief of raised intracranial pressure, not only is it somewhat thicker than before but it is resistant to erosion if the pressure rises again.

2 TRANSLUCENCIES AND EROSIONS OF THE VAULT

INTRODUCTION

The particular features of the vault of the skull which lead to peculiarities of its response to disease are as follows.
(1) The vault bones are thinned and flattened.
(2) They contain and are closely adjacent to the brain and are therefore subject to the stimulus of brain growth and transmitted pulsation.
(3) The vault bones have a highly vascular diploë, a very vascular covering in the scalp and a large collection of arteries and veins immediately below them in the meninges.
(4) Ossification takes place in the fibrous stage of the precursor of bone without the preliminary formation of cartilage.

(1) As might be expected in so flat a bone, destructive processes tend to affect its whole thickness at an early stage, and those informative margins where the interaction of normal tissue and disease may be studied are more limited in extent than they would be if the erosion were sunk in the depth of a large bone. Without most careful observation, one round translucency looks very much like another.

Although the bone may be placed so near the radiograph that its details should be clearer than is the case in most examinations of long bones, every *en face* picture is veiled by the more or less confusing shadows of the opposite part of the skull. Thus, the distinction between partial and complete bone destruction may sometimes be impossible, and in any case depends upon experience of the technique of radiography employed. This is the one part of the skull examination where a relatively short focus-film distance is of advantage since it tends to

preserve the features on the near side of the vault while blurring the shadows of those distant from the film. (For other reasons, however, a short focus-film is contra-indicated, 90–100 cm is now generally adopted.)

The distinction between complete and partial erosion may not always be solved by tangential views (*Figure 28*). Tangential views, on the other hand, will help with many other problems showing, for instance, the site of origin of an expanding process either (*Figures 29* and *84*) within the diploë causing expansion, (*Figure 85*) within the cranial cavity predominantly affecting the inner table, or (*Figure 88*) outside the skull, causing an indentation of the outer table. When interpreting a tangential view it must be borne in mind that the vault is more or less the surface of a sphere, and the peripheral part of any diseased area being studied if of even moderate size, dips down below the tangent and is viewed obliquely. It is easy to mistake the true thickness of an area of increased or decreased density, or to mistake the strands of dense bone on the surface for trabeculation running within.

(2) The proximity of the skin and brain and its developmental history are responsible for many of the lesions found. Intrusion of dermal tissue gives rise to dermoids and epidermoids while the failure of closure of the neural groove results in a meningocoele or an encephalocoele. Both are accompanied by defects in the bone through which they pass.

Dura, a closer neighbour still, is so tough a membrane that the sinusoidal veins held by it against the vault leave their impressions on the bones. As elsewhere in the skeleton, arteries running over the periosteum (but outside the deep layer of the dura) also cause clear-cut grooves, but apart from these obvious channels the vault, both normal and diseased, is moulded through the dura by underlying brain, particularly in the early years of

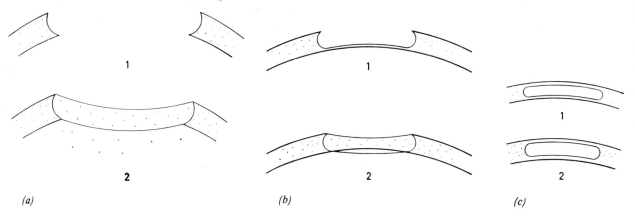

Figure 28. An erosion may be complete or partial. En face it is a circular translucency. In tangential views its appearance will depend upon its size and completeness as shown in these diagrams. (a) Complete erosion: (1) cross-section; (2) perspective drawing. A tangential radiograph would show the near side of the hole as well, superimposed on the far side which has been drawn. The curvature of the edges depends upon the size of the hole. (b) Erosion of the outer table and diploë: (1) cross-section; (2) perspective drawing. (c) Small erosion of diploë only: (1) cross-section; (2) tangential radiograph. This should usually be distinguishable from (a) or (b)

growth. The appearance of the vault thus becomes a guide to the state and history of the adjacent cranial contents. It seems probable that the ease which which such soft tissue affects the shape of the bone is the result of repeated intracranial pressure variation – arterial, respiratory (venous) and postural – transmitted to the inner table and either stimulating the osteoclasts or depressing osteoblastic action.

(3) The vascularity of the bone is probably responsible for the frequency with which metastases, particularly those requiring a good blood supply, are found. The vascularity must be at least partially responsible for the peculiarities of the response to osteomyelitis. There is an unexplained unwillingness of the vault to grow new periosteal bone or become sclerosed in response to injury and infection.

(4) Related to the developmental history of membranous bone may be the rarity of tumours derived from cartilage.

A list of the causes of translucent areas in the vault would include the following.

(1) Normal
(2) Developmental defects
    (*a*)   Meningocoele-encephalocoele
    (*b*)   Dermoid epidermoid
         Intradiploic
         Extracranial
         Intracranial
    (*c*)   Craniolacunia, craniofenestra
    (*d*)   Congenital parietal foraminae
    (*e*)   Symmetrical parietal thinning
    (*f*)   Symmetrical frontal fenestrae
    (*g*)   Fibrous dysplasia
    (*h*)   Arteriovenous malformation
    (*i*)   Haemangioma in bone
    (*j*)   Haemangioma of scalp
    (*k*)   Cranial dysostoses (*see* Chapter 11)
(3) Tumours
    (*a*)   Metastatic carcinoma
    (*b*)   Myeloma
    (*c*)   Chloroma
    (*d*)   Sarcoma, primary and secondary

    (*e*)   Neuroblastoma
    (*f*)   Leukaemic deposits
    (*g*)   Hodgkin's disease
    (*h*)   Neurofibroma in bone
    (*i*)   Meningioma
    (*j*)   Erosion by other intracranial tumours
    (*k*)   Extension from tumour of frontal sinuses
    (*l*)   Neurofibroma of scalp
    (*m*)   Invasion by tumours of skin
(4) Granuloma (lipoid and non-lipoid histiocytosis)
    (*a*)   Xanthomatosis (Hand–Schüller–Christian syndrome)
         (eosinophil granuloma) (Letterer–Siwe disease)
    (*b*)   Gaucher's disease
    (*c*)   Niemann–Pick disease
    (*d*)   Weber–Christian disease
(5) Boeck's sarcoid
(6) Infection–acute and chronic
(7) Hydatid cyst
(8) Aseptic necrosis
(9) Metabolic
    (*a*)   Rickets
    (*b*)   Hyperparathyroidism
    (*c*)   Hypophosphatasia
(10) Unknown aetiology
    (*a*)   Paget's disease and osteoporosis circumscripta
(11) Trauma
    (*a*)   Bone removal
    (*b*)   Bone absorption
         Secondary to cephalhaematoma
         Fibrosing osteitis
         Intradiploic haematoma
    (*c*)   Cephalhydrocoele (Leptomeningocoele cyst)

The plan followed is to group this enormous number of causes of translucency in the vault under the following headings.
(1) Normal vascular markings and their alteration by disease.
(2) Other normal translucencies.
(3) A generalized abnormal increase in translucency.
(4) Discrete abnormal translucencies which may be multiple and disseminated or sometimes single for a time (for example, metastases).

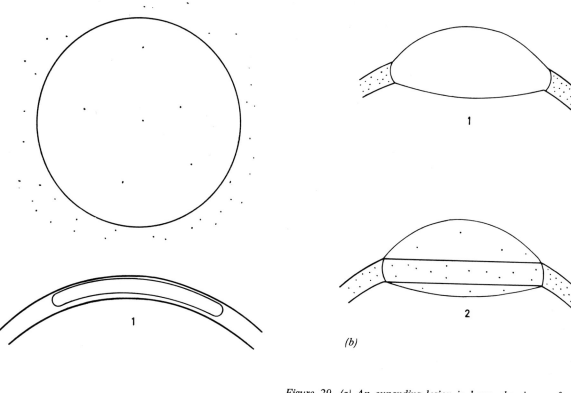

Figure 29. (a) An expanding lesion in bone, showing en face a large circular translucency, may also be distinguished in tangential view. (1) Cross-section of a large purely intradiploic translucency; (2) perspective drawing. (b) (1) Cross-section of a non-expanding intradiploic lesion; (2) tangential radiograph

(5) Discrete abnormal translucencies which are almost always single or confined to a small area.

NORMAL VASCULAR MARKINGS AND THEIR ALTERATION BY DISEASE

Dural sinuses, veins and arteries

The vault always shows numerous channels due to veins and arteries which run on its surfaces and through its structure. The majority of these are veins and the great variety of the appearance from one patient to the next or, indeed, on the two sides of the same skull is rarely of significance. However, the recognition, if possible, of channels which contain hypertrophied arteries is of the greatest importance, giving a clue to the presence, usually of a meningioma, sometimes of an angioma, and more rarely of some other vascular tumour.

Generally it is unwise to attach importance to the number and width of venous grooves, either dural or diploic, unless there is also evidence of an increase in the arterial supply.

However, on rare occasions, for example, some few falx meningiomas, almost all the arterial supply comes from the internal carotid while drainage is largely through the veins of the vault, particularly if the superior sagittal sinus is partially blocked by the tumour. Then the enlarged diploic and dural veins may be so numerous that their bony channels are obviously abnormal (*Figure 40*).

DURAL SINUSES

The dural sinuses (*Figures 30–32*), which are separated from bone by a thin membrane, but surrounded on their cephalic surface by a thick layer of dura, commonly cause visible impressions on the inner table. In this way the course of the superior sagittal, the transverse and sigmoid sinuses may be followed on plain radiographs. The terminal portions of superior cerebral veins may also cause thinning of the overlying vault where they gain a similar relationship to the dura before entering the superior sagittal sinus, and some of these impressions are widened where they correspond to lacunae laterales.

A vein running upwards near the coronal suture in company with the anterior branch of the middle meningeal artery often achieves the size and nature of a dural sinus, and has been called the spheno-parietal or spheno-bregmatic sinus. It frequently causes a prominent groove.

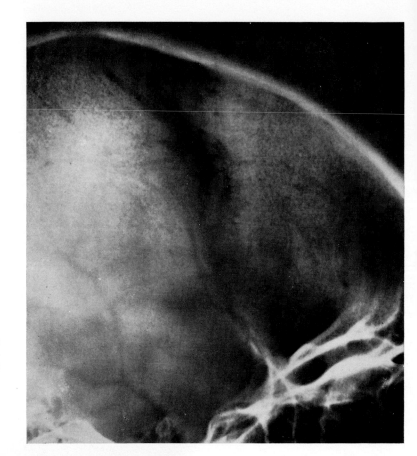

Figure 30. Spheno-bregmatic sinus. In this patient the anterior branch of the middle meningeal artery occupies the same groove as the spheno-bregmatic sinus for most of its course

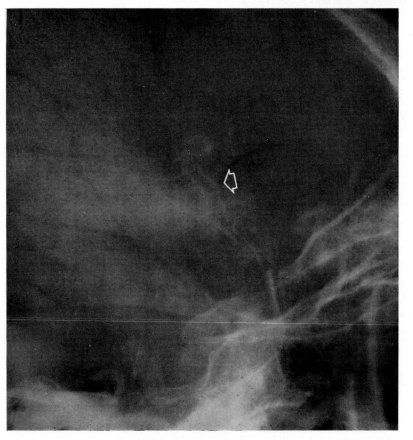

Figure 31. Sometimes both arterial and venous grooves may be very deep (as in this case where the bony wall is very obvious) or even for a short distance a tunnel

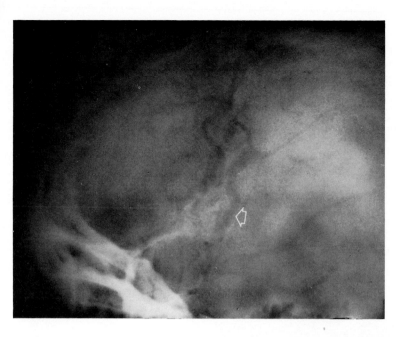

Figure 32. Occasionally the vein which runs with the anterior branch of the middle meningeal artery is neither dural nor extradural; but becomes for some distance diploic (having the usual characteristics of a diploic vein) before emerging again in the extradural plane

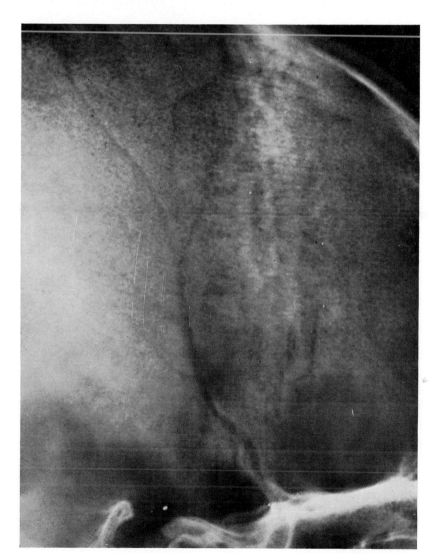

Figure 33. Normal arterial type of channel. The channel has a calibre which remains almost constant except where it diminishes by branching. The main component is an artery

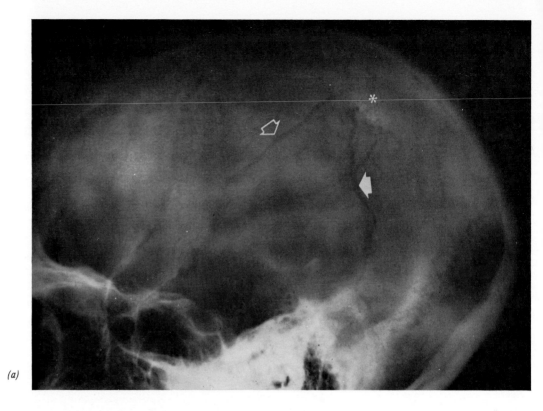

(a)

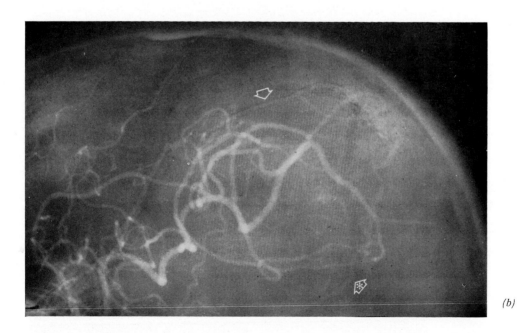

(b)

Figure 34. Meningioma. 'Venous' grooves may be of any size in the normal, but a wide 'arterial' type of groove indicates hypertrophy of an artery, and this is significant. (a) A parietal branch of the middle meningeal groove is arterial in type and too wide for a normal artery in this situation (open arrow). It runs towards a hyperostosis (asterisk). The channels leaving the region are for diploic veins (closed arrow) and by themselves would be of no significance. (b) The artery running in the 'arterial' groove is filled with contrast medium after angiography (open arrow). The diploic veins are not opacified. There is a second large artery behind the hyperostosis, but its groove is much less obvious on the plain radiograph (asterisk within arrow)

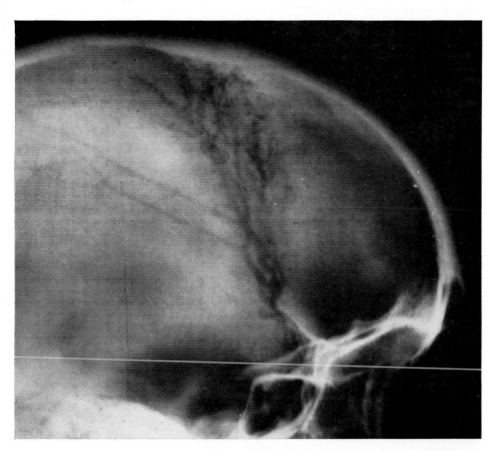

(a)

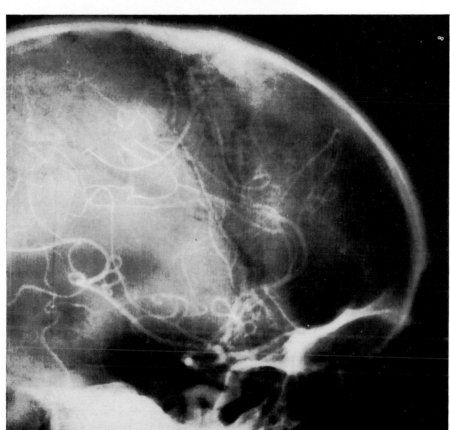

(b)

Figure 35. Meningioma. Vascular grooves. When hypertrophied arteries accompany the spheno-bregmatic sinus it may be much more difficult to recognize an increase in their size on the plain radiograph. (a) A leash of channels. On careful inspection some appear to have arterial characteristics. Although extremely tortuous they preserve their even calibre. (b) The arteries are filled with contrast medium; they seem narrower than the channels in which they run because only the lumen is outlined. Wide spaces not filled with contrast medium must be venous channels

DURAL VEINS

Other dural veins running by themselves do not, as a rule, produce any visible impression on the inner table of the vault.

ARTERIAL GROOVES

The anterior and posterior divisions of the middle meningeal artery, which lie in obvious grooves on the inner table (*Figure 33*), are frequently accompanied by one or more veins. This is particularly true of the anterior division of the middle meningeal artery (*see* above).

If a large vein shares such a groove with the artery, it will impart (possibly by transmitting arterial pulsation) venous characteristics to the groove (that is, an uneven calibre). The uneven calibre is of the greatest importance in making the distinction between a venous and an arterial type of canal. The groove where an artery is the major content, on the other hand, has walls which are parallel, however tortuous, and a calibre which remains constant on the turns, only diminished by branching. It is true that exceptions to this rule are seen, and that occasionally arteries are of irregular shape while some large veins may have parallel walls for considerable distances. These exceptions are unusual and an attempt to recognize 'arterial' from 'venous' markings is often of great help in diagnosis.

Thus, a wide groove having arterial characteristics is often evidence of a large artery, and its recognition is important in the search for tumours deriving their blood supply from branches of the external carotid (*Figures 34–37*).

Hypertrophied arteries also often become tortuous. Exaggerated tortuosity of an arterial groove is thus also of value in the diagnosis of tumours with an hypertrophied blood supply.

By far the commonest of such tumours are meningiomas. Arteriovenous malformations occasionally present a similar appearance. Very rarely metastases may acquire a sufficient blood supply to cause recognizable hypertrophy of vascular channels.

Meningioma (*Figures 34–36*)

One or more of the branches of the middle meningeal artery may be hypertrophied. Where such hypertrophied arterial channels are recognized they are usually seen to run towards a single small area of the vault, often marked by an hyperostosis or an erosion.

Sometimes numerous small arteries pierce the outer table to supply the tumour from external tributaries, and small round translucencies may be observed scattered around the attachment of the tumour representing paths for such perforating vessels.

Hypertrophy of one middle meningeal artery may, rather uncommonly, be confirmed by the presence of an enlarged foramen spinosum; but this foramen is inconstant in its size for many reasons and by itself is a most unreliable guide to the size of the middle meningeal artery.

(For a systematic study of meningiomas read on to the end of the section on Diploic Veins below, then turn to page 90.)

Arteriovenous malformation

An intracerebral arteriovenous malformation (*Figure 37*) may, though uncommonly, derive some blood supply from branches of the external carotid and in these cases hypertrophied meningeal arteries may leave prominent grooves in the overlying bones, and may be the only evidence on the vault of underlying pathology. More rarely still, an arteriovenous malformation may produce a similar radiological appearance when it affects the whole thickness of the scalp.

It will usually be found in arteriovenous malformations that the grooves for hypertrophied vessels are widespread, showing little tendency to come to one focal point. This and the absence of hyperostosis or erosion help to distinguish the appearance from that of the commoner cause of hypertrophied meningeal arteries — meningioma. Large arteriovenous malformations may enlarge the internal carotid or vertebral arteries to a degree great enough to cause recognizable expansion of the bony channels through which they run. There is occasionally localizing thinning of the vault overlying a superficially placed cerebral angioma (Rumbaugh and Potts, 1966).

For embryological reasons the majority of large angiomas which have a dual blood supply, from external and internal carotid (or from external carotid and vertebro-basilar system), are posteriorly placed. So-called 'dural' angiomas supplied by meningeal branches of the external and internal carotid may, however, be found in various other situations as well.

The capillary naevus of Sturge-Weber's syndrome is hardly every supplied by arteries which may be shown to be hypertrophied by radiological methods. The arterial channels and foramina are therefore nearly always normal. On the other hand, abnormally placed and unduly numerous venous channels caused by an excessive number of large dural veins is not so uncommon, particularly in adult life.

Sinus pericranii (Ohta *et al.*, 1975) is a collection of non-muscular blood vessels or a venous haemangioma adhering tightly to the outer surface of the skull bone and directly communicating with an intracranial venous sinus by way of many diploic veins of various sizes. It may show as an area of thinning with small defects in the outer table.

Diploic veins (*Figures 39* and *40*)

The majority of vascular channels which appear on radiographs of the vault are caused by veins ramifying in the diploë. Their number, distribution and width are very variable and of no established significance. They may, for instance, radiate from a common pool, producing a superficial resemblance to a translucent tumour with a large blood supply but their course is usually seen to have irregular hair-line trabeculae along their walls. They may also be distinguished from dural vein grooves in a tangential view which will show the oval hole caused by the vein within the diploic bone.

Diploic veins are rarely seen during the period of rapid skull growth in childhood before the age of 10 years. Thereafter they become more obvious and tend to grow larger with advancing years.

Before the sutures unite, each system of diploic veins is limited to a single bone, but after union, the systems join in a haphazard manner over the whole skull.

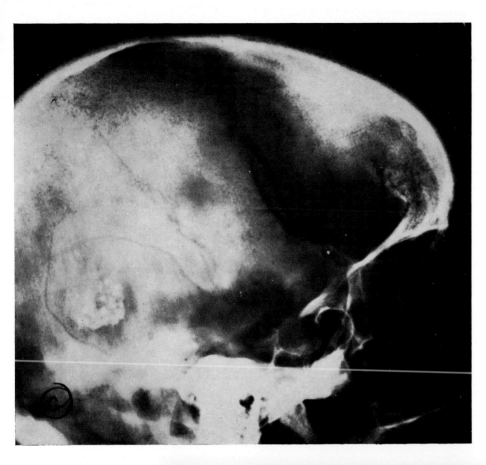

(a)

*Figure 36. Meningioma.
(a) Lateral radiograph
showing a frontal hyper-
ostosis towards which run
a number of 'arterial'
grooves. (b) A tomo-
gram during common
carotid angiography de-
monstrates the arteries
occupying the grooves
and running into the
abnormal bone*

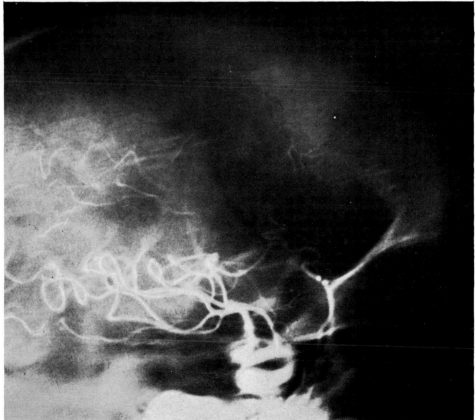

(b)

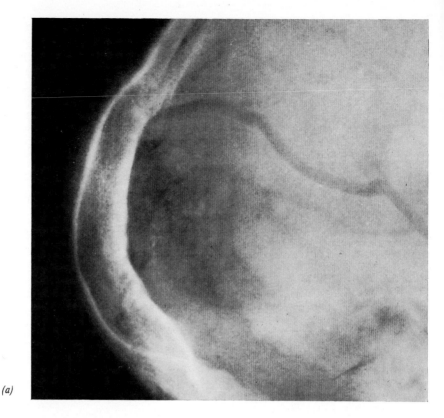

Figure 37. Angioma (A-V malformation). (a) The plain radiograph shows a number of dense flakes and spots of calcification. There is also a very wide arterial channel in the vault. (b) The angiogram demonstrates the angioma as well as a hypertrophied branch of the middle meningeal artery running in the bone channel

(a)

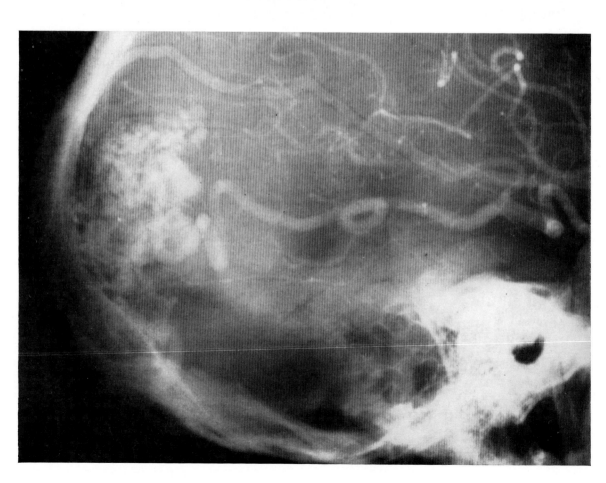

(b)

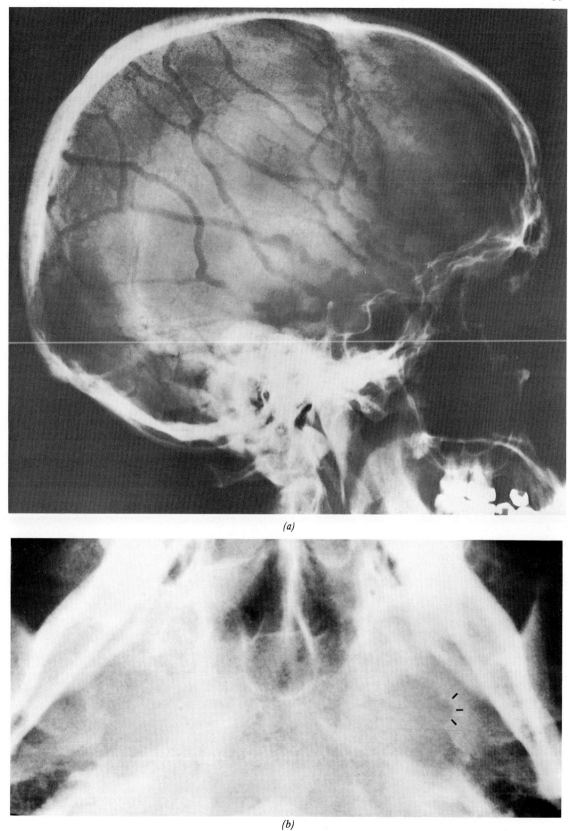

(a)

(b)

Figure 38. (a) Angiomas, when they are very large, may have hypertrophied arteries running to them from many sources, more than any meningioma. In this patient the anterior and posterior divisions of both middle meningeal arteries give branches supplying a midline meningeal and cerebral A-V malformation. (b) Both foramina spinosa were enlarged. This picture shows the left

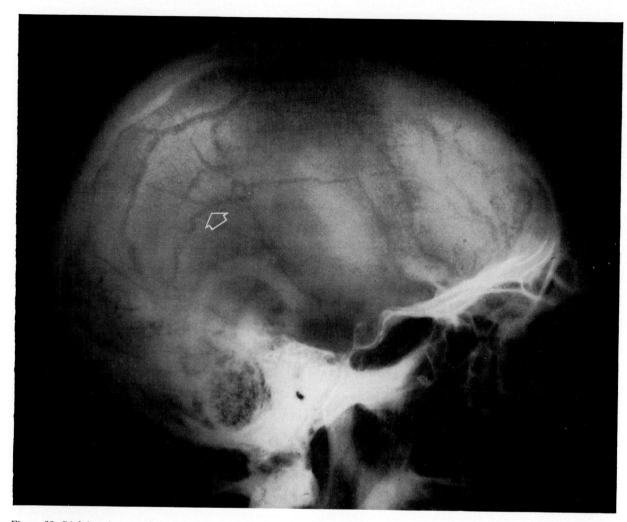

Figure 39. Diploic veins are of uneven calibre, have a wandering course with irregular confluences, and may not seem to drain into any main dural sinus. On close examination they are enclosed by a continuous fine white trabecular bony wall

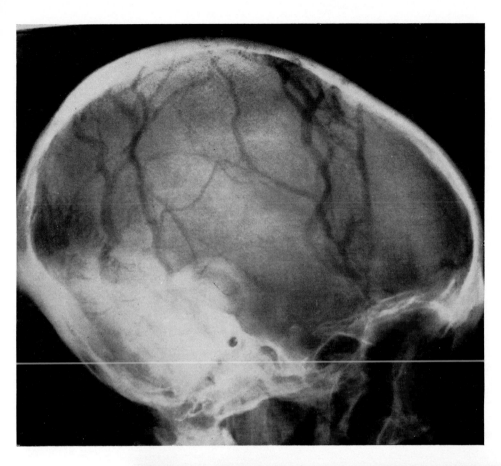

Figure 40. Hypertrophied diploic venous channels. A man aged 65 years who presented with Jacksonian epilepsy first on one side and then on the other. He had a very mild hemiparesis. (a) The lateral radiograph shows wide diploic channels joining the superior sagittal sinus to the transverse and sphenoparietal sinuses. There is no hypertrophy of any 'arterial' type of channel. Investigation revealed a falx meningioma deriving its blood supply from the anterior cerebral arteries. The patient's general condition contra-indicated operation (cont.)

(a)

(b) Six years later he was still active and had hardly any neurological signs. The hypertrophied anterior cerebral artery is shown, as well as the extreme vascularity of the tumour (cont.)

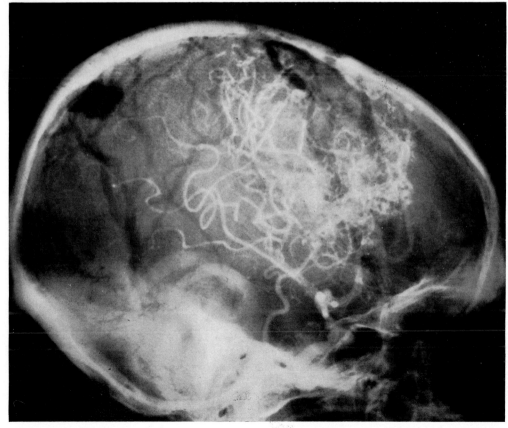

(b)

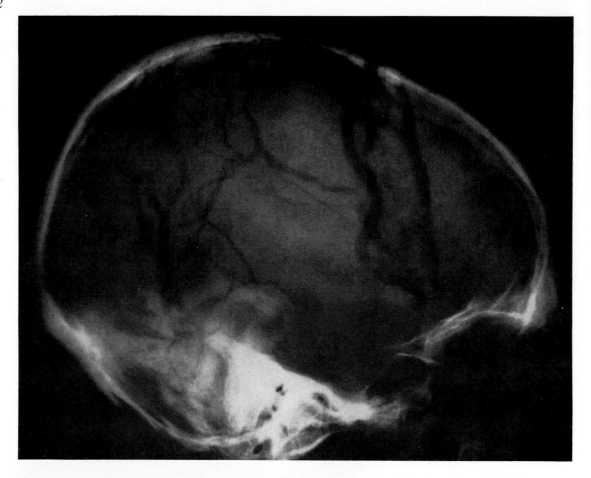

(c)

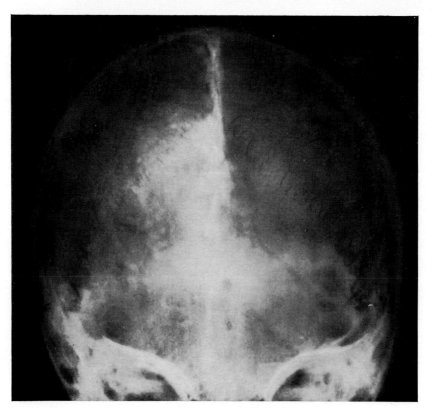

Figure 40 (cont.). (c) The plain radiograph at this time demonstrates further increase in the size of the venous channels and the question 'why?' cannot be answered with certainty. (d) Angiography showed that the superior sagittal sinus was not blocked. Presumably the great flow of blood through this very vascular tumour is responsible. The appearance of hypertrophied venous channels without evidence of enlargement of the middle meningeal artery has been seen in other cases of falx meningioma, but it is so uncommon that for practical purposes it is wise to ignore the venous markings of the vault unless there is also a suggestion of arterial hypertrophy

(d)

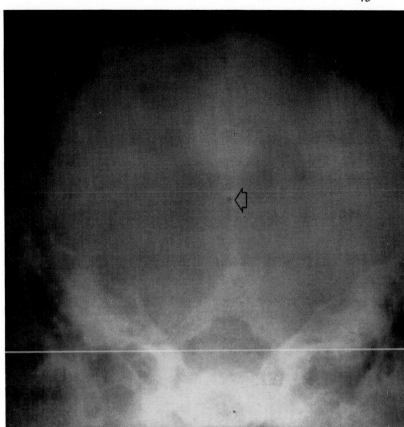

Figure 41. Emissary foramen. Note the blackness of the hole and its small diameter. There is a white line all round its edge. Very occasionally a dermoid sinus may have a similar appearance

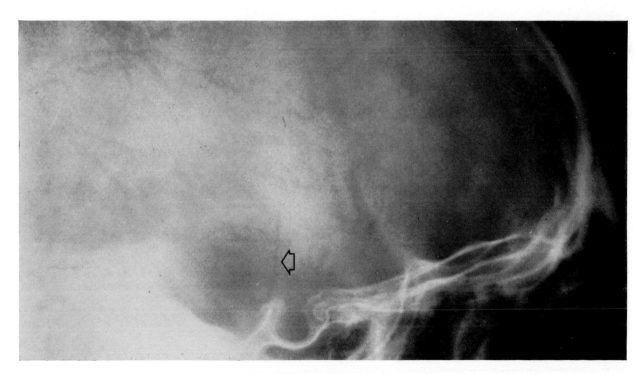

Figure 42. The groove on the outer table of the vault made by the deep branch of the middle temporal artery (arrow) closely resembles a fracture. It is sometimes possible to see that the line is not black enough to be a crack through the whole thickness of the vault

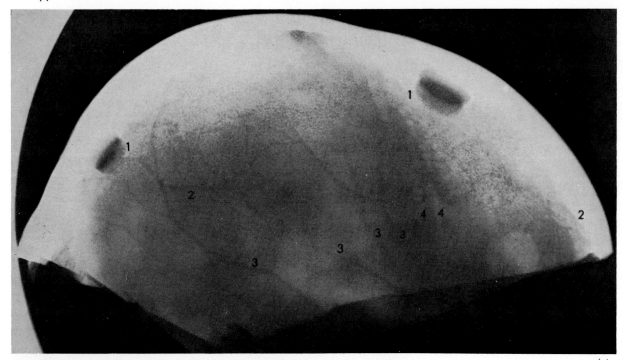

(a)

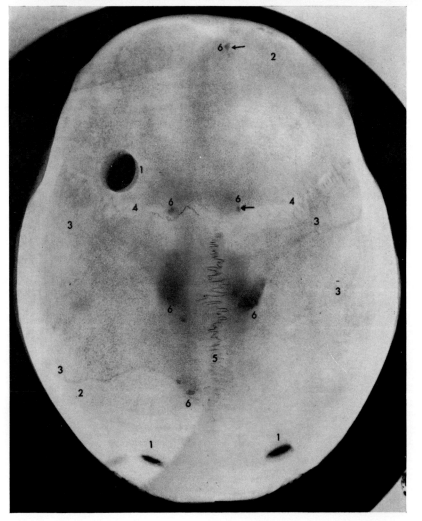

Figure 43. The skull vault. Much of the vault around the vertex is invisible in the lateral view, and its features may be indistinctly shown by other projections. (a) Lateral view of part of a fresh skull. Note: burr holes (1), diploic veins (2), middle meningeal grooves (3), the coronal suture (4). (b) Infero-superior view of the detached vault. The sagittal (5) and coronal sutures are clearly shown. Notice the dense bone through which they run. There are a number of depressions for Pacchionian granulations (6) which are quite invisible in the lateral view. Where their sloping edges are cut tangentially by the x-ray beam and the surroundings are diploic, a fine white line may be seen. This is the inner table of the vault (arrow). The larger ill-defined translucencies in which some of these depressions lie are caused by the lucunae laterales. Notice also how few of the Pacchionian depressions are connected with obvious venous channels in the vault

(b)

Emissary veins (*Figure 41*)

Foramina for emissary veins are often visible in the parasagittal area and near the torcula and are more obvious in the Towne's projection which gives a clear view of the occipital bone. They are rarely more than a millimetre or two in diameter, but occasionally may reach a larger size. They are recognizable by their depth (shown as translucency — blackness) compared with their narrow diameter and by their condensed margin of compact bone.

An emissary vein of rather large size (as much as 5 mm in diameter) often passes through the occipital bone just behind the sigmoid sinus. The foramen and the associated channel for this occipital emissary vein may be mistakenly ascribed to a pathological vascular enlargement.

Arterial grooves on the outer table of the skull (*Figure 42*)

Normal arteries run in the pericranium over the outer surface of the vault and form narrow straight channels which show as hair-lines easily mistaken for linear fractures. The most commonly seen — the deep temporal — runs upwards over the squamous temporal bone anterior to the shadow of the petrous in the lateral view. More anteriorly the supra-orbital may also be seen.

OTHER NORMAL TRANSLUCENCIES

Pacchionian granulations

Single or multiple translucencies up to 2 cm in diameter are commonly associated with Pacchionian or arachnoid granulations. Most of these are found in that part of the calvaria which covers the cerebral hemisphere, and they are most common in the parasagittal region (*Figure 43*).

They are more noticeable, however, when they occur far out in the fronto-parietal, temporal or occipital bones (*Figure 44*) where the presence of a round translucent area may be mistaken for a sign of local disease.

The collection of large arachnoid villi which forms the arachnoid granulation protrudes into a widened parietal vein. This vein, lying between the granulation and the vault, will be flattened, while the overlying vault is moulded to the general shape of the protuberance of the villi.

The bone thinning affects the inner and middle tables but not as a rule the outer table (*Figure 47*).

The diploë is absent or very much diminished in thickness. The inner table remains but lines the depression in the skull and may fuse towards the centre of the depression with the outer table. The appearance on a radiograph follows as might be expected from the anatomy. The thin area of bone is rounded or lobed. Careful study shows that its translucency is only relative and bone remains over its whole extent. Where the x-ray beam passes at a tangent to the dip of the inner table the

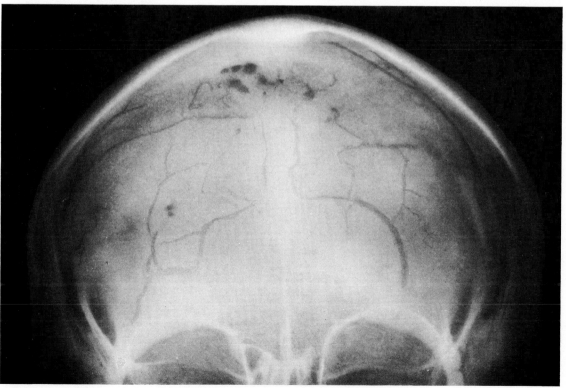

Figure 44. Typical parasagittal Pacchionian granulations

46

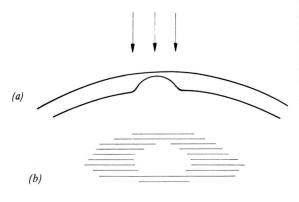

(a)

(b)

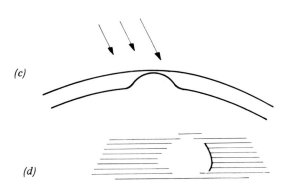

(c)

(d)

Figure 45. A depression in the inner table with a well-preserved inner table, for example, a depression for Pacchionian granulations. (a) Showing direction of rays. (b) En face radiograph. (c) Rays tangential to one slope of depression. (d) En face view shows a white edge

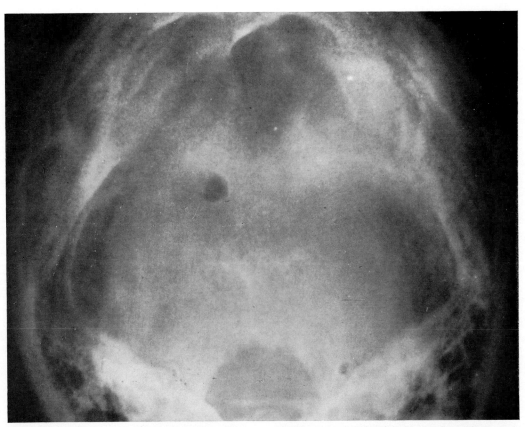

Figure 46. Pacchionian granulations. A single deep depression may resemble or be associated with an emissary foramen, but emissary veins are usually small. Note the slightly lobulated appearance of this depression, and the white line representing the inner table of the skull seen around only that part of the border where the slope of the depression and the direction of the rays coincide

picture shows a cortical shell next to the translucency. Views tangential to the vault reveal the impression from within the skull to be rather steep-walled (*Figures 45–47*).

In the parasagittal region the thinning of the vault may have more shallow sloping walls where it corresponds to the situation of a venous lacuna lateralis into which the granulation protrudes. Elsewhere it is uncommon to see a bony channel leading from the translucency, but when seen it is usually due to a diploic vein which has arisen from anastomosis with the dural vein serving the arachnoid granulation.

In the posterior fossa, very large granulations are sometimes encountered, particularly after middle life. They may be scattered transversely across the occiput below the groove for the transverse sinus or grouped below the confluence of the sinus.

Convolutional impressions

In childhood the growing vault moulds itself to the shape of the underlying convolutions (*Figure 8*). The translucency of the resulting thin areas of bone should not give rise to confusion. In adults these translucent areas are usually absent over the upper part of the vault, but are constantly present in the lower parts. (Long recumbency in childhood may cause unusual degrees of convolutional impressions under the most dependent part of the cerebrum.) Translucency due to deep impressions on the temporal bone may mask the presence of an erosion.

In children and young adults, a marked increase of convolutional impressions over the vertex may accompany very long-standing raised intracranial pressure. These impressions are really the evidence of bone growth attempting to keep pace with brain expansion. In fact, a balance may be achieved as in some cases of craniostenosis in which the intracranial pressure is not seriously raised, but the convolutional impressions are nevertheless great.

A GENERALIZED ABNORMAL INCREASE IN TRANSLUCENCY

These are all manifestations of widespread disease which will probably be found elsewhere in the skeleton as well as in the skull: rickets; primary and secondary hyperparathyroidism; hypophosphatasia; Paget's disease and osteoporosis circumscripta; osteogenesis imperfecta.

Rickets

In infants suffering from rickets, the bones of the skull may be very thin, and in some such cases fine traversing lines suggest multiple fractures. In others there may be areas in which ossification is lacking altogether. Rickets of this severity is now very uncommon in England.

Hyperparathyroidism (primary and secondary) (*Figures 48* and *49*)

The usual change encountered in the vault is a diffuse osteoporosis of granular pattern, but about 1 case in 10

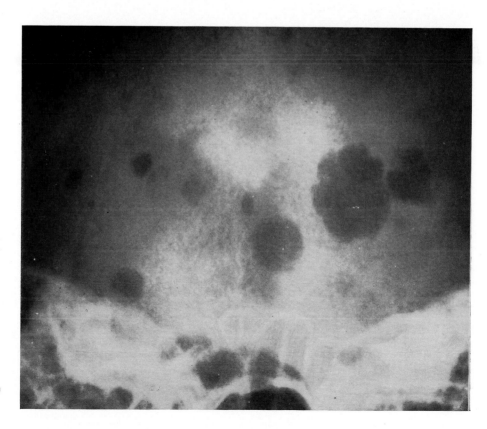

Figure 47. Pacchionian granulations. (a) Large depressions are sometimes seen scattered across the occipital bone below the transverse sinuses. They are more common after middle age, and are normal. The largest of the translucent areas shown in this radiograph was surgically explored (cont.)

(a)

48

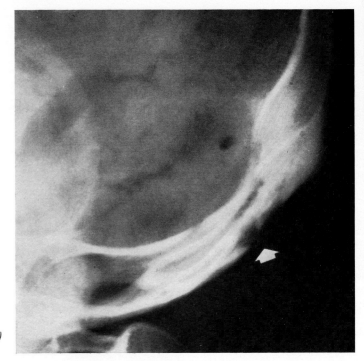

(b)

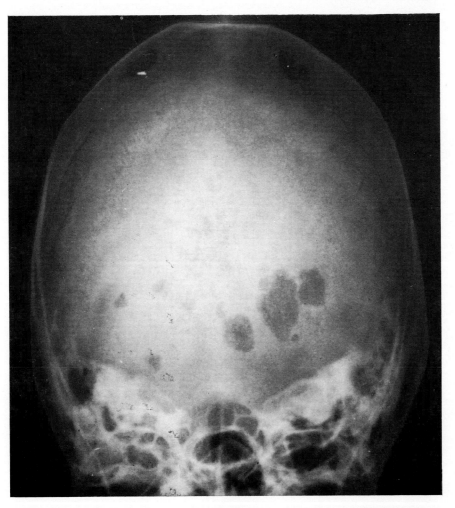

Figure 47 (cont.). (b) Lateral view showing how even the outer table may bulge over a sufficiently large collection of arachnoid villi (arrow). (c) Five years later: apart from the surgical defect, no change can be seen

(c)

also shows cystic areas with slight expansion. These 'cysts' may seem here and there to have an apparently corticated edge, though in other places their borders are indefinite. They may have a multiloculated appearance and may be multiple (scattered) or solitary. The whole vault is always abnormal.

Hypophosphatasia (*Figure 50*)

Early in life the bones of the skull in patients with this condition may be entirely uncalcified and their growth delayed so that the sutures are wide and the anterior fontanelle bulges. Later, as ossification catches up, if the child survives, premature fusion of sutures may occur, and the skull exhibits the features of craniostenosis. The

bone texture is a peculiar mixture of dense and translucent regions; and the outer table exhibits the most marked deficiency of normal growth and structure.

Paget's disease and osteoporosis circumscripta

Paget's disease in some patients (probably early in the disease) produces a more or less marked, rather patchy translucency of the whole vault which is, nevertheless, abnormally thickened. Very rarely, in Paget's disease proper, only part of the vault is affected. Osteoporosis circumscripta is a different manifestation of Paget's disease, causing total radiographic disappearance of bone, and always stopping short of involving the whole.

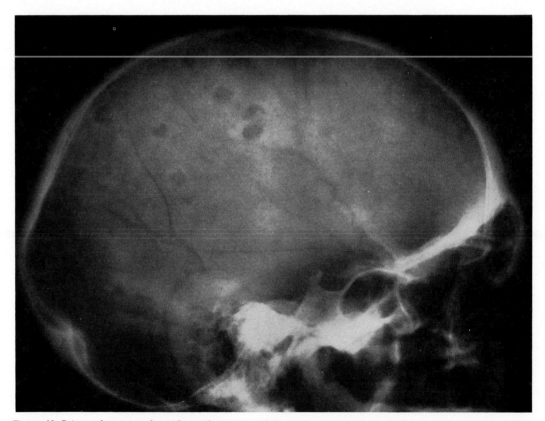

Figure 48. Primary hyperparathyroidism. The texture of the whole vault is abnormal. There is a loss of bone detail and hypertranslucency. In addition, in this case, there are a number of small 'cystic' areas

(Reproduced by courtesy of Dr Hodson)

50

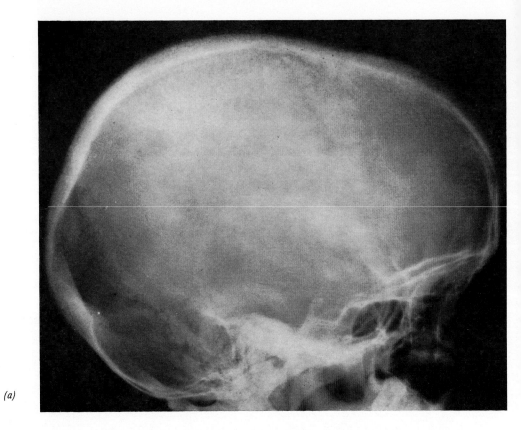

(a)

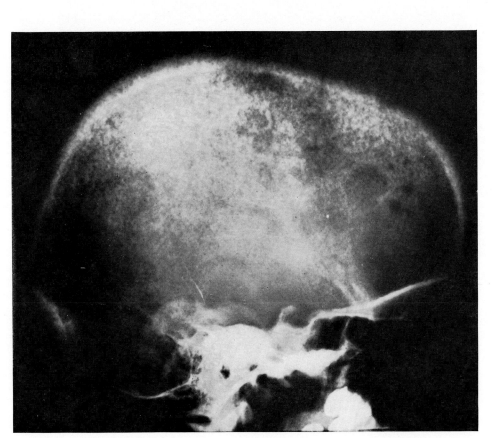

Figure 49. Renal osteo-dystrophy. (a) At the age of 14 years there was slight loss of definition of all bones radiographed, including the vault of the skull. (b) At 17 years the skull bones show a typical rather granular appearance. They are hypertranslucent as well as thickened. Round areas of greater translucency are seen in this patient (who also at this time showed many 'cysts' in the long bones and pelvis). The porosis of the lower part of the vault, greater than that of the vertex, is a little reminiscent of osteoporosis circumscripta

(b)

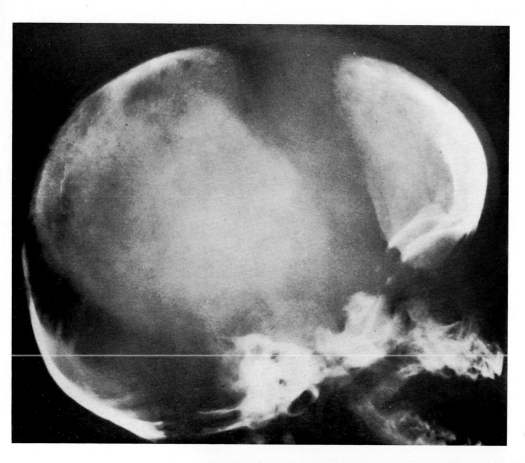

(a)

Figure 50a and b. Hypophosphatasia in a child who subsequently died. The radiographs show deficiency of ossification leading to very wide sutural gaps, together with an abnormal texture of the bone that has been formed. It is dense but full of rounded defects. The periosteal surface is irregular

(Reproduced by courtesy of Dr Strarer)

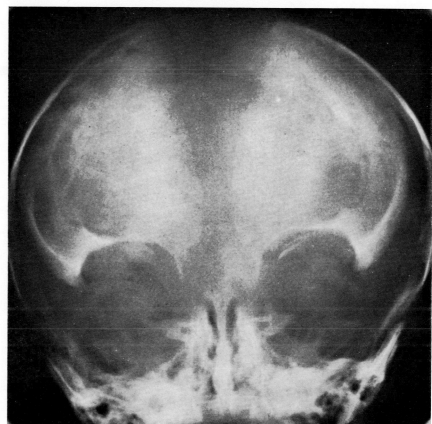

(b)

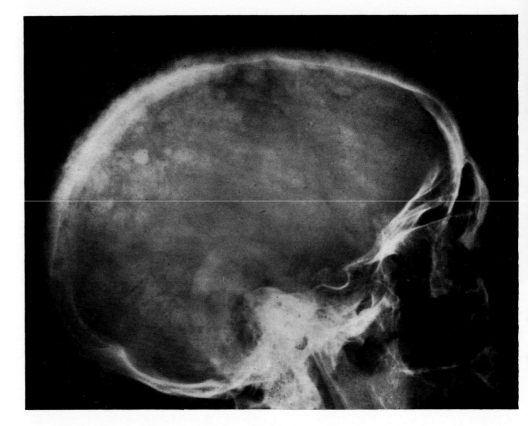

Figure 51. Paget's disease in a man aged 58 years. The typical mixture of lytic and sclerotic areas is shown. The skull is thick where it is affected—predominantly over the vertex

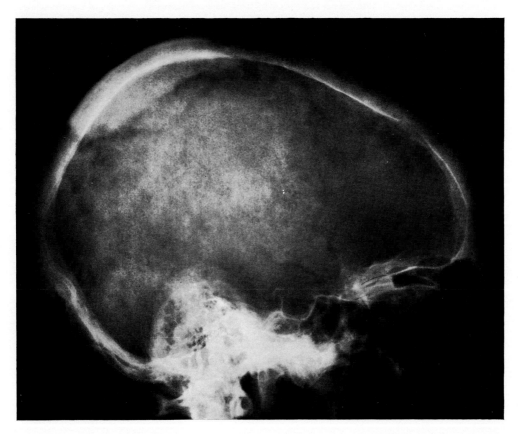

Figure 52. Paget's disease. (a) Lateral view. Translucent stage in a man aged 70 years who also had a subdural haematoma (cont.)

(a)

PAGET'S DISEASE (*Figures 51–53*)

The typical appearance of Paget's disease of the vault is of a wide area of thickening in which the middle and outer tables take the most prominent part. The bone shows a disorganized mixture of translucent and dense patches which fade one into another. Some coarse trabeculae are nearly always visible except in the most advanced cases with the densest skulls. The pathological process which this appearance represents is of overactive and uncontrolled bone remodelling. Osteoclastic action has destroyed the normal bone architecture and osteoblasts are actively laying down thick spicules of new bone which is not allowed to re-form into a normal pattern because of the further osteoclastic attack. Filling all spaces in the bone is a very vascular connective tissue.

The relationship between the hypervascularity and the activity of osteoclasts and osteoblasts is not clearly understood. It seems probable that an explanation of the cause for the great increase in capillary and sinusoidal blood vessels would go far towards explaining the cause for this condition.

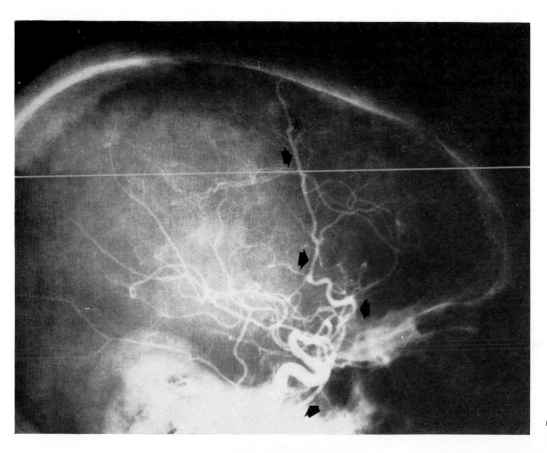

(b)

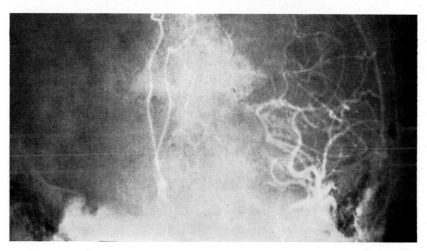

Figure 52 (cont.) (b) Lateral view. (c) Half axial view. Paget's bone is very vascular. These extracts from an arteriogram show the middle meningeal artery (arrows) sending branches into the bone

(c)

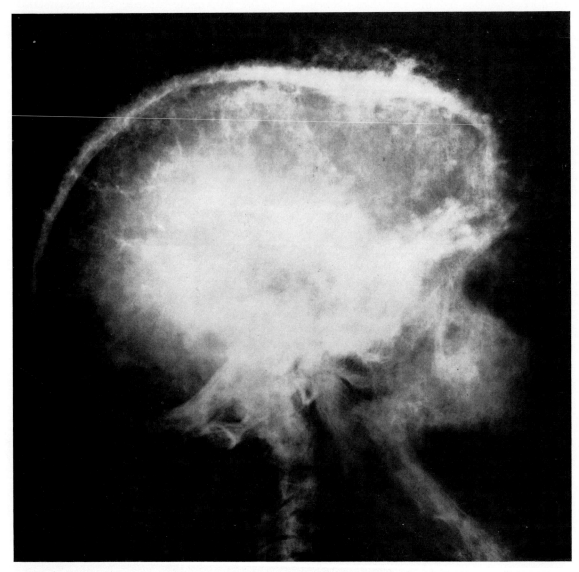

Figure 53. Paget's disease. The patient, aged 66 years, has extremely severe and widespread disease. The skull, although enormously thick, is hypertranslucent and shows coarse trabeculae rather than the more common woolly appearance. Note the relatively normal squamous occiput, and basilar invagination. The paranasal sinuses are obliterated. The patient is deaf and is going blind

The skull is sometimes, but not often, the only bone showing evidence of the disease. Paget's disease is commoner in men, rare before middle age, and there is some familial predilection (*see also* Osteosarcoma on page 97).

OSTEOPOROSIS CIRCUMSCRIPTA (*Figures 54* and *55*)

Schüller's second disease (osteoporosis circumscripta) is frequently associated with typical Paget's disease elsewhere in the skeleton and even in other parts of the same skull. It may develop later into typical Paget's disease; its microscopic pattern is similar but lacks new bone.

The radiological appearance is of a sharply defined translucent zone, usually large and sometimes involving more than half of the whole vault. The margins are rounded and show no sharp 'headlands', but there may be some large rounded 'bays' and 'peninsulars'.

This bone, like that of Paget's disease proper, is soft and bends so that the skull may be deformed.

The only serious difficulty in diagnosis is from xanthomatosis which is nearly always a disease of younger people. The presence of Paget's disease elsewhere in the skeleton may add weight to the diagnosis.

It is interesting to note that osteoporosis circumscripta as a form of Paget's disease is found nowhere but in the vault; and to compare the effects of infection and of trauma, both of which sometimes produce destruction in the vault without as much new bone formation as is seen in other parts of the skeleton.

In all cases of osteoporosis circumscripta seen by the author areas of translucency appear to begin low down in the vault, near the skull base, and from there extend upwards. Commonly, the first parts of the vault to be affected are the squamous occipital and the area round the pterion. It is tempting to speculate about the means by which the disease reaches the skull (Perhaps at points of major venous drainage?) (For systematic reading about Paget's disease turn to page 98.)

Osteogenesis imperfecta (*Figure 56, 57 and 244*)

All the bones of the vault are thin as part of a fragile construction of the whole skeleton. In early childhood the sutures may be abnormally wide, and as ossification proceeds a number of wormian bones may develop in the sutural gaps. In some cases, basilar impression takes place. The more severe cases present with multiple fractures in infancy or at birth, but milder forms (although showing slender bones more liable to fracture than normal) may first be found by chance in adult life.

In childhood, the wide sutures might suggest a diagnosis of raised intracranial pressure, but other evidence of this will be lacking and the appearance of the rest of the skeleton, including the base of the skull, provides confirmatory evidence of the true diagnosis.

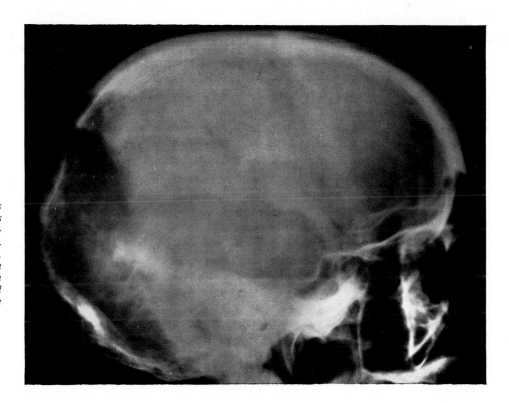

Figure 54. Osteoporosis circumscripta. (Paget's disease). Note the very extensive area of translucency. Like all the author's cases, the area of destruction seems to begin right down near the base of the skull and spread upwards into the rest of the vault

56

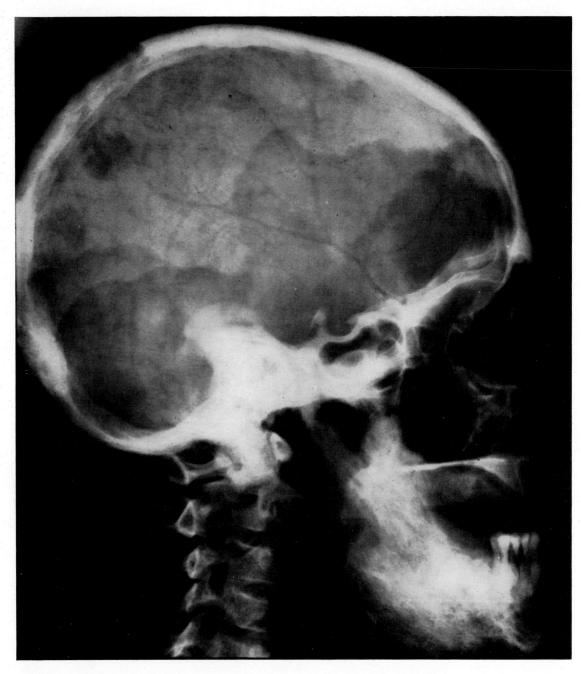

Figure 55. Osteoporosis circumscripta (Paget's disease). The typical distribution of the lytic areas is show as if spreading upwards from the lowest parts of the vault. The patient, a woman aged 48 years, has typical Paget's disease of the mandible

DISCRETE ABNORMAL TRANSLUCENCIES WHICH MAY BE MULTIPLE AND DISSEMINATED, OR SOMETIMES SINGLE FOR A TIME

Included in this section are descriptions of the following conditions: (1) metastases; (2) lipoid and non-lipoid histiocytosis and related diseases; (3) osteomyelitis; (4) radiation necrosis; (5) craniolacunia; (6) congenital parietal foramina; (7) symmetrical parietal thinning; (8) symmetrical frontal fenestrae; and (9) cranial dysostosis.

Metastases

Blood-borne metastases are common in the vault. They are usually osteolytic and are often multiple. When numerous, they are likely to be first recognized while less than 5 mm in diameter and lying in the diploë. They then present relative but not complete translucency and are rounded. There is no sclerosis or cortical edge to the erosion (*Figure 59*). Distinction from multiple myeloma is difficult or impossible (*Figures 58 and 63*). As soon as they break through the outer table they may give rise to small soft-tissue swellings, visible in tangential view with a bright light and frequently containing some areas of spicular new bone formation.

A solitary metastasis may present as a larger area of bone destruction. The outer and inner tables may then also be involved and therefore the translucency more marked. The edge of the erosion will be most irregular (*Figure 62*) and there may be evidence of small satellite erosions due to spread under the pericranium or through the vascular spaces. Under observation these coalesce. In many ways the radiological appearance of this type of lesion resembles acute osteomyelitis.

Solitary metastases are sometimes seen which are highly vascular and cause hypertrophy of adventitious supplying arteries. A typical, fairly slow-growing tumour of this sort arises from the thyroid gland (*Figure 60*). In such a case (because of the large vascular channels in the bone), a distinction must be made from meningioma. A metastasis may be suggested by the exuberant spread of bone destruction. (For a systematic study of malignant disease it may be as well to read on to the end of Radiation Necrosis and then refer to the section on Erosion by other Intracranial Tumours on page 94.)

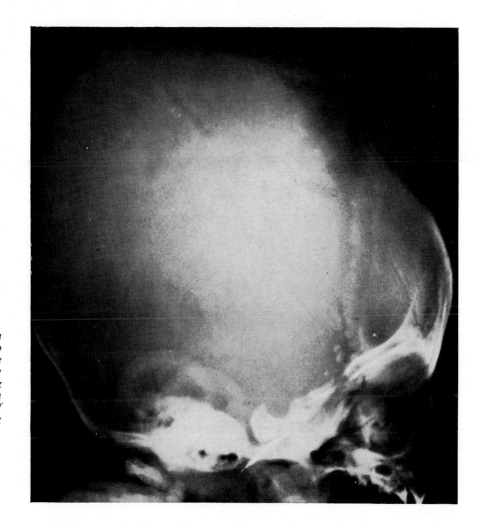

Figure 56. Osteogenesis imperfecta in an infant aged 5 months who had had multiple fractures. The parietal bone in particular is very imperfectly ossified, showing radiating tongues of paper-thin bone. There is a number of wormian bones and a gaping fracture

58

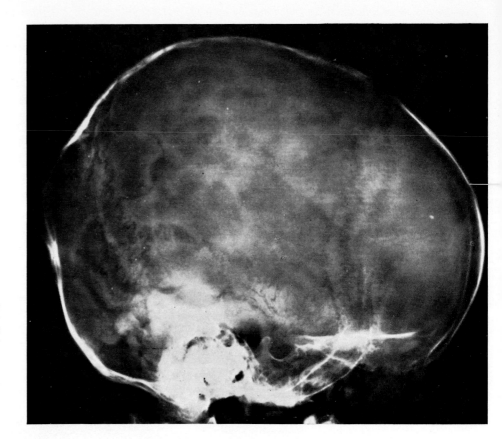

Figure 57. Osteogenesis imperfecta in a child. The extreme fragility of the vault is shown. There is a large number of Wormian bones

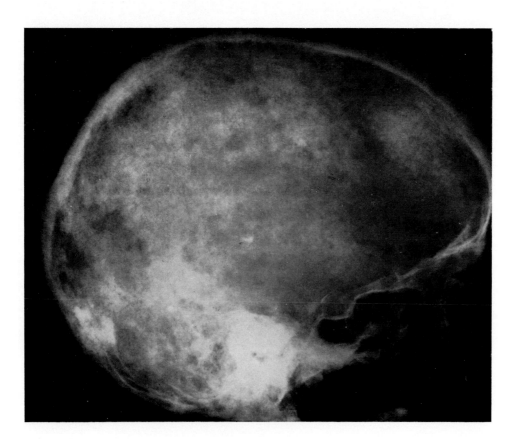

Figure 58. Metastasis from carcinoma of the breast. It was impossible to be certain of the presence of secondaries elsewhere in the skeleton, and the lungs were clear. The lateral view shows ill-defined confluent translucencies, some of them still small, scattered throughout the vault. There are no palpable scalp nodules; but the original radiograph shows many small erosions of the outer table of the skull

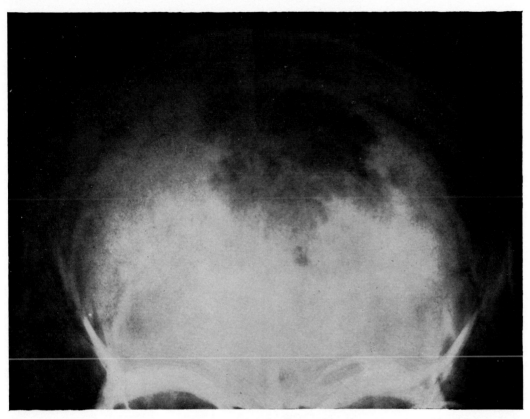

Figure 59. Metastasis from carcinoma of the breast. It is hardly surprising that metastases and osteomyelitis should sometimes appear identical when their exactly similar methods of spread through and round the bones of the vault are remembered

MYELOMA (*Figures 63–65*)

The single or multiple, rounded, sharply circumscribed translucencies of myeloma deposits may be of any size up to several centimetres in diameter and are usually recognized for what they are (with the reservation, however, that some secondary carcinoma deposits produce an identical picture).

The typical translucency is due to the deposit expanding but retaining its rounded contour and coherent edge beyond which, in the bone, there is no osteoblastic stimulation. At the same time, no macroscopic spicules of bone remain in the tumour itself.

Occasionally, myeloma, like other metastatic deposits, may grow under and through the pericranium, stimulating it in such a way that there is some new bone formation around the edge of the tumour with erosion of the outer table towards the centre of the mass.

In good radiographs it is usually possible to distinguish malignant deposits from normal translucencies, particularly depressions for Pacchionian granulations which have an apparently corticated edge where the ray strikes the in-turned table tangentially (*see* page 46).

NEUROBLASTOMA

Metastatic deposits from neuroblastoma may be found in the skull and present a variety of appearance (*Figures 66* and *301*).
(1) Diploic bone deposits which are not very destructive and may show as a large number of small discrete or confluent, rather irregular and veiled translucencies. They resemble early osteomyelitis but are likely to be more widespread than osteomyelitis at a similar stage.
(2) Extradural (subperiosteal) deposits, possibly of considerable size, causing raised intracranial pressure and suture diastasis.
(3) Subpericranial deposits presenting as palpable lumps and so stimulating the pericranium that fine radial bone spiculation is seen.
(4) Sutural deposits possibly analogous to metaphysial deposits in long bones. These add to or cause confusion with the appearance of suture diastasis.
(5) Occasionally, larger deposits causing complete bone destruction over an area of an inch or more in diameter. The orbit is not uncommonly affected.

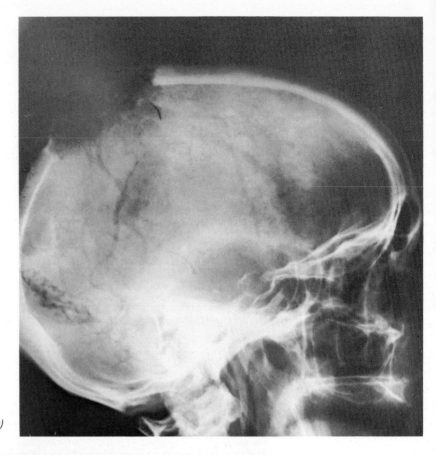

(a)

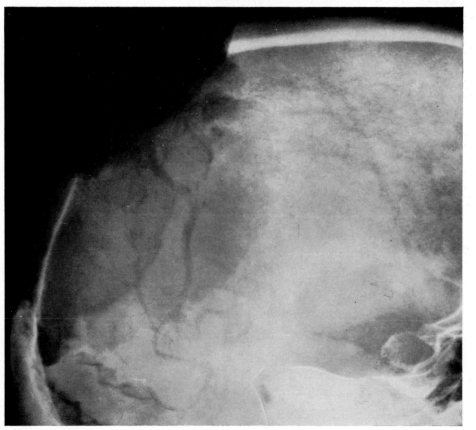

Figure 60. Metastatic thyroid-gland carcinoma. There was a large pulsating tumour on the top of the head. It grew very slowly. (a) An area of total bone destruction is surrounded by a much wider zone in which only the outer table of the skull has been eroded (arrows). (b) One year later, there has been only a moderate increase in the bone destruction

(b)

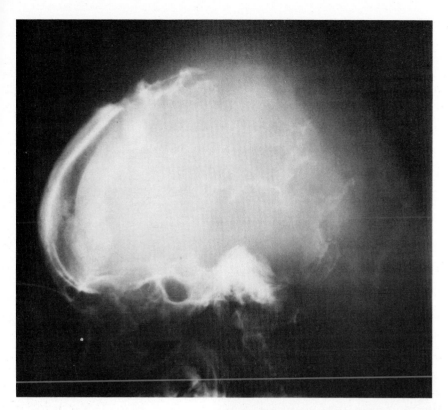

(a)

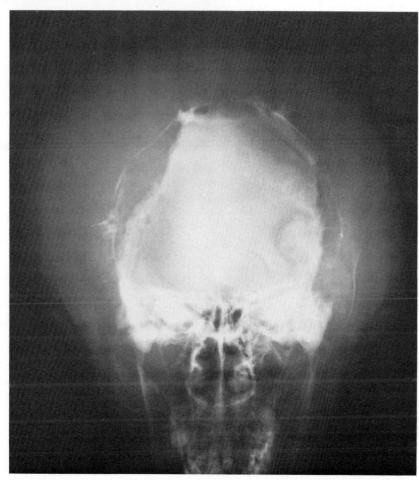

Figure 61. Metastases from carcinoma of the thyroid may reach enormous proportions as in this patient whose head appeared to be almost twice its normal size due to the expanding soft tissues. Very little bone remains. (a) Lateral view. (b) Antero-posterior view

(b)

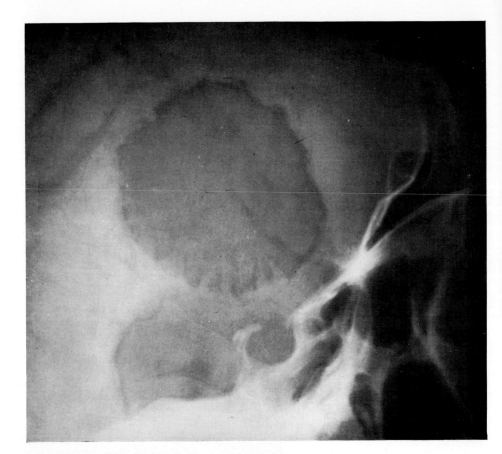

Figure 62. Metastasis from a haemangio-endothelioma. The patient, aged 69 years, has other metastases in the femur and ribs. The radiograph shows complete bone destruction; the edges, though for the most part clear-cut, are irregular

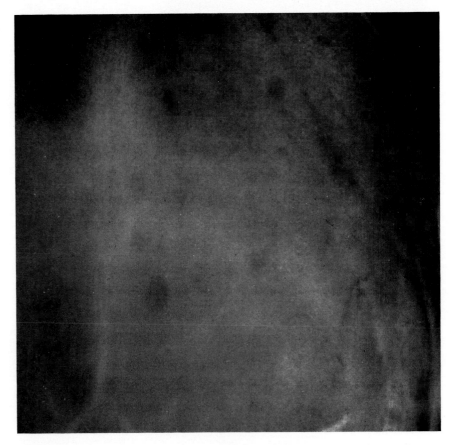

Figure 63. Multiple myeloma. Well-defined circular and oval translucencies. None appears to have a corticated edge. Tangential views confirm that they are intradiploic. They might equally be carcinoma metastases

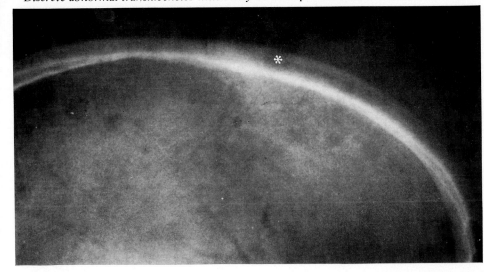

Figure 64. Myelomatosis in a woman aged 62 years. In the tangential view deposits are seen in the middle table. One is beginning to erode the outer table from within (asterisk)

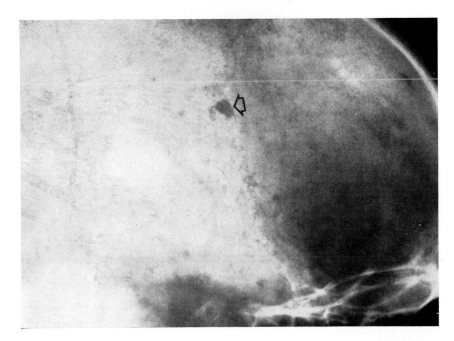

Figure 65. Myelomatosis in a man aged 60 years with no complaint about his head, but with a history of back pain for 16 months. There were widespread deposits elsewhere. In the skull the lesions are small, very translucent for their size, and unequal in volume. They are not unevenly distributed. Note also a depression caused by a collection of Pacchionian granulations (arrow). The diagnosis of isolated deposits may be very difficult because of their resemblance to Pacchionian depression, but tangential and oblique views will usually show the difference between an intradiploic erosion and a depression in the inner table and thus solve the problem

LEUKAEMIC DEPOSITS

It is extremely uncommon to find leukaemic bone deposits in the skulls of adults. When they occur they resemble the picture of Hodgkin's disease (*Figure 67*). In children with acute leukaemia changes are rather more frequently seen and the appearance is identical with that due to metastatic neuroblastoma (*Figure 66*).

HODGKIN'S DISEASE (*Figure 67*)

Bone deposits in the skull are not very common in Hodgkin's disease, but when they do occur they are usually predominantly osteoblastic. Even when erosions form the bulk of the lesion there is usually some sur-

rounding sclerosis. Since bony invasion takes place in the late stages of the disease, the differential diagnosis will in all probability have been solved by the clinical findings before radiological changes in the vault are examined, and resemblance to other metastatic deposits or to chronic osteomyelitis noted.

Lipoid and non-lipoid histiocytosis and related diseases (*Figures 68 and 69*)

XANTHOMATOSIS

The amount of bone destruction which can occur in xanthomatosis with the fully developed Hand–Schüller–Christian syndrome is most striking. Isolated eosinophil

Figure 66. Neuro-blastoma metastases 18 months after the beginning of the known illness in a boy aged 4½ years who died a few weeks later with widely disseminated metastases. He originally presented with multiple glandular enlargement, palor, pyrexia, and loss of weight. At the time of this radiograph he had papilloedema. The radiograph shows widespread ill-defined erosions of the vault, and of the sphenoid bone. There is severe suture diastasis, no doubt due partly to intracranial metastases and partly to deposits in the region of the sutures. With a bright light fine spiculation was visible in the soft tissues around the bregma

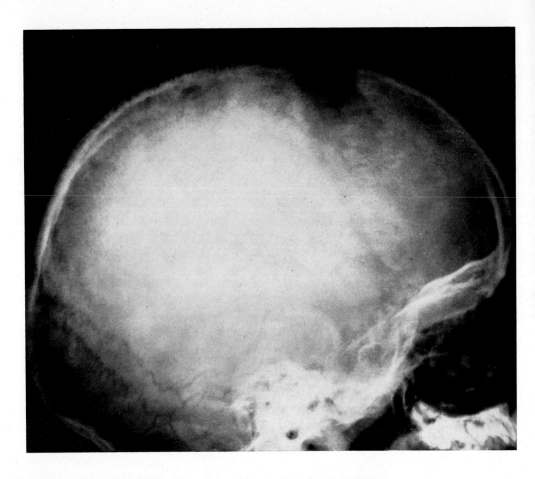

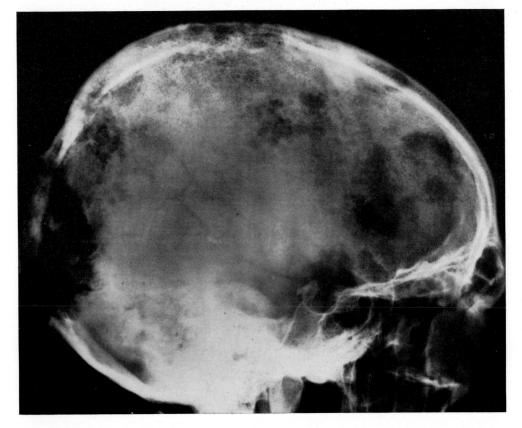

Figure 67. Hodgkin's disease. A man aged 42 years with disseminated Hodgkin's disease first diagnosed a few months before this radiograph was taken. There were tender scalp nodules. At necropsy 2 years later there were numerous deposits of tumour tissue in the calvaria. The largest of these were 4 cm in diameter and showed bony regeneration at its periphery. The radiograph shows confluent erosions of all tables, and some new bone formation extending into the soft tissues

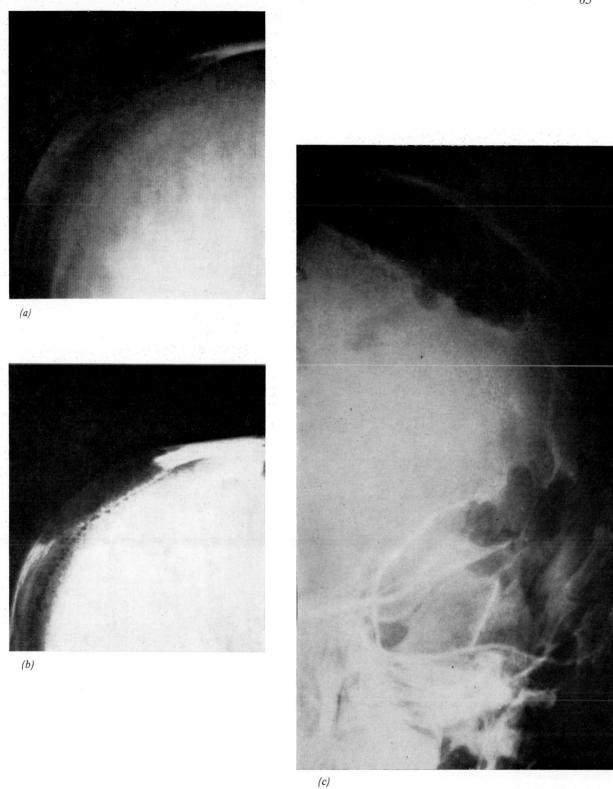

(a)

(b)

(c)

Figure 68. Eosinophil granuloma in a boy aged 3 years who came under observation when, after a blow on the head, a soft lump persisted. (a) Local tangential view of one of the many lesions suggests that it may have begun as an extradural deposit. The outer lump is slightly displaced and is beginning to be eroded. (b) Nine months later. (c) The left side of the same skull. There are erosions of the vault, and the orbital plate of the frontal bone, extending into the greater wing of the sphenoid. A fine white line may be seen around some parts of these erosions, probably due more to eversion of the bone edges than to reactive sclerosis

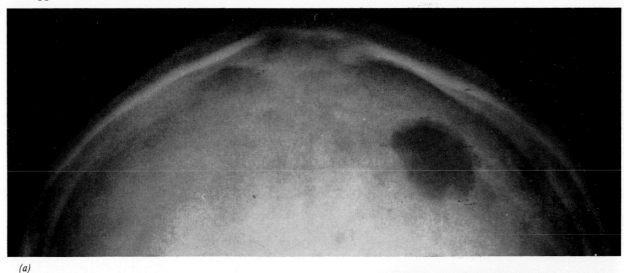

(a)

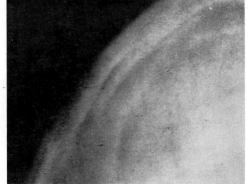

Figure 69. Eosinophil granuloma in a girl aged 2 years. (a) The area of destruction has heavily scalloped edges and affects inner and outer tables to different degrees. In the centre there is complete bone loss. As usual, no sclerosis is shown. (b) In this patient the 'intradiploic' nature of the deposit is apparent from the tangential view; but in others the main destruction may suggest a subperiosteal origin

(b)

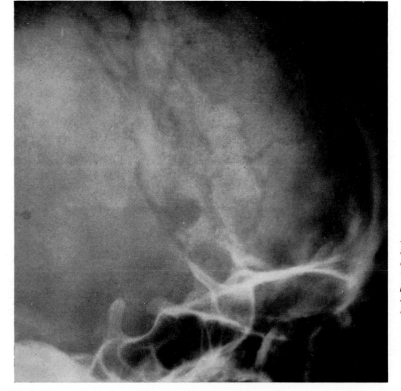

Figure 70. Acute haematogenous osteomyelitis; a rare condition in the skull. A single, fairly well-defined circular translucency appeared within 3 weeks below a tender swelling of the scalp. The patient developed an extradural abscess, and in spite of surgical treatment and antibiotics died of meningitis

granulomata may show destruction, but the lesions are not always so obvious.

The deposits in the vault usually begin in the diploë, and from this site they may expand to destroy the whole thickness of the skull over a wide area. There may, on the other hand, be pericranial and extradural extensions connected with the diploic deposit through very small erosions in the outer or inner tables. It is most unusual in the Hand—Schüller—Christian syndrome to find isolated lesions in the skull without some deposit elsewhere.

In Letterer—Siwe disease, similar bone defects have been described, usually, but not always, of small size.

The usual characteristic features of these diseases in the vault are that the bone replacement appears irregular in shape (unlike that of neoplastic erosion, which is usually round) and there is no sclerosis of remaining bone around the erosion. The edge of the defect is usually sharp (but this must depend to some extent on the thickness of the vault and the angle of ray). Bone in the immediate vicinity of the deposit appears radiologically of normal texture.

GAUCHER'S DISEASE

There is some doubt as to whether vault bone defects are ever found in Gaucher's disease. A diffuse osteoporosis has been described. Evidence of the disease will be found elsewhere.

NIEMANN—PICK DISEASE

Multiple defects have been described in the vault in very rare cases of this disease.

WEBER—CHRISTIAN DISEASE

In a very few cases of this rare diffuse panniculitis when the marrow spaces are involved and the condition is advanced to myelo-fibrous, multiple round translucencies may appear in the diploë, closely resembling multiple myeloma deposits.

Sarcoidosis

As in other parts of the skeleton, sarcoidosis may occasionally give rise to rounded areas of translucency with sclerotic margins. The lesions may expand beyond the bone and form scalp nodules.

Osteomyelitis (*Figures 70–77*)

ACUTE

Osteomyelitis of the vault is roughly divisible into only two types — acute and chronic — regardless of the

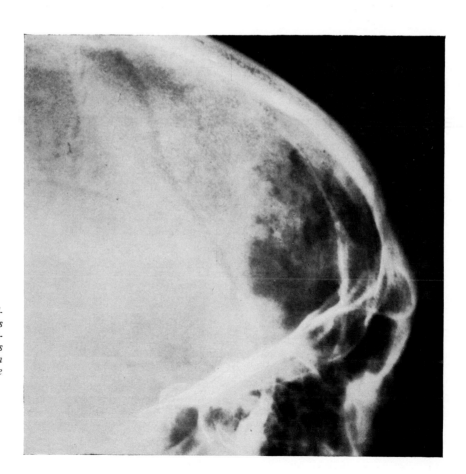

Figure 71. Acute osteomyelitis spreading from the frontal sinuses. There is a wide area of confluent erosions. Infection and granulation tissue has spread under the pericranium and in the extradural space destroying the bone

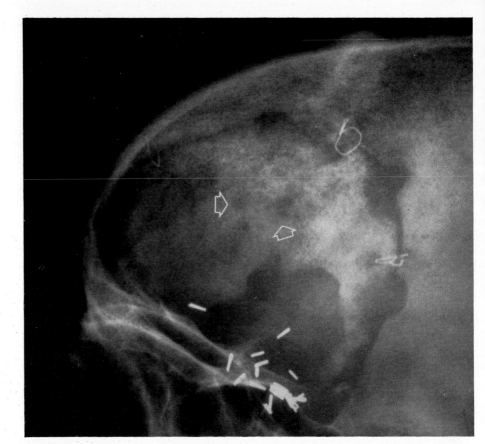

Figure 72. Osteomyelitis of a bone flap. There are very early small erosions (not to be confused with the relatively large areas removed surgically)

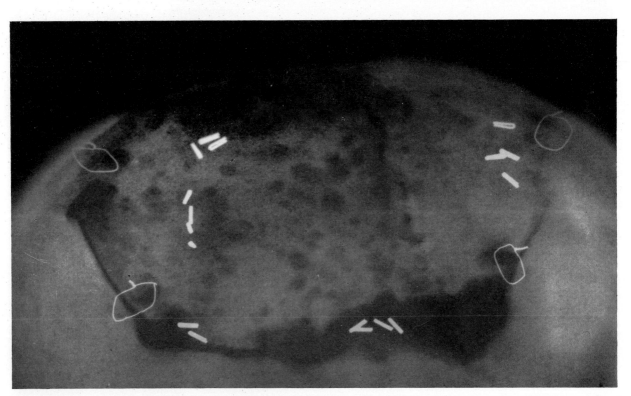

Figure 73. Osteomyelitis of a bone flap. The blood supply of this bone flap was probably inadequate. Low-grade infection has occurred and the bone is now being destroyed by subpericranial granulation tissue. An exactly similar change may follow avascular necrosis of a bone flap without infection. The process may or may not stop short of total bone destruction

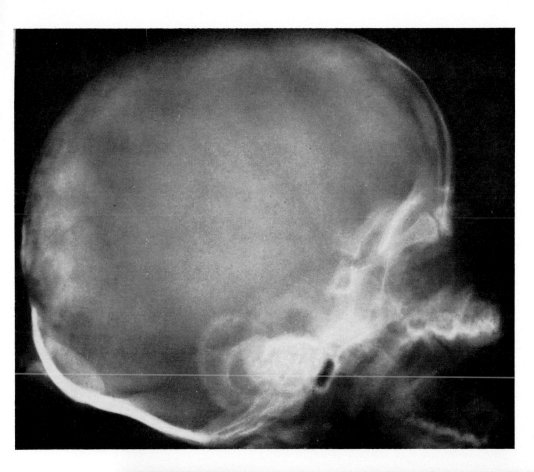

(a)

Figure 74. Congenital syphilitic osteitis in an infant. (a) There is widespread destruction of the thin bones of the vault. (b) At the age of 10 years, after adequate treatment, the skull is normal

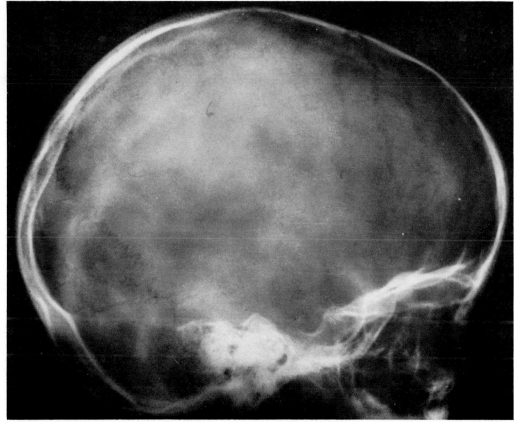

(b)

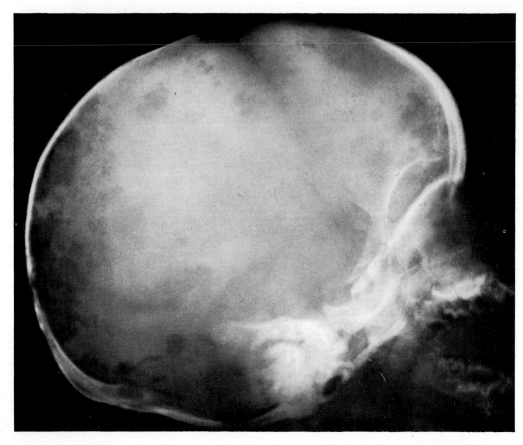

Figure 75. Congenital syphilitic osteitis. There are widespread areas of confluent bone destruction

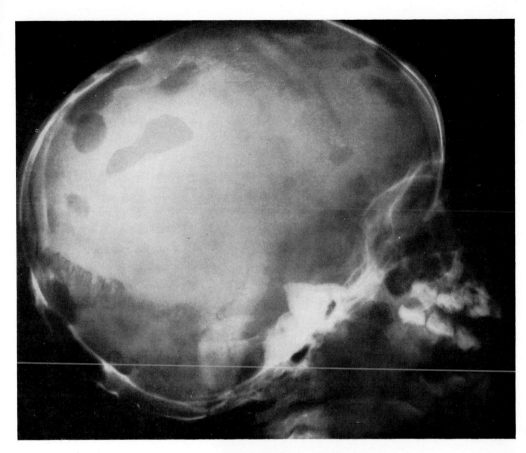

(a)

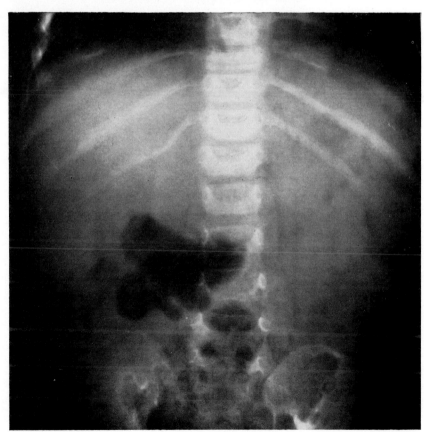

Figure 76. Acute tuberculous osteo-myelitis. An unusual manifestation in a child from Hong Kong. (a) The skull radiograph is indistinguishable from xanthomatosis. (b) There are similar lesions elsewhere in the skeleton

(b)

72

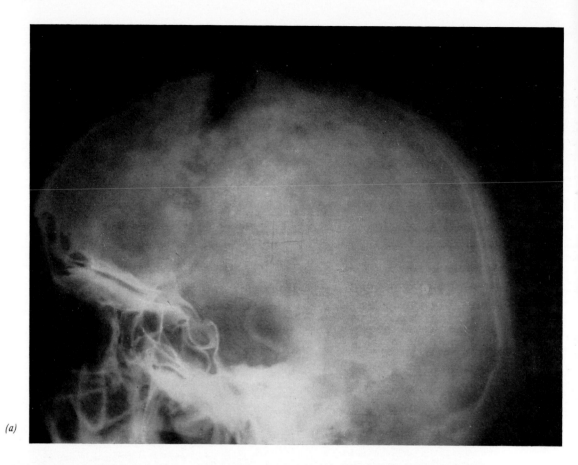

(a)

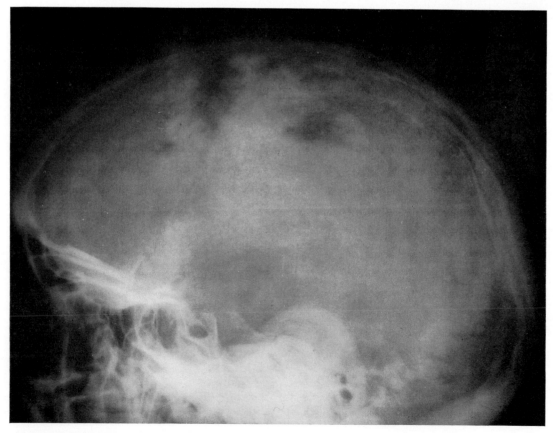

Figure 77.
See legend
under (e)

(b)

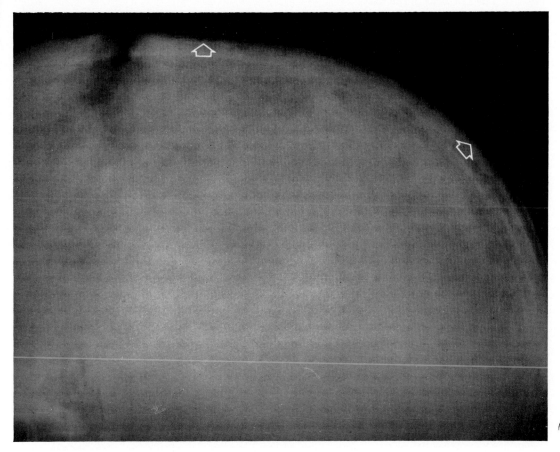

(c)

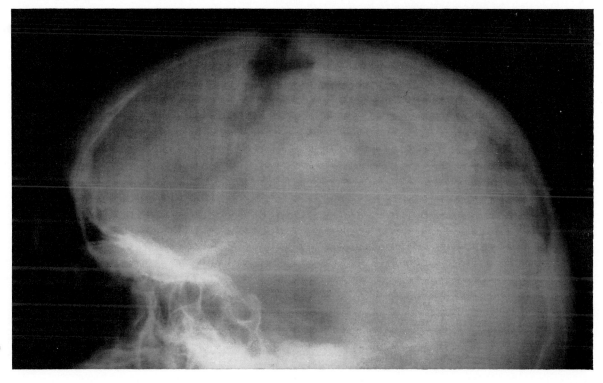

(d)

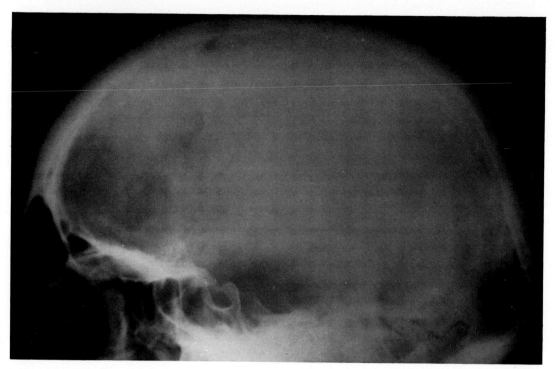

(e)

Figure 77. Acute leading to chronic osteomyelitis. The patient suffered a small puncture wound and thereafter a low-grade inflammatory process with discharging sinuses. Surgical exploration is responsible for one of the bone defects, but the remainder are due to bone removal by the subpericranial granulation tissue. Note the erosion of the outer table in (c) (arrows). After more than a year the skull has returned to an almost normal appearance. There is little sclerosis at any time. (a) After several weeks of infection. (b) Three weeks later. (c) Another fortnight. (d) A further fortnight later. (e) Fourteen months afterwards

organism responsible. In the acute phase of infection the process is almost exclusively lytic and it is only in more long-standing disease that sclerosis tends to occur. The appearance of osteomyelitis in the vault therefore, differs somewhat from the appearance in osteomyelitis of other bones. In the skull vault, new subperiosteal bone is less readily formed. Sequestra are uncommon and, except following operation, tend to be small and spontaneously absorbed — the excellent blood supply of the skull and scalp probably being responsible for this.

Pus from the diseased bone has little difficulty in making its way into and opening up a subpericranial space, the bone being too thin to encourage chronic bone abscess formation. Having reached these planes there is little barrier to further spread over the surface of the outer (and inner) table, and the disease may extend widely (*Figure 77*).

Osteomyelitis of the vault may be the result of a spread of infection from the frontal sinus or rarely from the mastoid air cells. It follows sepsis in puncture wounds of the scalp and sometimes interferes with the healing of a craniotomy.

Blood-borne infection is uncommon but may present as a moderately well-defined round translucency involving the full thickness of the bone below a tender swelling of the scalp (*Figure 70*). The ease with which skull bone texture can be shown sometimes allows bone destruction to be demonstrated very early in the course of the infection. The size of the translucency is likely to increase rapidly if untreated. The presence of an extradural abscess may complicate the clinical picture but the signs of local infection will probably relieve the radiologist from having to distinguish this erosion from one due to a new growth.

Infection introduced at operation, by puncture wounds or spreading from a neighbouring acutely infected frontal sinus usually first shows itself as multiple, irregularly rounded areas of slightly greater translucency than the surrounding vault (*Figures 71* and *72*). As they grow in size and number they coalesce quite rapidly and become more translucent. Only after several weeks of infection does an ill-defined sclerosis begin to appear in the neighbourhood, and even then tangential views show little periosteal new bone.

After a craniotomy wound has become infected, there is a tendency for infection to be confined to the hypo-vascular or avascular piece of bone (*Figures 72* and *73*) and in this way, because of the ease with which granulation tissue can grow from the scalp tissues, very considerable areas of dead bone flap may be absorbed and disappear.

CHRONIC

Very low-grade infection, coccal, fungoid, syphilitic, tuberculous, leprous, and so on, may, however, provoke an osteoblastic reaction in which the thickness of the vault is increased by deposition of bone from the periosteum. Lytic areas are few and only large ones are visible. Sclerosis dominates the picture and is widespread.

Radiation necrosis (*Figures 78* and *79*)

Aseptic necrosis of areas of the vault, particularly bone flaps, may occur after irradiation of intracranial tumours. Often the appearance in every way resembles osteo-myelitis in which many foci of destruction coalesce without evidence of sclerosis or periosteal new bone formation, but is slow in its development, sometimes taking years to appear and many, many years to develop fully. It is unaccompanied by clinical evidence of infection. Several parts of the vault may be affected.

Subsequent healing may occur and the vault return almost to normal.

Radiation necrosis is sometimes accompanied by sclerosis in addition to areas of erosion, but in the author's experience this is a rare manifestation. The distribution of the abnormal bone is consistent with the radiation fields and may be symmetrical.

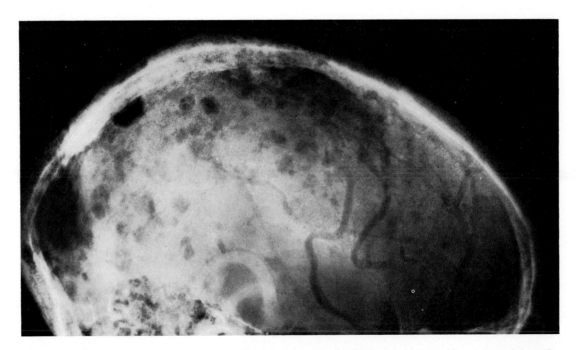

Figure 78. Radiation necrosis in a patient aged 49 years who received radiotherapy for a cirsoid aneurysm of the scalp 22 years before. In addition to the widespread erosions of the diploë, there are two parietal burr holes and a number of very wide vascular channels

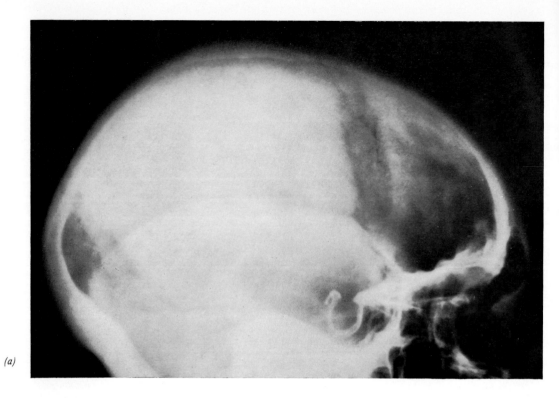

(a)

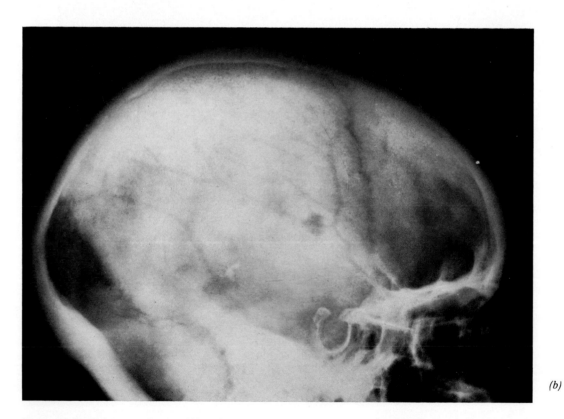

(b)

Figure 79. Radiation necrosis. In 1943, when the patient was aged 46 years, she received a course of irradiation to the pituitary. (a) Lateral view 1948, normal except for the pituitary fossa. (b) (1953) There are a number of rather irregular-shaped translucencies in the vault, only one of these is obvious (cont.)

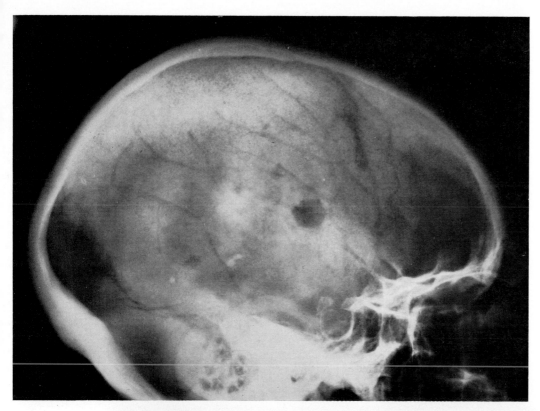

(c)

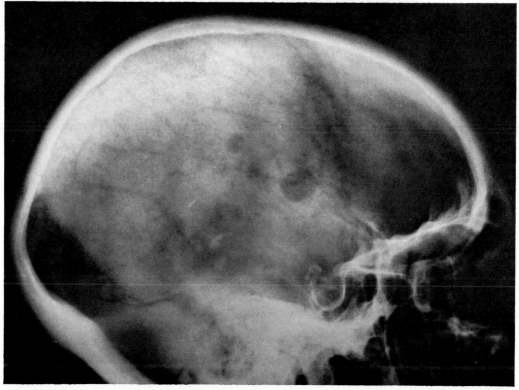

(d)

Figure 79 (cont.). (c) (1958) The translucencies have enlarged, but there is no evidence of surrounding sclerosis. The large one has well-defined edges and a rather angular profile. These erosions are on both sides of the head, distributed over symmetrical fields. (d) (1960) Further enlargement; still little or no sclerosis (note also the steady increase in calcification of the carotid siphon). Sclerosis is uncommon in post-irradiation necrosis of the vault. The appearance is indistinguishable from osteomyelitis and metastasis; but the symmetrical distribution, the history of irradiation, and the slow progress establish the diagnosis. There is no clinical evidence of disease of the vault

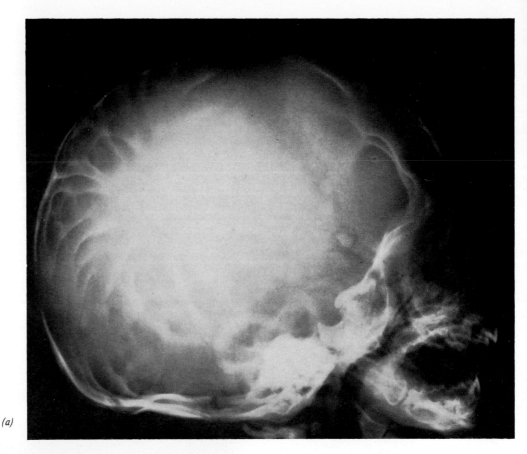

(a)

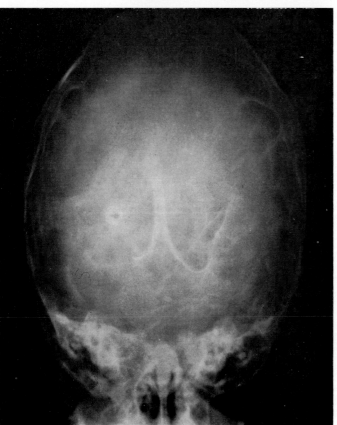

(b)

Figure 80. Craniolacunia in a child aged 2¾ years who had a meningomyelocoele and for whom a ventriculo-caval shunt was performed for hydrocephalus. It is said in the literature that craniolacunia disappears by the age of 8 months, though it may be followed by the radiological signs of hydrocephalus. Here is a child in whom the pattern is intermediate between cranio-lacunia as seen at birth and increased convolutional impressions as seen later

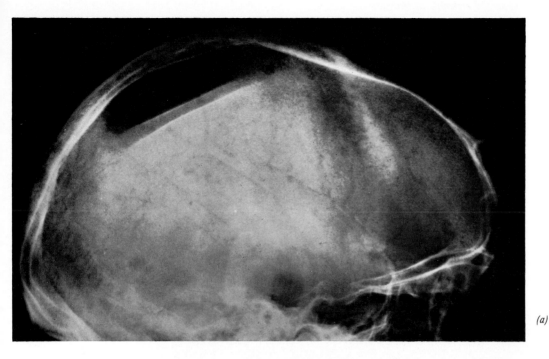

(a)

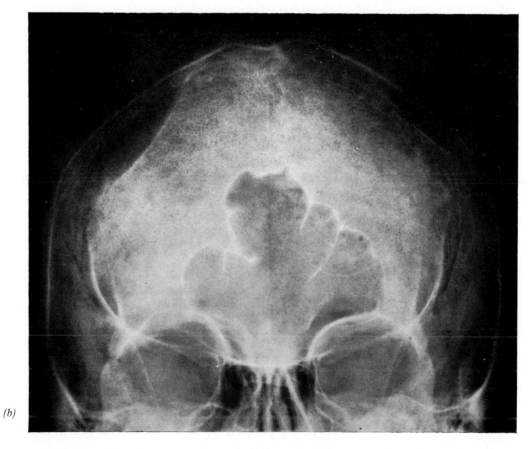

(b)

Figure 81. Symmetrical parietal thinning, sometimes said to be due to senility, certainly becomes obvious with the onset of baldness. The age of onset in the majority of cases is not known, but the appearance has occasionally been reported in young men. It tends to be confused with congenital parietal foraminae. Less severe degrees of thinning may easily be overlooked in skull radiographs. (a) Lateral view at the age of 75 years. Note the straight white line of the outer table viewed tangentially at the lower margin of the thin area. (b) Postero-anterior view (cont.)

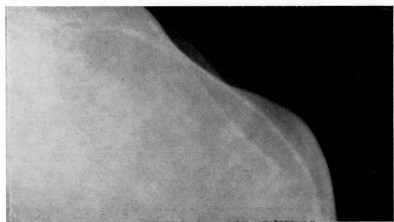

(c)

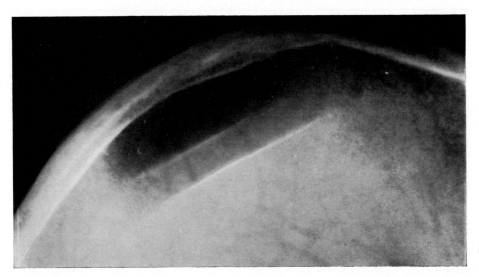

Figure 81 (cont.). (c) Tangential view to show how the abnormality of shape is confined to outer and middle tables. (d) The same patient at the age of 61 years. A portion of the lateral view

(d)

Craniolacunia (lüchenschädel: craniofenestra) (*Figure 80*)

There is confusion in the literature between two causes of a similar appearance.

(1) In newborn babies and infants, the vault may sometimes show widespread areas of extreme thinning (craniolacunia) or even complete defects (craniofenestra) which in their general arrangement suggest an exaggerated form of convolutional impressions. In the majority of cases there is also an abnormality such as meningocoele or an Arnold–Chiari malformation which is likely to give rise to hydrocephalus (*see also* page 1).

(2) Failure of normal ossification (as a manifestation of generalized osteodystrophy) may also result in large areas of translucency limited by narrow bands of bone in the skulls of newborn babies.

Examination of the skulls will show that the outer table of the skull presents a more or less regular surface, though in some places it may be paper-thin. The inner table, on the other hand, is indented and in the floor of the dents distinction between the three tables is lost in the thin area of bone.

It would seem certain that whatever the cause of deficient ossification, the pressure of growth of the brain and its vessels must play a considerable part in shaping the form of the defects, and it is understandable that excessive pressure plus a normal ossification stimulus should produce a similar appearance to that which arises from normal pressure plus deficient ossification.

Congenital parietal foramina (*Figure 82*)

A small foramen for an emissary vein is usually found in the upper part of the parietal bone about 4 cm in front of the lambda and 1 cm from the midline. This represents the last stage of a membranous defect where ossification spreading from the anterior and posterior centres delays in meeting. The defect initially extends to the midline and in infants in whom ossification is unusually slow, the interval will be felt or seen radiologically as a lozenge-shaped translucency. It is then described as the sagittal fontanelle. During the first few months or years of life, the fontanelle is further partially obliterated by a midline bar of bone. The lozenge-shaped area thus becomes transformed into two round defects, one on either side of the midline, and these are the enlarged parietal foramina which sometimes persist into adult life. The abnormality may be inherited as an autosomal dominant.

Symmetrical parietal thinning (*Figure 81*)

In this condition, the cause of which is unknown, the skull is thin over the middle of the upper parts of the parietal bones. The thinning consists of flattening of outer table and diploë over a roughly circular area, or an oval whose long diameter is parasagittal.

Symmetrical parietal thinning has been described in a number of people under the age of 30 years, but there is evidence that the thin areas may increase or become more obvious or turn into true defects with advance of age and the condition merges with that described as concentric circumscribed senile atrophy.

Symmetrical frontal fenestrae

These have also been described on one occasion in an infant. They appear to have arisen as a result of an abnormal spread of ossification from the primary centres.

Cranial dysostosis and cleidocranial dysostosis (*Figures 250* and *251*)

A wide spectrum of disease of variable severity is covered by these two names. Both membranous and cartilaginous bone are involved. The vault is thin and the sutures, especially the metopic suture, are wide in childhood. They gradually close with the formation of many wormian bones, but the vault may be deformed so that a degree of basilar invagination takes place. The mandible and maxilla may be hypoplastic and many of the patients present with malocclusion. In cleidocranial dysostosis there is also hypoplasia of the clavicles and there may be hypoplasia of the pubic bones.

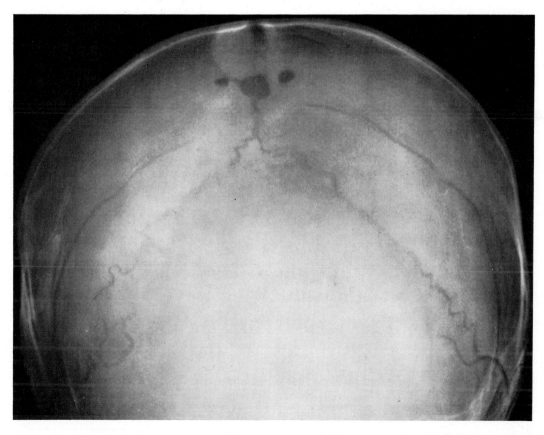

Figure 82. A small meningocoele with congenital parietal foramina on either side

DISCRETE ABNORMAL TRANSLUCENCIES WHICH ARE ALMOST ALWAYS SINGLE OR CONFINED TO A SMALL AREA

These may be due to: meningocoele or encephalocoele; dermoid and epidermoid; haemangioma; meningioma; rarely other intracranial tumours; osteoclastoma; neurofibroma; sarcoma; malignant skin ulcers.

Meningocoele or encephalocoele (cranium bifidum)
(Figures 82 and 83)

The combination of a midline bone defect with a congenital swelling of the soft tissues may be due to a meningocoele, an encephalocoele or a dermoid cyst.

Encephalocoeles are usually of large size, but defects up to about 2.5 cm in diameter with clear-cut margins are identical whether the structure passing through them is a meningocoele or a dermoid. Both may cause a pressure deformity of the outer profile of the skull around the edges of the defect where the cystic space is trapped beneath the galea.

Similar congenital defects in the bony walls of the orbit also occur (*see* page 289).

Difficulty in recognizing the presence of a meningocoele may arise when the midline failure of fusion is far anterior and the swelling lost in a general deformity of the root of the nose. In severe cases, however, the radiological picture is characteristic. Small nasal meningocoeles may defy diagnosis.

MEDIAN CLEFT FACE

Under this general heading are included all those conditions like cleft nose, cleft palate and orbital hypertelorism which follow the failure of medial migration and union of the embryonal precursors of structures in the median facial region. They are dealt with at greater length in Chapter 11. The associated median frontal defect is cranium bifidum occultum frontalis. This defect is filled by dura and pericranium and if the child survives it eventually tends to ossify.

Epidermoid and dermoid

INTRADIPLOIC DERMOIDS *(Figures 84, 86 and 87)*

These are found in all bones of the vault, but particularly in the squamous parts of the occipital and temporal bones and in the frontal bone in relation to the frontal sinuses and orbits.

They present clear, more-or-less round, well-demarcated translucencies, but a shell (possibly incomplete) of inner or outer table (or both) remains over the surface of the tumour. The expansion of the bone may be very great and in tangential view will be obvious if much of the outer and inner tables remain, and it will then usually be seen that the tumour is expanding chiefly outwards. Much more rarely the expansion is inwards to form an intracranial space-occupying lesion.

Growth and remoulding over the mass may finally remove most traces of one or other layer and then the

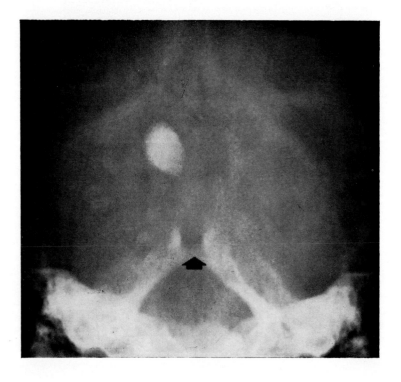

Figure 83. Occipital meningocoele. A small pedunculated swelling had been present on the back of the head since birth. This was found to communicate via a narrow channel full of cerebrospinal fluid with the subarachnoid space. The bone channel is visible some way below the soft-tissue lump. Such a communication may also occur between a superficial dermoid and an intracranial portion of the cyst

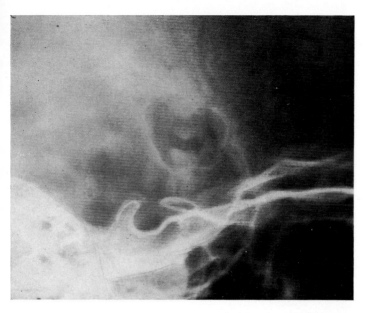

(a)

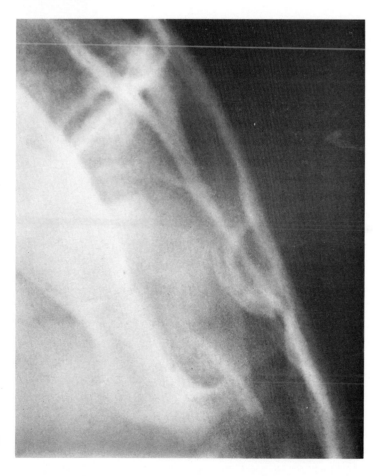

(b)

Figure 84. Intradiploic dermoid in a girl aged 5 years with a 2½-year history of a left temporal swelling. It was about 2 cm in diameter, had a rubbery consistency, and felt as if there were a bony margin surrounding it. (a) The lateral view shows a translucency with scalloped edges apparently affecting one table of the skull much more than the other since there is a darker central zone. The edges are all sharp and appear condensed. This condensation represents, at least in part, the tangentially viewed skull table as it turns around the edge of the mass. (b) An axial view shows the inner table pushed inwards. The outer table was almost completely destroyed, but the original radiograph shows an edge of it everted, thus confirming the intradiploic position of the mass. Operation revealed a dermoid cyst. The differential diagnosis on radiological grounds is virtually limited to dermoid and epidermoid

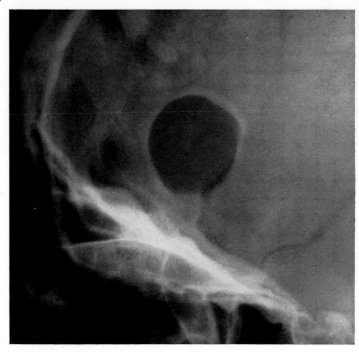

(a)

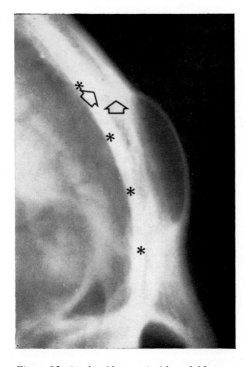

(b)

Figure 85. Arachnoid cyst. A girl aged 19 years complained of headaches and a lump on the head. (a) There is a very sharply localized translucency. (b) This tangential view shows that the bone is bulged (arrows) and thinned over a sharply restricted area by something inside the head. Do not be confused by superimposed shadows (asterisks). Note also air in the cerebral sulci after pneumoencephalography. By far the most likely diagnosis—in this case correct—is of an arachnoid cyst. This cyst lay in the subdural space

clue to the intradiploic nature of the tumour is in the everted tables at the edges of the erosion when seen tangentially.

These tumours are reported to have been calcified on occasion, the type of calcification illustrated being that of a thin shell over the tumour surface, so that whether originating from epidermoid itself or displaced bone tissue is uncertain.

It should be possible by radiological means to establish

that the tumour is intradiploic. Other rarer causes of circumscribed, slowly expanding masses in this situation are fibrous dysplasia, fibrosing osteitis and neurofibroma, in all of which the surrounding bone commonly shows some other evidence of abnormality. Osteoclastoma should also perhaps be considered, but if it occurs at all in the vault it must be much more rare than was at one time believed.

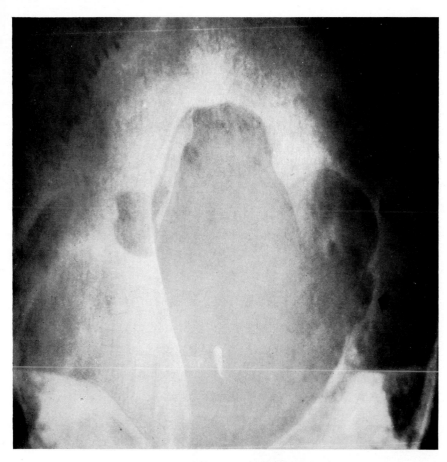

(a)

Figure 86. Intradiploic dermoid.
(a) Over much of the affected
area the whole thickness of the
skull is eroded. A 'sclerotic'
edge is seen where the inner or
outer table of the skull is turned
edge-on to the beam of x-rays
(closed arrow). (b) In the lateral
view a thin shell of bone is visible
in one place where the inner
table is preserved although displaced inwards (open arrow).
Other radiographs show out-
ward displacement of the outer
table, thus confirming the intradiploic position of the expanding
lesion

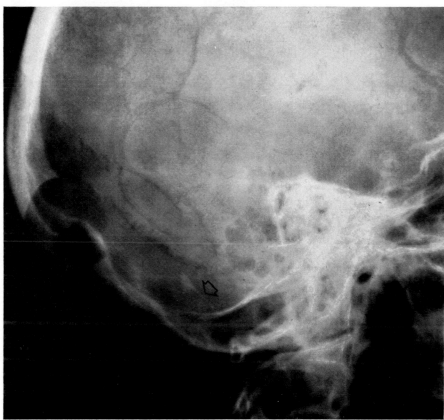

(b)

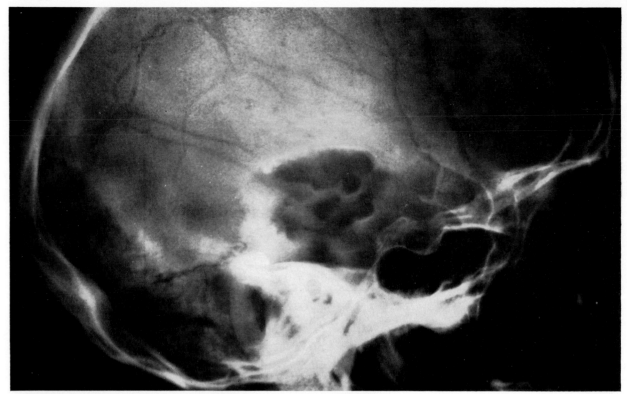

(a)

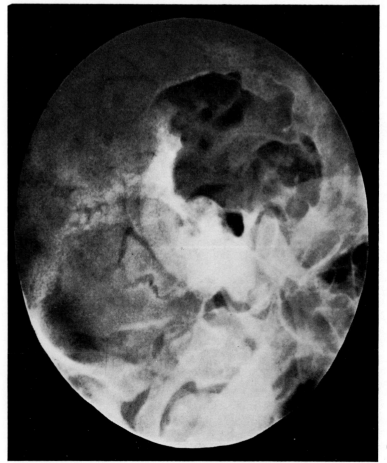

Figure 87. Epidermoid. The upward extension of a huge extradural mass of cholesteatoma from the petrous bone has caused a patchy thinning of the squamous temporal. The aetiology of this cholesteatoma remains in some doubt. The patient had a discharging ear and developed a temporal lobe abscess, but most of the cholesteatomatous tissue showed no sign of infection

(b)

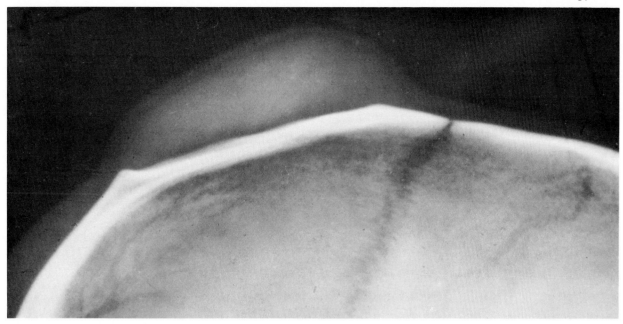

(a)

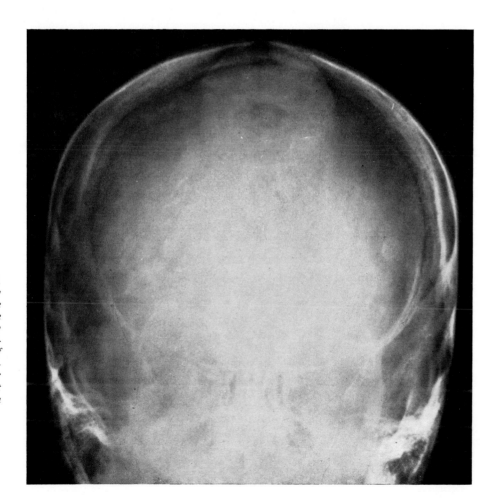

Figure 88. A frontal dermoid. (a) The defect is extremely difficult to see but this, the lateral, shows flattening of the outer profile of the skull by the dermoid under the pericranium, and overgrowth of bone at the pericranium attachment. (b) A postero-anterior view shows the skull defect which was occupied by a portion of the cyst

(b)

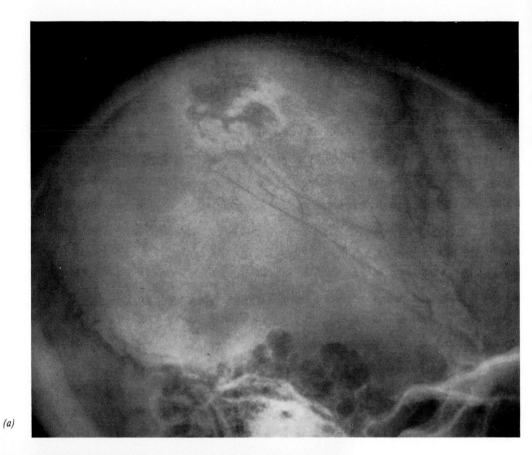

(a)

(b)

Figure 89. Fibrous dysplasia. A 'blister' type of lesion in which translucency is the predominant feature. There is, nevertheless, a peripheral region of structureless sclerosed bone

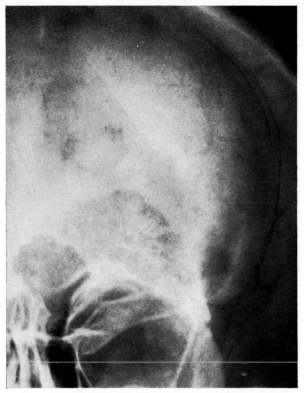
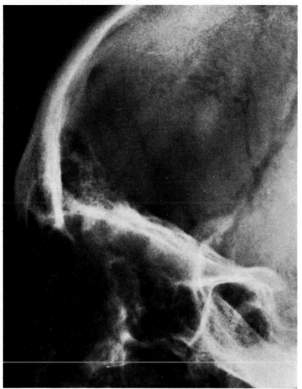

(a)   *(b)*

Figure 90. A cavernous haemangioma in bone in the skull of a woman aged 61 years. It increased slightly in size during 5 years following a second biopsy, but had shown little change for 6 years before. There is a visible swelling. (a) The radiograph shows that there are trabeculae throughout, arranged around more or less circular translucencies towards the centre of the mass, but radiating at the periphery. A more definitely radial spiculation is seen in some cases. (b) The lateral view shows a 'soap-bubble' appearance

INTRACRANIAL AND EXTRACRANIAL DERMOIDS
(*Figure 88*)

Dermoid cysts are sometimes found lying on the midline beneath the galea and may then cause a pressure deformity of the outer table of the skull. They may also intrude into the cranial cavity and some of these will show a narrow channel in the bone (compare with *Figure 83*).

Arteriovenous malformation

Rumbaugh and Potts (1966) have pointed out that there may sometimes (2 out of their 61 cases) be an area of vault thinning or thickening overlying a superficial intracranial angioma.

Fibrous dysplasia (*Figure 89*)

Fibrous dysplasia may be monostotic or polyostotic and when combined with endocrine dysfunction and cutaneous pigmentation is known as Albright's syndrome.

In the skull several types of the disease have been described, but they merge one into another and it is more helpful to restrict sub-classification into: (1) the sclerotic

form in which the base and facial bones are most commonly affected, and (2) the 'cystic' form which tends to produce a 'blister' upon the contour of the vault (*see* page 118).

All intermediates of the purely sclerotic and the lytic types are encountered, and in most there is a large proportion of dense non-trabeculated bone.

The translucency of the 'cysts' (which are formed of fibrous tissue) is only relative because they are always surrounded by disorganized dense woven bone. They expand the vault at the expense of the outer table.

In the mixed form, the dense areas are interspersed with irregular zones of translucency showing a characteristic amorphous texture.

The amorphous dense areas in fibrous dysplasia in the vault alongside areas of translucency resemble the shadows of ossification in relation to fibrous tissue in other skeletal lesions, such as osteogenic or ossifying fibromas.

This does not necessarily indicate a common pathology but draws attention to the similarity of the tissues found in the different conditions. The blood supply to fibrous dysplasia is greater than that to normal bone. This may manifest itself as a large arterial groove in the inner table resembling the sign of middle meningeal hypertrophy in some cases of meningioma.

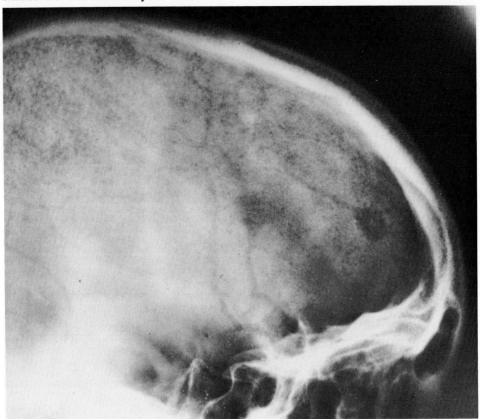

Figure 91. A very common appearance in haemangioma of bone. A circumscribed translucency with radiating trabecular structure

The term 'doughnut lesion' is descriptive not denoting a particular pathology but indicating a ring density with a translucent centre. Some seem to be cases of fibrosing osteitis (Keates and Holt, 1969). Other cases may be familial (Bartlett and Kishore, 1976) but their essential pathology is obscure.

Traumatic and post-traumatic conditions (*Figure 98*)

A translucency may be found immediately after injury to the vault due to a fracture, or may develop later as a result of cephalhaematoma, fibrosing osteitis, intra-diploic haematoma or cephalhydrocoele. These conditions are described elsewhere.

Similar appearances may be found when a small sequestrum is left by radiation treatment or in tuberculous osteomyelitis or eosinophil granuloma. These have been called 'button sequestra' (Meng and Wu, 1942; Wells, 1956; Rosen and Nadel, 1969).

Cephalhydrocoele may manifest as a 'growing fracture'.

Haemangioma of the vault (*Figures 90* and *91*)

Cavernous haemangioma of the vault, usually but not always solitary, produces a circular translucency often about 1.3 cm in diameter in which some spicules of bone remain. There may be expansion of the middle table, the texture of which is changed to a soap-bubble appearance (but the bubbles are small ones). In tangential views the outer table may not be distinguishable and diploë may be replaced by vertical trabeculae the outer pointed ends of which are free. The lesion may then be mistaken for an osteogenic metastasis but in haemangioma the spiculation is carried into the depth of the translucency. The spicules are less closely packed than in the typical sun-ray shadow of an osteogenic sarcoma.

Meningioma (*Figures 92–94*)

Apart from the vascular grooves already described, the reaction of bone to an underlying meningioma is due to the presence of meningioma cells in its lacunae and vascular spaces. By far the most common effect is stimulation of the osteoblasts, but from time to time a purely osteolytic reaction is set up. This effect upon bone has not been found to depend upon the cell type of the tumour, not even closely upon its malignancy.

Thus, somewhat irregular bone erosion may be found over a benign slow-growing meningioma when for some unknown reason the cells have failed to stimulate an osteoblastic reaction. Inspection of such a case in

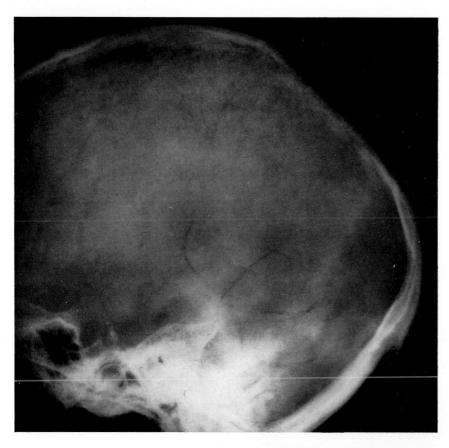

(a)

Figure 92. Meningioma. From time to time a meningioma is seen which has infiltrated the bone but caused erosion rather than hyperostosis. The type of reaction gives no clue to the vascularity or cellularity of the tumour. In this case the wide area of erosion has slightly irregular edges showing the infiltrating nature of the lesion. Note also the large depression for Pacchionian granulations

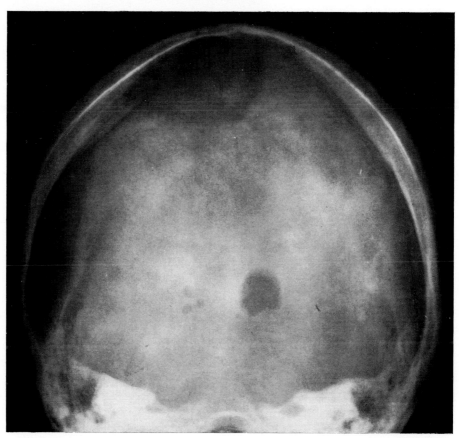

(b)

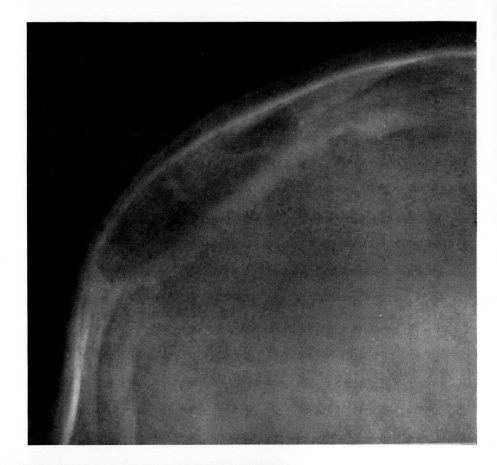

(a)

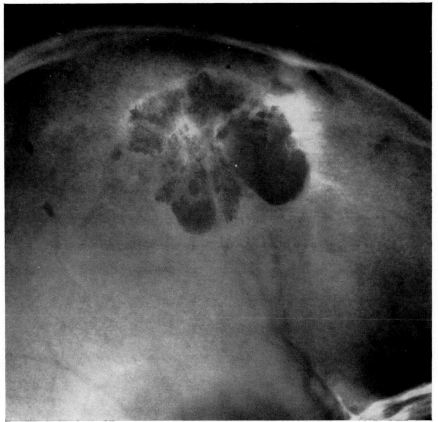

Figure 93. 'Intradiploic meningioma in a young man who complained only of a lump on the head. At operation a meningioma was found extending through the bone from the dura, but not into the cranial cavity. The radiographs show erosion and sclerosis with a few well-defined trabecular strands of bone which clearly distinguish the condition from fibrous dysplasia

(b)

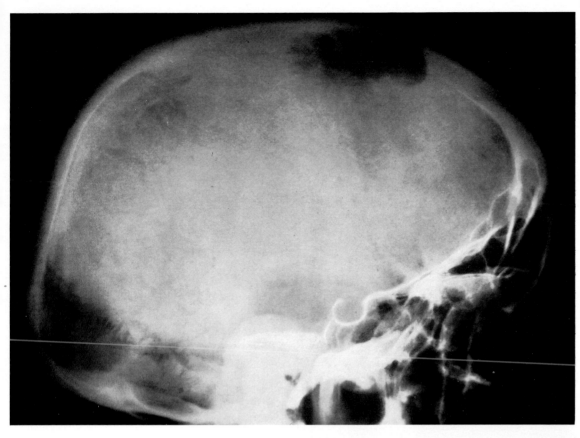

(a)

Figure 94. 'Malignant' meningioma. There was a history suggesting the presence of an intracranial tumour for many years with recent deterioration of the patient's condition. A lump was visible over the skull erosion. The tumour was enormous, very cellular, and had transgressed the barrier of the pia mater and invaded the brain. It recurred rapidly after removal. The radiographs show a large erosion with moderately sharp edges and no evidence of hyperostosis

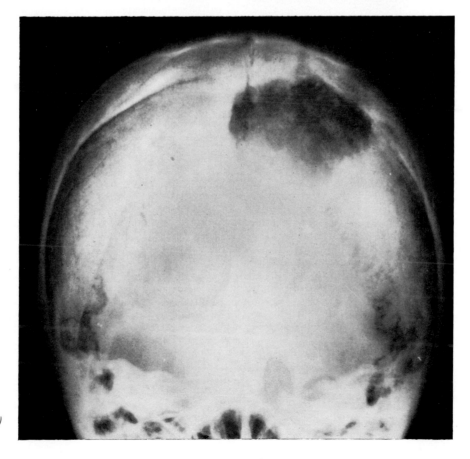

(b)

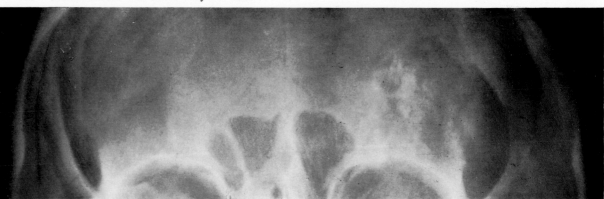

(a)

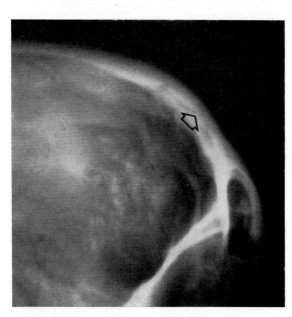

(b)

Figure 95. Bone erosion due to oligodendroglioma. Erosion of bone by intracerebral tumours is very uncommon; but in this case it is due to an oligodendroglioma which was found to have infiltrated the dura over an area of 5 × 2.5 cm. There is calcification in the tumour. The clinical history began 2 years before with fits. By the time of investigation the patient had severely raised intracranial pressure. After a frontal lobectomy and radiotherapy the patient remained well for 6½ years. Notice the irregular erosion of the inner table of the skull seen tangentially in the lateral view (arrow)

tangential view will usually reveal a remaining ghost of the vault and even slight exterior new-bone formation where the meningioma cells, having grown through the thickness of the skull, are raising or stimulating the pericranium. *En face*, the erosion is likely to show small radiating tongues and islands of translucency.

Complete replacement of an area of vault by tumour (which may present as a palpable lump under the scalp) seems to be a feature more commonly of the rare malignant meningioma. The edge of this sort of erosion may be remarkably clear-cut and even partly corticated.

It is a paradox that the malignant tumour sometimes produces a hole with a clear-cut edge, while the benign tumour forms an erosion whose edge shows evidence of free infiltration. The explanation lies partly in the fact that there is complete bone destruction in one case while in the other there is bone reaction to slow invasion. 'Malignant' may mean 'recurrent', 'rapidly growing', 'metastasizing', 'locally infiltrating', or simply 'difficult to extirpate'. A change in rate of growth may follow operation. A meningioma said to be malignant may have any of these characteristics and few of them can be dem-

onstrated radiographically, but it may be noted that the tumour which passes through the bone, destroying every vestige, leaving a clean hole, is likely to be the tumour which passes through the pia and infiltrates the brain.

Very rarely, a meningioma may present the appearance of an intradiploic tumour, the major portion forming an expanding translucent mass between the inner and outer tables.

The appearance differs from that of an intradiploic epidermoid in the greater amount of surrounding bone reaction, and in that the tumour appears from the tangential film to have extended into the bone from deep to the inner table, and it differs from fibrous dysplasia because of the presence of sharply defined bone trabeculae (for a systematic study of meningiomas turn now to page 115).

Erosion due to other intracranial tumours
(Figure 95)

On rare occasion, erosion of the vault may take place due to a carcinoma metastasis in the brain and meninges.

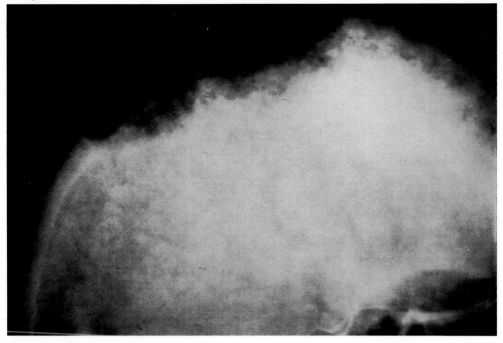

Figure 96. Sarcoma on Paget's disease. The usual manifestation of sarcomatous change in Paget's disease is, as in this patient, the appearance of a soft-tissue lump with destruction of the underlying abnormal bone

The bone destruction is not likely to be more than an indistinct and patchy increase in translucency before the intracranial mass brings life to an end, except in cases of carcinoma of the prostate metastasizing to the bone, in which an osseous reaction very like that to meningioma may develop. At operation the soft-tissue mass protruding from the inner aspect of the cranium may prolong the illusion of a meningioma. The signs of an intracranial tumour will dominate the picture. In carcinomatous meningitis definite bone erosion is exceedingly uncommon. Other slow-growing meningeal deposits, for example, of lymphoma, may also cause slight inner table bone erosion.

Destruction of the overlying bone by other cerebral tumours is very uncommon. A few single cases have been reported (as that of an ependymoblastoma which caused gross erosion). The author has seen a few cases of oligodendroglioma in which slight overlying bone erosion followed the spread of the tumour through the dura.

Chondroma and chondrosarcoma

These tumours hardly ever arise in the vault. When they do they may present as translucencies with some faint calcification in the soft-tissue mass within or outside the skull cavity.

Osteoclastoma

It is very doubtful whether osteoclastoma ever arises in the bones of the vault although very rarely it may spread thence from the temporal bone, sphenoid or lower part of the occipital bone. The appearance will then be like that of an epidermoid expanding between the two tables.

Remoulding of bone takes place around the tumour and thus a partial bony wall is retained outlining the expansion in tangential views, and in *en face* views sometimes giving the impression of coarse trabeculation.

Periosteal fibrosarcoma

Fibrosarcoma affecting the vault is exceedingly uncommon. When seen there is a soft-tissue tumour and the underlying bone change is usually suggestive of pressure erosion rather than infiltration, until a late stage when obvious destruction of bone takes place.

In the earlier stages tangential views may show no abnormality. A little later they show flattening of the outer table below the tumour, and there may be some new-bone formation at the periphery of the flat area.

Ewing's tumour

This is very rarely a primary tumour in the vault. The appearance described is of an osteolytic lesion surrounded by well-marked sclerosis of the inner and outer tables. The sclerotic bone is later eroded by expansion of the tumour.

Metastatic Ewing's tumour is more likely to be almost purely osteolytic. The appearance is of multiple rounded translucencies and very closely resembles some cases of multiple myeloma.

Chloroma

This produces an erosion identical with that of solitary myeloma.

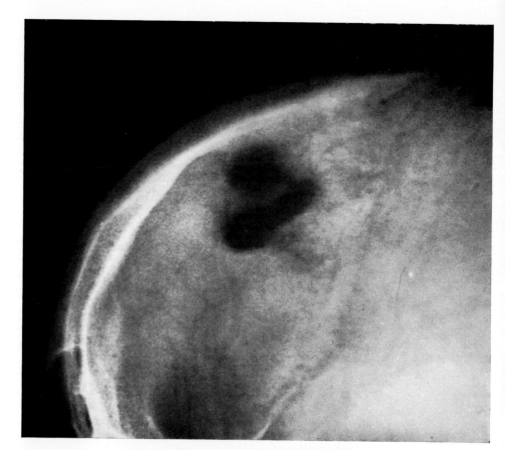

Figure 97. Erosion of bone below a large rodent ulcer of the scalp

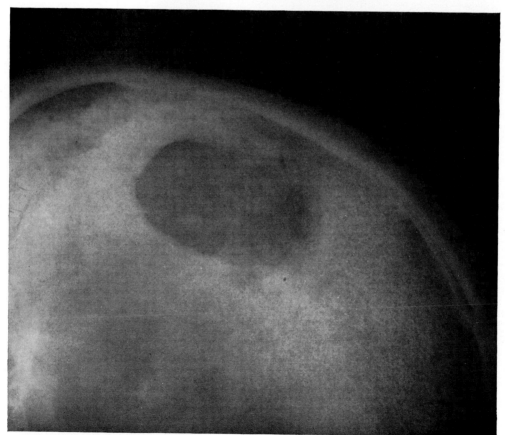

Figure 98. Surgical defect (after injury in an adult). Note the blurring of bone edges which occurs after a number of years

Neurofibroma

Irregular bone defects are occasionally seen in neurofibromatosis (characteristically of the lower part of the lambdoid suture).

Osteosarcoma (*Figure 96*)

Osteogenic sarcoma is sometimes found arising from the bones of the vault. Its appearance is fairly characteristic — a soft-tissue mass with rapidly developing underlying bone erosion.

There will probably be some spicules of new-bone formation around the edge of the erosion but the proportion of sclerosis to erosion varies from case to case. A few show sun-ray spiculation.

Sarcomatous degeneration in Paget's disease may be diagnosed when an erosion appears and extends rapidly through a previously dense area.

Skin malignancy (*Figure 97*)

Malignant tumours of the skin may extend to destroy the underlying vault, affecting first the outer table. The cause of the lesion is of course not in doubt, although malignant subpericranial deposits of, for instance, myeloma may produce large tumours also with relatively greater destruction of the outer table than the inner parts of the vault. (For systematic study of malignant disease, turn to page 123.)

Hydatid disease

Extensive areas of bone thinning and actual destruction, with deformity of neighbouring parts of the skull, may result from the presence of an hydatid cyst, presumably because of the extreme chronicity of the condition. They are very rarely seen in England. Bonakdarpour (1967) has reported from a very large collection of material that the primarily intradiploic cysts may be unilocular or multilocular. The multilocular cysts usually break through the bone resulting in erosion and destruction and invasion of the cranial cavity, but the unilocular ones may make enormous expanding lesions with walls covered in impressions like convolutional atrophy. Of the cases of hydatid disease 1—2 per cent have skeletal lesions. Of these only 3—4 per cent are in the skull.

Defects of unknown cause

Irregular areas of thinning of the vault, even complete defects, are sometimes found without clinical evidence of local disease, and without the association of neurofibromatosis or any other condition of which defective ossification is a known feature. Contrast examinations fail to show any intracranial mass or abnormal vascularity although the plain radiographs may demonstrate unusually large venous channels in the vicinity in some cases.

The causes of this probably heterogeneous collection remain dubious. Some, no doubt, are the late results of forgotten head injury, others of congenital origin. Even these categories do not cover all cases, for defects of unknown cause may appear occasionally during the course of severe childhood illness and steadily increase in size.

3 INCREASED DENSITY OF THE VAULT

The vault may appear dense either because the bones are thickened or because they contain an unusual concentration of calcium salts. (The latter usually also involves conversion of the diploë to a more compact form of bone.) The changes may affect the whole or only a localized part and this provides the simplest method of classification under which increased density of the vault may be discussed.

In a few conditions the skull may be thickened although it remains abnormally translucent. Such diseases are referred to in the previous chapter.

The variation in both thickness and density of the vault is very great in the normal. One or more of the following criteria must therefore be fulfilled before the appearance can be ascribed to disease: (1) the texture of the bone must be obviously altered; (2) the area of thickening or density must be very sharply localized; (3) there may be other changes present in the skull (as in acromegaly) to suggest that the thickening is pathological.

Hyperostosis frontalis interna is so common that it appears to be a normal feature when present in a mild degree.

GENERALIZED INCREASE IN DENSITY

Paget's disease (*Figure 99*)

After a prolonged period the vault becomes dense and by the time the first radiographs are taken the changes are usually found throughout the affected skull. The outstanding feature is the thickness of the bone which loses its differentiation into the normal three tables and usually acquires a granular appearance. The inner table is less severely affected than the others. In addition to the change in density, texture and thickness, there may be an alteration of shape in the most severely affected cases, brought about by the diminution in strength of the bone; this results in basilar invagination.

Other parts of the skeleton will also be affected but, even without this diagnostic assistance, Paget's disease of the vault of the skull where it has reached the stage of sclerosis is always recognizable. (For a systematic study of Paget's disease turn now to page 125.)

Acromegaly (*Figure 100*)

The vault in acromegaly is often thick, but only occasionally does it grow definitely beyond the limits of the normal in this respect and the texture and shape of the bones are not disturbed. Additional evidence which may support the diagnosis of acromegaly is an enlargement of the frontal sinuses and overgrowth of the mandible. The mandibular angle becomes widened, the teeth are widely spaced, and the anterior part of the lower jaw protrudes beyond the limits of the normal profile. The eosinphil adenoma of the pituitary almost invariably enlarges the sella turcica. However, the radiological features of acromegaly are often indeterminate in those cases in which the diagnosis cannot be established on clinical grounds — so that the recognition of acromegaly on the skull radiograph is more of academic than practical interest.

In rare cases of giantism the skull bones may also be thick though more usually the skull does not grow in proportion to the general increase in body size.

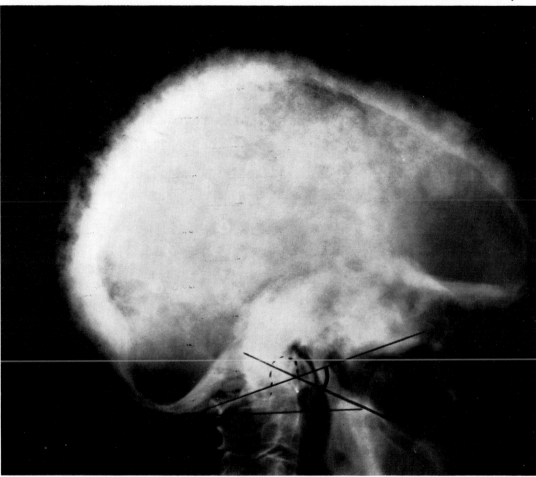

Figure 99. Paget's disease in a patient aged 71 years. There is a great thickening of the whole vault and much of the base, sparing only part of the squamous occiput (and parts of the squamous temporals). The vault has a typically woolly appearance, and a thin shell of inner table cortex is preserved as usual. In spite of its thickness the bone is not much less radiolucent than normal. Thickening of the upper part of the vault combined with basilar invagination (here extreme) causes the 'tam-o-shanter' skull deformity. Bull's angle and the modified Chamberlain's line have been drawn

Cerebral atrophy

The vault may be unusually thick compared with the general skeletal habitus of the patient in some cases of cerebral atrophy, particularly in later childhood. The bones are not only rather massive but their inner tables exhibit few and shallow convolutional impressions. This alteration in thickness from the strictly normal is more easily recognized when it affects only one half of the vault of the skull (*see* Hemi-atrophy on page 126).

Dystrophia myotonica (*Figure 101*)

A high proportion of patients suffering from this rare condition are found to have thick skulls with large frontal sinuses and small pituitary fossae. The appearance, however, is not diagnostic.

Arteriovenous malformation

Very rarely a large arteriovenous shunt seems to result in some generalized thickening of the vault, perhaps related to changes in intracranial pressure.

Relief of raised intracranial pressure (*Figures 25, 26* and *102*)

When chronic raised intracranial pressure is dropped to normal levels in infancy and childhood after successful operation for hydrocephalus, the thickness of the vault of the skull may suddenly increase. The vault in these cases may grow merely to a thickness consistent with the age of the patient. Less commonly it changes from being abnormally thin under the influence of the raised intracranial pressure to being abnormally thick when the

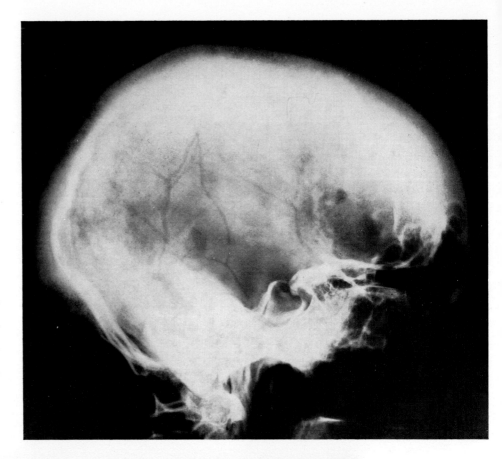

Figure 100. Acromegaly in a woman aged 50 years with a 30-year history of slowly advancing disease. The sella is enlarged, particularly in a downward direction. The bones are dense and massive and the frontal sinuses very well developed. Thickening of the bones of the vault is by no means always present in acromegaly

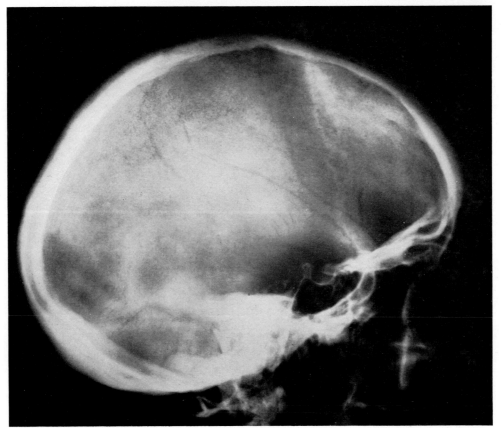

Figure 101. Dystrophia myotonica. In many cases of dystrophia myotonica the skull vault is thick, the sella small, and the frontal sinuses well developed

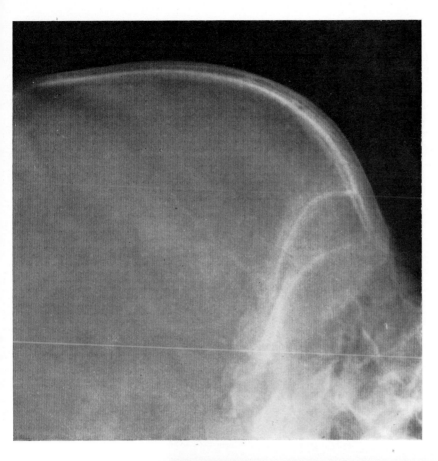

Figure 102. Cerebral atrophy or abiotrophy in a child aged 4 months who failed to develop normally. His twin was a stillborn hydrocephalic. The head is small and some of the bones are thick. All sutures remain visible. On close examination the frontal bone appears 'laminated' in the same way as it may afer the successful relief of raised intracranial pressure in childhood. Presumably the diminished stimulus to absorption of the inner table results in an increase of skull thickness by growth inwards as well as deposition on the outer table. The persistent ghost-like shadow of the previous inner table may be analogous to Harrison's lines. The interaction of skeletal growth, brain growth and intracranial pressure changes are also seen in craniolacunia, in convolutional impressions, and possibly in the sella of the hydrocephalic

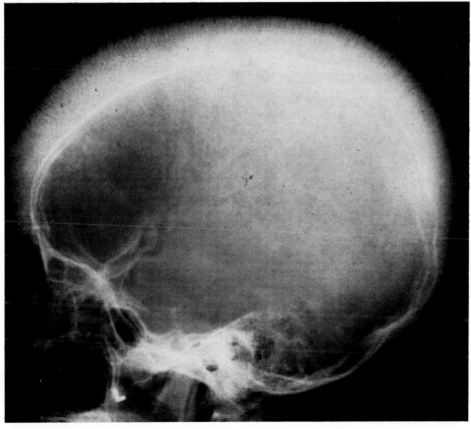

Figure 103. Cooley's anaemia. In this case the whole of the vault except for the squamous occiput is seriously affected. The outer table has disappeared

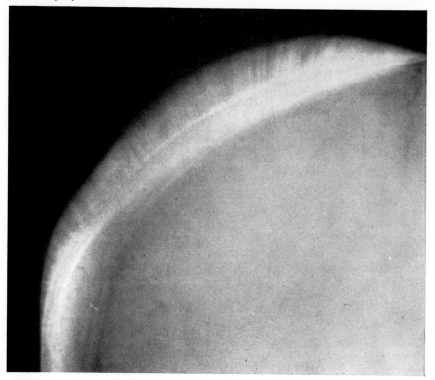

Figure 104. Severe chronic anaemia. A detail of the vault of another case. The outer table has been absorbed. The diploic thickening takes the form of radiating spicules

obstruction is removed. During the first few months of relief, careful examination of the bones of the vault where they are seen tangentially in these cases often reveals a laminated appearance consisting of one or more fine lines of dense bone parallel to the inner table lying within the general thickness of the bone. It seems probable that this is due to the deposition of a new-bone layer over the inner surface of the calvaria.

Some adults who have had very long-standing raised intracranial pressure also have unusually thick skulls. The cause of the raised intracranial pressure is then found to be a congenital obstruction which may be intermittent.

Prolonged medication for epilepsy

Kattan (1970) has recorded a moderate generalized calvarial thickening after several years medication with Dilantin.

Severe chronic anaemias (*Figures 103–106*)

In Cooley's anaemia and in sickle-cell anaemia the increase in bone marrow may eventually result in great thickening of the diploë of the child's skull. In such cases the middle table appears as if replaced by close-packed radiating spicules and may be over an inch in thickness. The outer table becomes absorbed.

Earlier in the disease there may only be some widening of the diploë, particularly of frontal and parietal bones, without obvious alteration in the trabecular pattern.

Some chronic, iron-deficiency anaemias cause a slight degree of the same appearance and it may also be seen in mild form in secondary polycythaemia.

Myelosclerosis (*Figures 107* and *108*)

In some cases of myelosclerosis the diploë is replaced by dense amorphous bone. This appearance may be found when other parts of the skeleton show relatively mild changes.

Marble bones (Albers–Schönberg disease) (*Figure 109a*)

In this rare disease the whole skeleton is usually affected. The increase in density is usually accompanied by only a moderate increase in thickness, but in the bones of the base this may be sufficient to cause compression of nerve roots as they pass through bony foramina. The features of the bones of the vault are invisible because of the extreme density of the shadow cast. The differential diagnosis includes Englemann's disease, osteomyelosclerosis and hyperostosis generalisata with pachydermia (*Figure 109b*). There are probably also other rare forms of osteopetrosis such as the familial cases of idiopathic osteosclerosis described by Russell *et al.* (1968).

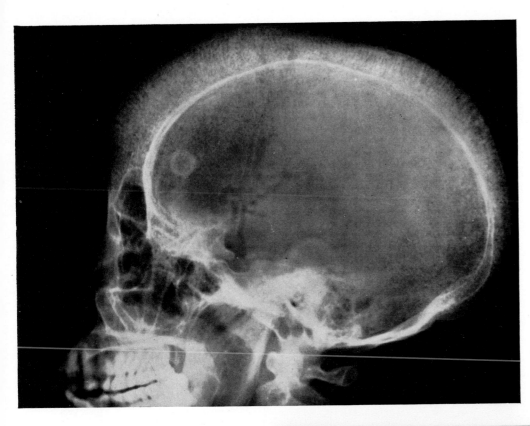

(a)

Figure 105. Sickle-cell anaemia. The middle table of the calvaria is greatly increased in thickness. This change appears slowly in chronic severe cases. Eventually the outer table may be completely absorbed

(Reproduced by courtesy of Dr Lehmann)

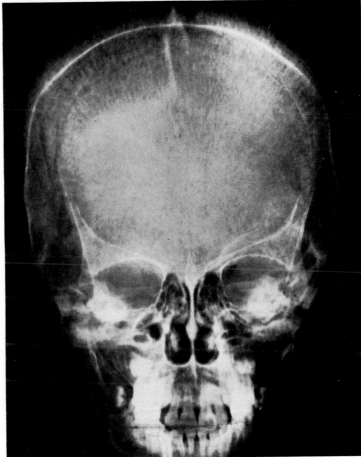

(b)

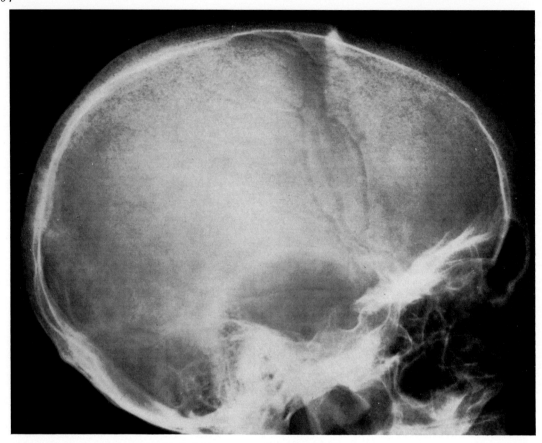

Figure 106. Haemolytic anaemia in a child aged 12 years who had had recurrent palor and jaundice since infancy. Haemoglobin 6·5 g. The red cells showed low osmotic fragility. The skull vault is thick, but because it is almost entirely composed of diploic bone full of marrow spaces, it shows increased translucency. The squamous temporal is a very thin bone and stands out as a black shadow even in this translucent skull

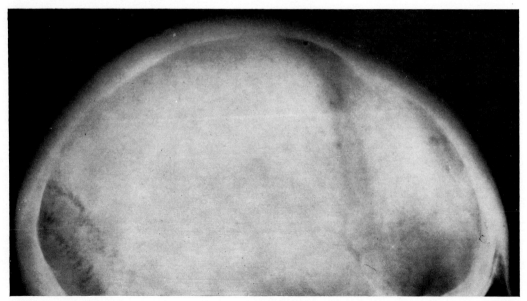

Figure 107. Myelosclerosis in a man aged 56 years after at least 1 year of clinical illness. The patient died 3 years later and was found to have myelofibrosis, myelosclerosis and widespread extramedullary erythropoiesis at autopsy. Up to the time of his death there were marrow spaces in long bones on ordinary radiography, but some rather diffuse sclerosis of bones, particularly the pelvis, was apparent. The skull shows almost complete absence of normal diploë

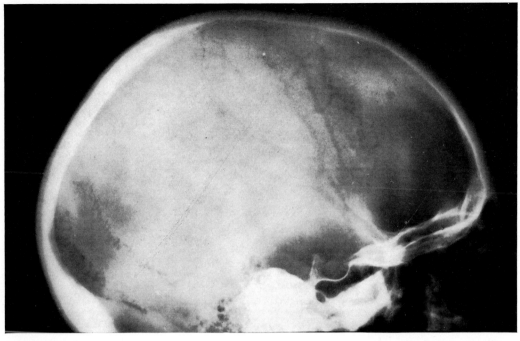

Figure 108. Myelosclerosis in a woman aged 61 years with a 6-year history of hepato-splenomegaly. A rib biopsy showed myelosclerosis. Other bones exhibited a mild diffuse sclerosis. The vault shows complete absence of diploë

Progressive diaphysial dysplasia (Englemann's disease)

The appearance of the skull in Englemann's disease is similar to that in Albers–Schönberg disease, and the cranial nerves may be similarly affected.

Hyperostosis generalisata with pachydermia (Uehlinger's disease)

Bone thickening may be extensive (*Figure 109b*) and as in osteopetrosis (Albers–Schönberg disease) may result in deformity and cranial nerve palsies. The skin lesion establishes the diagnosis.

Dwarfism with dense bones

Caffey (1967) described a mother and son who were proportionate dwarfs showing dense calvariae and fibular bones with narrow medullary cavities. They had bouts of tetany with hypocalcaemia and hyperphosphataemia.

Hyperostosis corticalis generalisata familiaris (von Buchem's disease)

There is severe sclerosis of the whole skull including the mandible as well as the ribs, clavicles and diaphyses of the long bones. The serum alkaline phosphatase is always increased and it has been suggested that this is the late form of hyperphosphatasia (Rubin, 1965). Halliday's disease (Halliday, 1949) appears to be another name for the same condition.

Craniometaphysial dysplasia

This is a recently described dysplasia in which rather patchy thickening of the occipital and frontal bones occurs and the diploë disappears. The base is also affected and the sinuses and mastoids are obliterated. It may be one manifestation of a more pleomorphic syndrome (*see* Chapter 11).

Melorrheostosis

In melorrheostosis, a very rare condition, part of the skull (both vault and base) may show a diffuse featureless increase in density. The condition also affects other bones.

Toulouse–Lautrec syndrome (pyknodysostosis)

The entire skeleton shows increased density. The sutures are wide and the fontanelle tends to remain open. There may be excess wormian bones. Though dense, the skull bones are also thin (*see* Chapter 11).

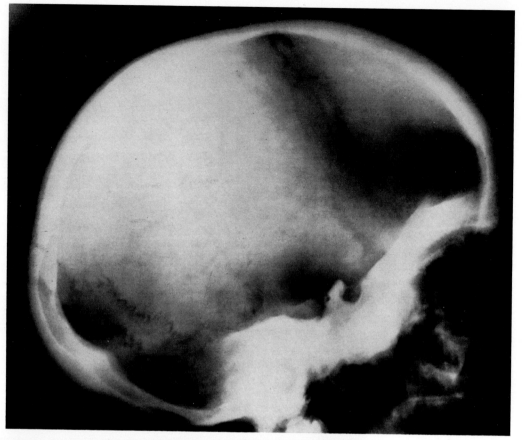

(a)

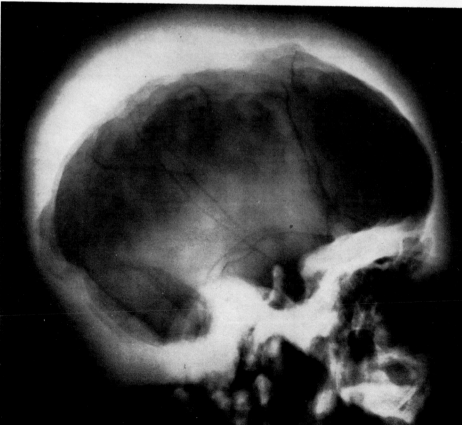

(b)

Figure 109. Osteopetrosis (Albers-Schönberg disease). (a) A woman aged 45 years. Both the vault and the base are abnormally dense, but the bones are little, if at all, increased in thickness. The structure is that of compact bone except in the frontal regions where some diploë is still visible. (b) Hyperostosis generalisata with pachydermia. The remainder of the skeleton showed mild changes. This condition generally affects males and may be first observed at or a little before adolescence. It may be inherited and it can go on to cause neurological disturbance by nerve-root compression. This patient, a man aged 38 years, was symptomless

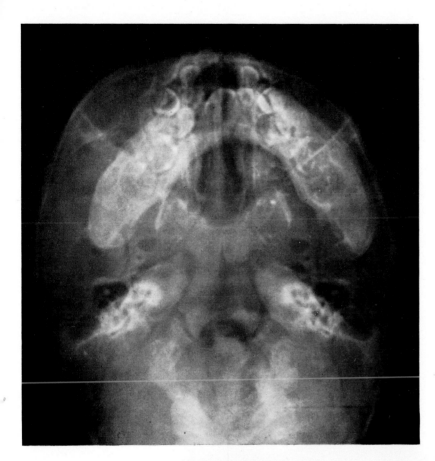

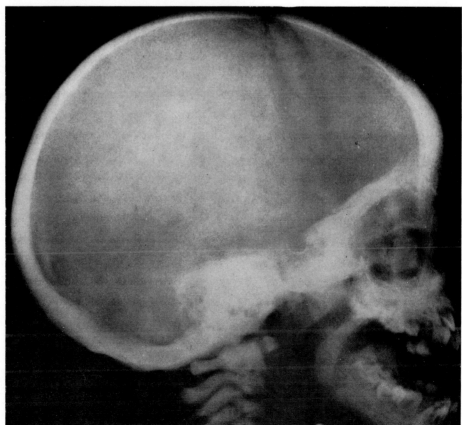

Figure 111. Vitamin D resistant rickets. The patient has an excessive urinary loss of phosphates and has been treated with very large doses of vitamin D. Both he and his father have bowed legs. (a) Aged 8 months. The skull bones are thick and dense. The lambdoid suture is difficult to see, but the coronal suture is open (cont.)

(a)

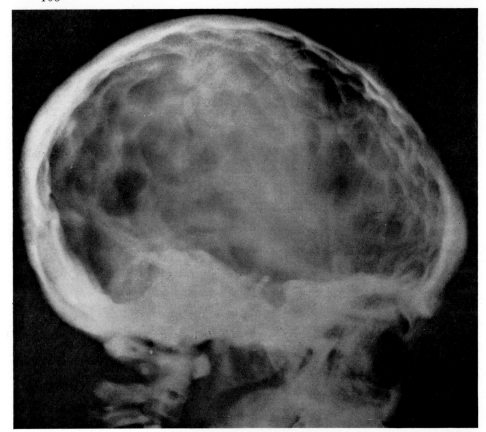

(b)

Figure 111 (cont.). (b) The patient at the age of 4½ years. The remaining sutures have been closed for some time, and excessive convolutional impressions show the skull's attempt to keep pace with underlying brain growth. The bones of the base remain dense and too massive for the age of this patient. (c) The patient's sister, aged 2 years, is similarly affected

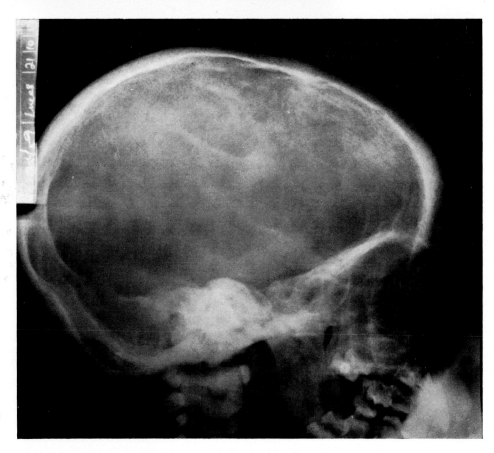

(c)

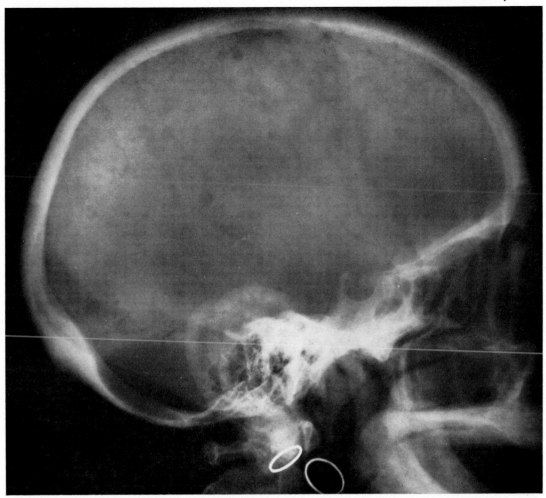

Figure 112. Renal osteodystrophy with secondary hyperparathyroidism. A middle-aged woman with pronounced bone disease throughout the skeleton, including increased density, decreased density, 'cystic' areas and fractures. The skull bones have lost their normal texture. They are, overall, denser than normal. The vault shows a number of round translucencies as well. The sella has very little recognizable cortex

Chronic fluorine poisoning

Some cases of chronic fluorine poisoning show a diffuse increase in bone density, usually of a mild degree, affecting the whole skeleton, including both the vault and base of the skull.

Caffey's syndrome (infantile cortical hyperostosis) (*Figure 110*)

Caffey's syndrome is a rare condition of unknown aetiology. Hyperostoses are found on many bones of the skeleton due to subperiosteal new bone formation, and in some cases areas of thickening of the vault have been observed. The disease only affects infants and young children and has to be distinguished from the effects of injury. Other conditions which give rise to periosteal new bone formation in long bones, for example, osteomyelitis, rarely do so in the vault.

Chronic syphilitic osteitis

Occasional widespread increase in density and thickness of the bones of the vault and has been found to be due to syphilis — in childhood, due to congenital syphilis.

Vitamin D poisoning

Hypervitaminosis D, due either to overdosage or to abnormal vitamin D metabolism, may lead to a generalized increase in bone density of the whole skull. Some patients show premature synostosis of the sutures.

Hyperostosis corticalis generalisata congenita

This is a condition which does not disable the patient in whom the entire skeleton shows the changed cortical bone largely at the expense of the medullary cavity. The mandible may be so dense that the tooth roots are obscured.

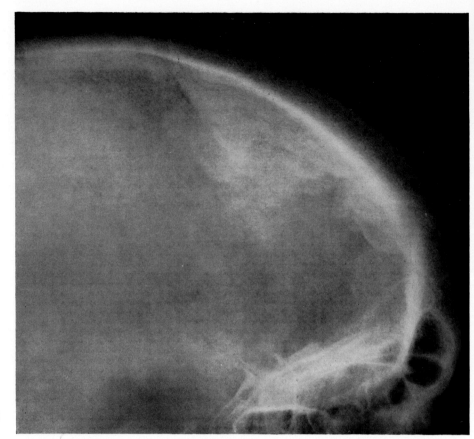

(a)

Figure 113. a and b. Hyperostosis frontalis interna in an elderly woman. The bone thickening is more or less symmetrical

(b)

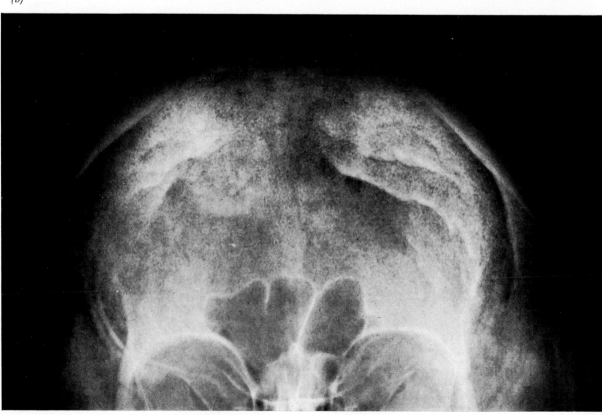

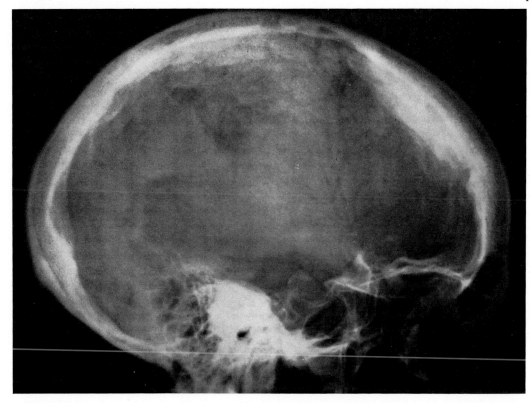

Figure 114. Hyperostosis fronto-parietalis

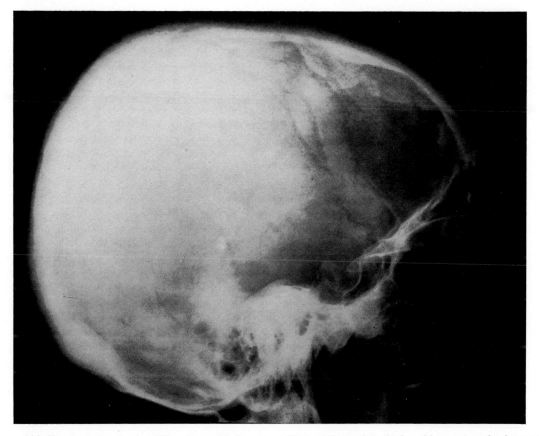

Figure 115. Hyperostosis calvariae diffusa in an elderly woman. Most of the vault is thick and has an irregular inner table

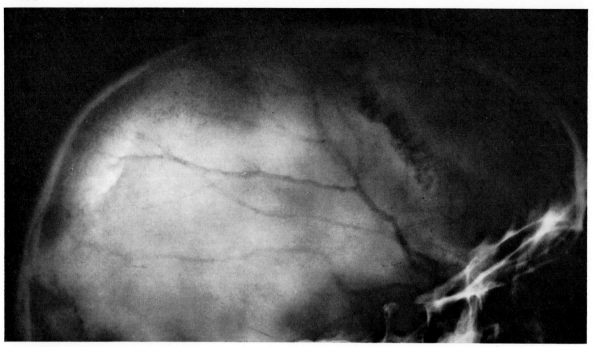

(a)

(b)

Figure 116. Meningioma in a woman aged 45 years with an 8-month history of left Jacksonian epilepsy and early papilloedema. There is a small but obvious hyperotosis affecting principally the inner table. In the lateral view (a) note also the hypertrophied arterial channels. In the half axial view (b) the thickening of the inner table is seen clearly in profile

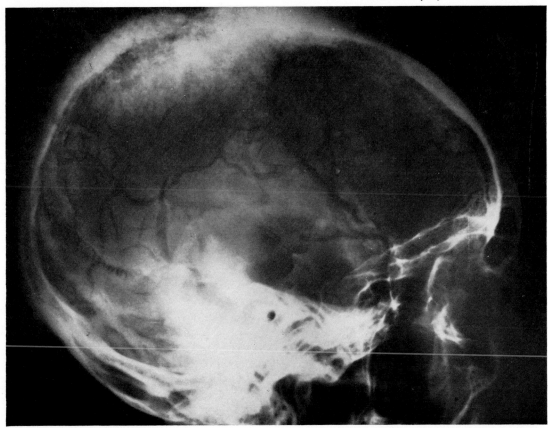

Figure 117. Meningioma hyperostosis. The whole thickness of the vault is affected over a wide area. The hyperostosis is very dense and has a granular texture in this case. In the centre of the hyperostosis there is an erosion. This tumour was observed over a number of years and the hyperostosis increased further in size before operation

Chronic idiopathic hypercalcaemia (*Figure 225*)

The skull in chronic idiopathic hypercalcaemia shows an exactly similar change to that in hypervitaminosis D.

Vitamin D resistant rickets (*Figure 111*)

Under treatment the porotic bones may become dense, and premature fusion of sutures is sometimes seen.

Primary hyperparathyroidism (under treatment)

A patchy but widespread increased bone density may occur in this condition, but it is a very unusual manifestation, hypertranslucency being more common.

Renal rickets (under treatment) (*Figure 112*)

In some patients with renal rickets, particularly under treatment, skull changes are seen which may occasionally include increase in density.

Hypoparathyroidism

Occasionally the increase in density, sometimes found elsewhere in the skeleton in hypoparathyroidism and in pseudohypoparathyroidism, also affects the skull.

LOCALIZED INCREASE IN DENSITY OF THE SKULL VAULT

There are a large number of conditions in which part of the vault of the skull becomes abnormally dense. In many the appearance is characteristic, and after consideration of the clinical and associated radiological findings a diagnosis may be suggested.

An attempt is made to arrange the cause in order of frequency, but there is little objective evidence to support the order chosen and it should be regarded only as a rough guide.

Hyperotosis frontalis interna (*Figure 113*)

The inner table of both halves of the frontal bone is irregularly thickened to produce a surface resembling

114

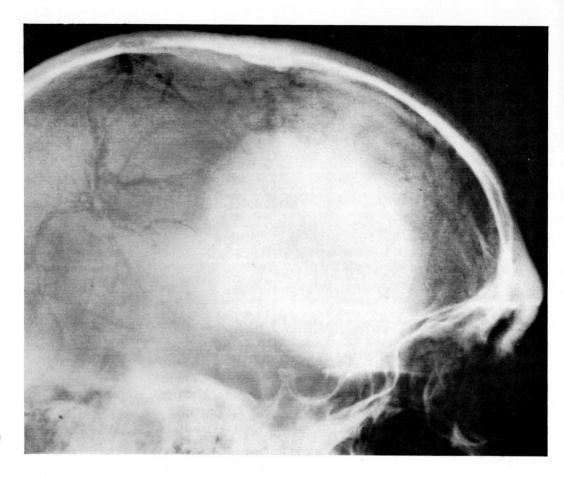

(a)

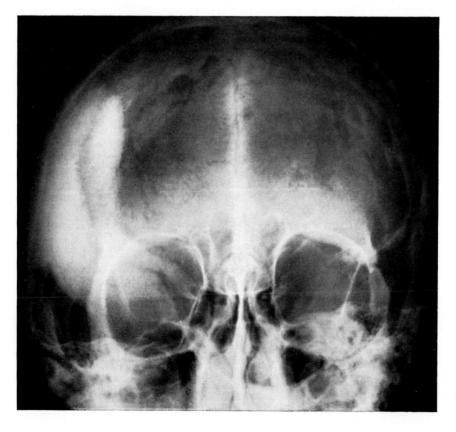

(b)

Figure 118. Meningioma. There is a wide area around the pterion in which the vault shows great thickening and density. The edge of the hyperostosis consists of radiating trabeculae and pin-head translucencies. It tails off into normal bone. There is no convincing evidence of a hypertrophied arterial supply. The hyperostosis spreads into both sphenoid wings. The patient, a man aged 33 years, complained of a lump on the head; there were no abnormal neurological signs but a substantial intracranial soft-tissue tumour was present. The appearance of the hyperostosis is not to be confused with fibrous dysplasia

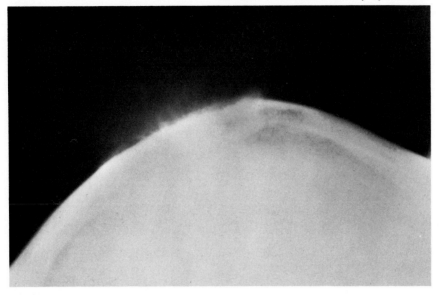

Figure 119. Meningioma. A soft-tissue radiograph to show the superficial lump of a tumour which has passed through the vault and is causing a visible protuberance. Note the tumour mass, radiating spicules of bone and 'Codman's triangle' which would mean a sarcoma seen in a long bone but may result in the skull, as in this case, from a completely benign meningioma. It may only be possible to distinguish a sarcoma from a meningioma of the vault by the course of the disease; but sarcomas of the vault are extremely rare, and it is better to err on the hopeful side

that of a choppy sea, and this is more or less a mould of the underlying convolutions. Some degree of hyperostosis frontalis interna may be a normal feature of the skull in middle age. It is, however, particularly associated with slight mental retardation and obesity in Morgagni's syndrome which affects women at the menopause. The main importance of hyperostosis frontalis interna is the resemblance of the changes to hyperostosis due to meningioma. Hyperostosis frontalis interna is symmetrical in degree on the two sides and is not associated with an increase in arterial grooves on the inner table. Nevertheless, it is a very common condition and since it renders the bone dense, making structural details difficult to see, an additional hyperostosis due to the presence of a meningioma may be very well masked.

Hyperostosis fronto-parietalis (*Figure 114*)

Sometimes thickening of the inner table of the vault, as described in the last paragraph, also affects the parietal bones; the condition is then known as hyperostosis fronto-parietalis. There may be a region of more normal skull along the line of the coronal suture separating the areas of hyperostosis.

Hyperostosis calvariae diffusa (*Figure 115*)

An irregular thickening of the inner table of the vault producing an exaggerated convolutional pattern is rarely seen to affect the whole of the supratentorial part of the skull. Its significance is unknown. (It is included here with more localized disease in the interests of tidiness.)

Nebula frontalis

A triangular dense area in the lateral view, with its base towards the bregma and the apex near the lower part of the coronal suture, is called nebula frontalis. It is due to thickening of the skull in this region and is an anatomical feature.

Meningioma (*Figures 116–119*)

Hyperostosis is the commonest manifestation on skull radiographs of the presence of a meningioma. Since many of these tumours may be completely removed at operation and some present with clinical signs insufficient in themselves to warrant CT or γ-scanning, the recognition of hyperostosis due to a meningioma is of great importance.

The area of bone involved may be large or small. It may be confined to the vault or extend to the bones of the base. Meningiomas are commoner in the parasagittal region than over the convexity, but hyperostosis is more difficult to recognize near the vertex than further out on the vault. Another common site is in the region of the pterion.

The increase in density of the affected part of the vault is due partly to an increase in thickness of the bone and partly to alteration of structure. Although the inner table is nearly always the most severely affected, it is common to find that part of the diploic layer has been changed into compact bone, and not infrequently the outer table is also increased in width. Sometimes an extension of tumour through the bone raises a palpable lump under the scalp. In such cases tangential views may show spicular new-bone formation outside the outer table.

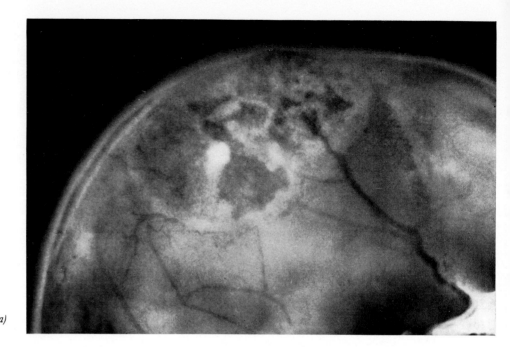

(a)

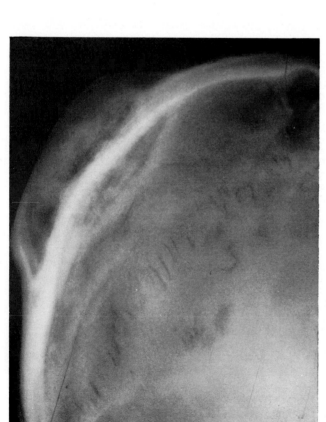

*Figure 120 a and b. Fibrous dysplasia. A localized 'blister'.
The vault is expanded outwards and the affected bone shows
a mixture of translucency and sclerosis in which no trabeculae
are visible. A ring of dense bone lies around the whole abnormal area. Do not be confused by the vascular channel;
this could not be a meningioma*

(b)

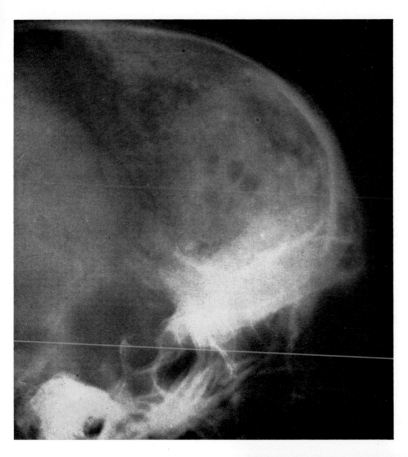

(a)

Figure 121 a and b. Fibrous dysplasia. The bone is expanded and dense but not with the opacity of ivory bone. There are a few translucent areas. The diseased regions appear structureless

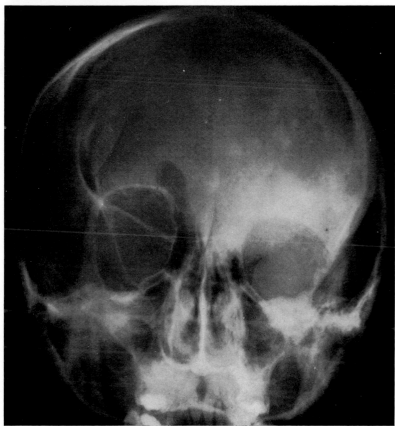

(b)

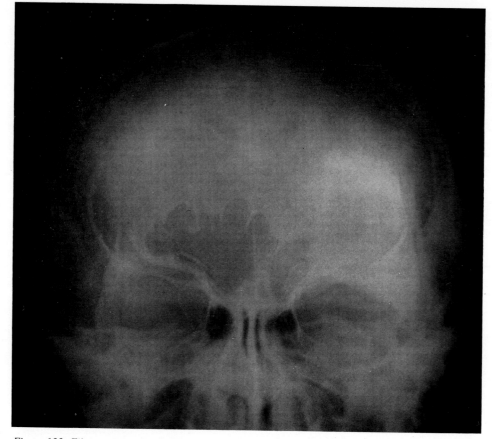

Figure 122. Fibrous dysplasia (sclerotic form). In the central region there is less sclerosis, but no truly translucent areas are shown

Calcification and bone formation may also take place within the intracranial portion of the tumour as described in Chapter 9, and in these cases the opacity in the tumour usually blends with the shadow of the hyperostosis itself. The centre of the point of attachment of the tumour is often indicated by the maximum prominence of the hyperostosis of the inner table.

Sometimes (as described in Chapter 2) a meningioma causes an osteoclastic reaction in the bone rather than the more typical hyperostosis. At other times a mixed response is observed and, in these, areas of sclerosis and areas of erosion may lie side by side in a manner the reason for which is difficult to understand. Some of the erosions are filled by a solid mass of tumour, but in other cases the area of porosis appears to be an osteoclastic response to the presence of a very few meningioma cells in much the same way that the hyperostosis is an osteoblastic reaction which may extend far beyond the macroscopic spread of the tumour.

Most meningiomas derive part of their blood supply from hypertrophied branches of the external carotid at their point of attachment to the meninges, and the channels and foramina in the vault in and around the hyperostosis may produce a characteristic appearance (*see* Vascular channels in the skull, page 36).

The extent of the hyperostosis gives no indication of the size of any intracranial portion of the tumour nor does the presence of hyperostosis rather than erosion give any indication of the exact histological picture. The most prolific and extensive thickening of the vault with spicular new-bone formation beneath the periosteum may be seen in patients whose tumours show no evidence of malignancy. The only really good radiological evidence upon which sarcomatous change may be suggested is the rapid development of an erosion or of a soft-tissue tumour.

The term 'hemicraniosis' has been used to indicate multiple hyperostoses on the one side of the head in cases of multiple unilateral meningiomas. The condition is extremely uncommon. (For systematic reading about meningiomas turn now to page 164).

Fibrous dysplasia (localized fibro-cystic disease of bone) (*Figures 120–124* and *236*)

Fibrous dysplasia may affect the skull alone or the skull condition may be part of a more generalized skeletal disease. When other bones are involved — with or without endocrine disturbance — it is usual to find that the base of the skull shows fibrous dysplasia as well as the vault. Even when only the skull is affected the disease may be fairly extensive and spread from the base and facial bones. However, localized areas of fibrous dysplasia affecting the vault alone are encountered

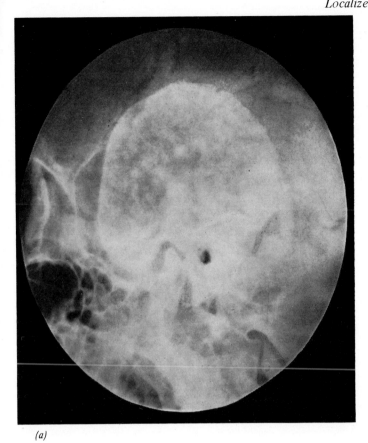

(a)

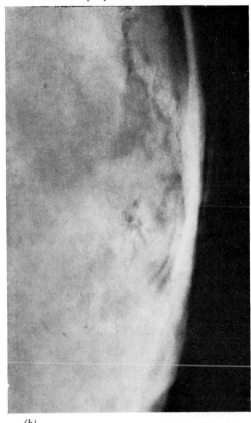

(b)

Figure 123. Fibrous dysplasia of the temporal bone in a young woman complaining of a lump on the head. There was a suggestion that it had enlarged recently, but the evidence for this was open to doubt. (a) The texture of the abnormal bone is typical of fibrous dysplasia. The disease is confined to the temporal bone. (b) In the half axial, and in other views, a false impression is given of the superimposition of abnormal bone over a normal vault. This is due to the lie of the squamoparietal suture. The edge of the squamous temporal normally overrides the parietal. The suture is clearly seen here, and the dense vault apparently medial to it is formed by the frontal and parietal bones much nearer the observer's eye

from time to time. The involved bone presents one of two main types of appearance, and the details of the radiological pathology do not depend upon the presence or absence of endocrine changes, nor is there any obvious difference in the individual lesions between the monostotic and the polyostotic form.

The radiological appearances have been given a variety of names, but it may be more satisfactory to refer to them simply as the 'sclerotic' form and the 'cystic' form. The cystic form as it affects the vault is described in detail in the chapter concerned with translucencies in the bones of the vault. It forms a blister-like expansion, but although the centre of the lesion is usually of abnormal translucency, areas of formless sclerosis are often seen lying in the transparent area, while the periphery of the lesion is nearly always an area of abnormally dense bone. Normal trabeculae are not visible within the sclerosis and this reflects the microscopic picture of an intimate mixture of fibrous tissue and woven bone. The lesion is entirely characteristic and should not be mistaken for any other.

The sclerotic form of fibrous dysplasia is more commonly seen in the base and facial bones than as an isolated disease of the vault, but it may extend to the vault from the other bones of the skull and then appears as a very extensive and often very dense deformity. Most cases of leontiasis ossea are the result of fibrous dysplasia of this type. The vault may be as much as an inch in thickness and because of the histological structure of the bone presents a featureless ground-glass appearance.

Arteriovenous malformation

Dural arteriovenous malformation may sometimes be covered by a somewhat thickened area of vault, in which there may be excess vascular channels.

Chronic osteomyelitis (*Figures 125* and *126*)

It is only in more long-standing disease that sclerosis tends to occur. The appearance of the vault in osteomyelitis, therefore, differs somewhat from the appearance in osteomyelitis of other bones. In the skull vault, new

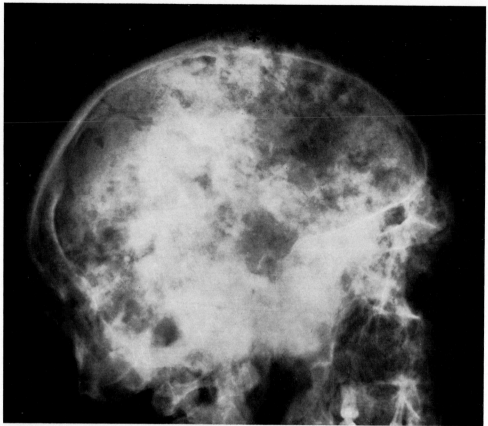

(a)

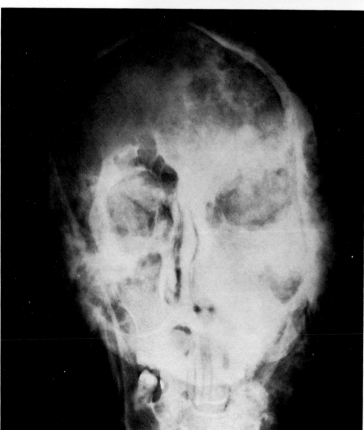

(b)

Figure 124 a and b. Fibrous dysplasia in a man aged 42 years who has had asymmetry of the face since the age of 7 years. Elsewhere he has very widespread changes almost completely confined to the left side of the body. In the skull the abnormality spreads across the midline, particularly in the sphenoid and temporal bones. There is no endocrine disturbance and no cutaneous pigmentation. The mixture of sclerosis and translucency is a little like Paget's disease, but the areas of sclerosis have better defined margins and are more homogeneous in their texture. In the lateral view there is a blister-like expansion on the vertex which is entirely typical of fibrous dysplasia

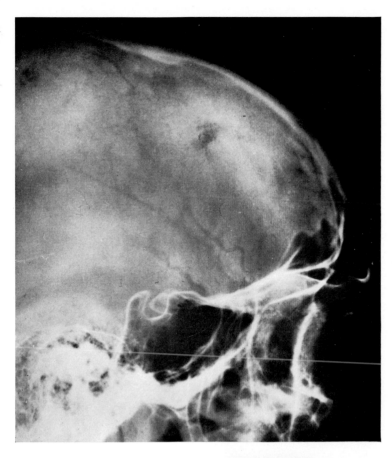

Figure 125. Chronic (tuberculous) osteomyelitis. There is an erosion with surrounding sclerosis. It is indistinguishable from the reaction due to a meningioma

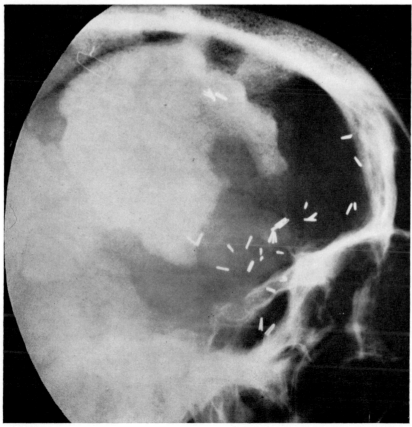

Figure 126. Ischaemic bone flap. A period of ischaemia may result in a bone flap which is denser than the surrounding skull. Eventually such a potential sequestrum may recover or die and show evidence of lysis by surrounding granulation tissue. The anterior part of this flap was found to be avascular. The posterior part bled and was left in situ

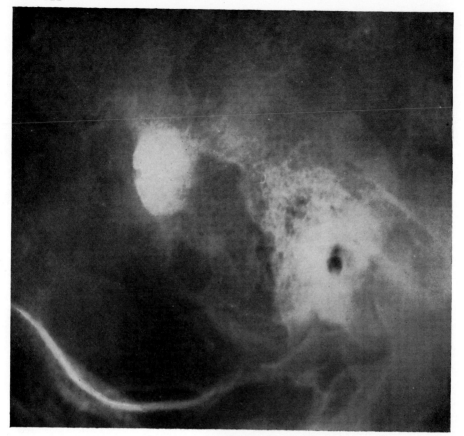

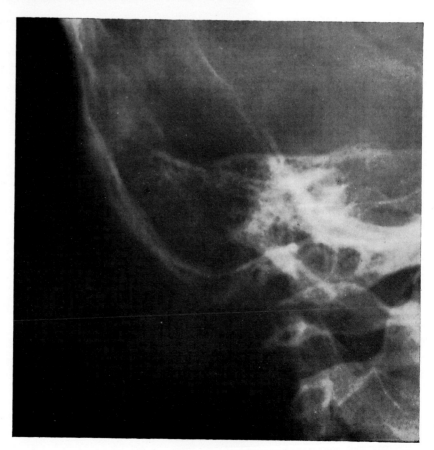

Figure 127. Osteoma. A dense osteoma of the temporal bone in a boy aged 11 years. It is symptomless. Tangential views showed that it protruded from the outer table

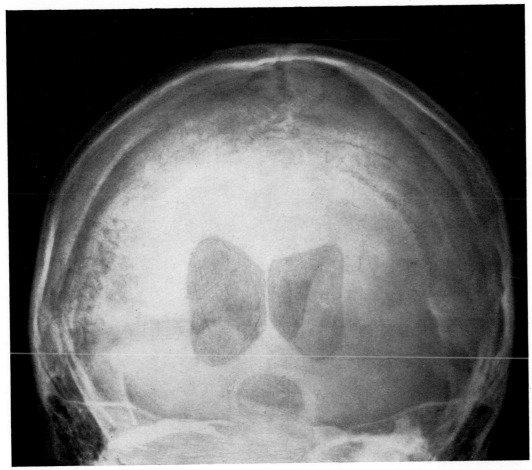

Figure 128. Hemiatrophy (mild) in a boy aged 7 years. The history is one of slow development and the onset of epileptic attacks (left-sided) each followed by transitory loss of power in the left arm. Two months before the examination the paralysis failed to clear up after an attack. At operation a parietal cortical scar was found and excised. The antero-posterior skull view at pneumoencephalography shows that the right side of the vault is thicker than the left side and lacks convolutional markings. The lateral ventricle is dilated on this side

subperiosteal bone is less readily formed, sequestra are uncommon and, except following operation, tend to be small and spontaneously absorbed.

Very low-grade infection due to any organism may, however, provoke an osteoblastic reaction in which the thickness of the vault is increased by deposition of bone from the periosteum. Lytic areas are few and only large ones are visible. Sclerosis then dominates the picture and is widespread.

A grossly abnormal vault can, however, revert to an almost normal appearance even after months of infection. This power of reparation is probably the result of the excellent blood supply.

Since there is no easy radiological distinction between infection due to different organisms, the only clinical entity which is easily separated from the others is the sclerosing low-grade osteomyelitis or osteitis which complicates some cases of long-standing frontal sinusitis and in which the increase in thickness and density of the bone extends from the region of the sinuses.

Metastatic carcinoma

Secondary deposits in the vault of the skull usually show as areas of osteoporosis, but from time to time sclerotic metastases occur either alone or mixed with areas of bone destruction. There will almost certainly be evidence of metastatic disease elsewhere in the skeleton. The typical sclerotic secondary deposit in the vault appears only a little denser than surrounding bone. It has a very ill-defined edge, is rarely more than a centimetre in diameter and the areas are nearly always multiple. Tangential radiographs may demonstrate localized thickening of the bone due to subperiosteal accretion and there is sometimes soft-tissue thickening over the affected area. (For a systematic study of malignant disease of the skull turn now to page 158.)

Paget's disease

Although it is common to find the whole of the vault as well as a large part of the base of the skull involved at the

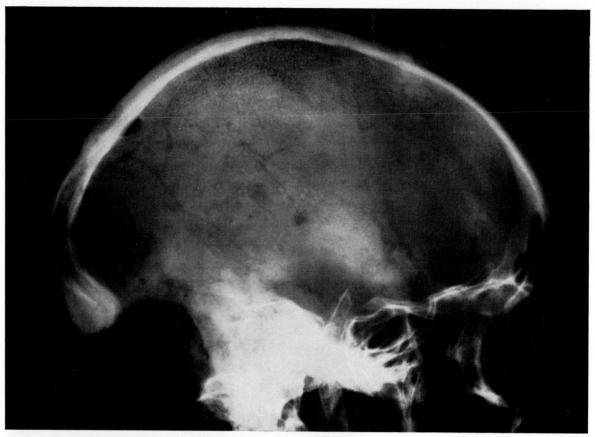

(a)

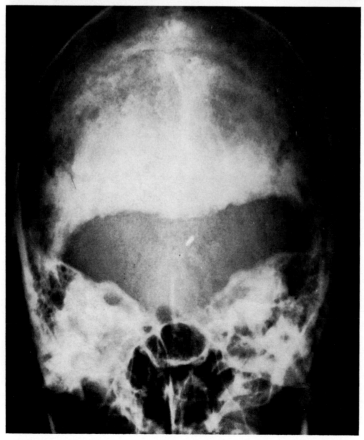

Figure 129 a and b. Radiation necrosis (plus infection) in a man aged 47 years who 15 years before had had a partial excision of a posterior fossa tumour followed by irradiation. He had remained well until 6 weeks before this radiograph was taken when he developed signs of local inflammation of the craniotomy wound. At operation several inches of the bone edge around the purulent area appeared totally avascular and were extremely hard and dense. There was no clear line of demarcation between dead and living bone, but when all the dead bone had been removed the subsequent radiograph showed that the sclerotic part had been taken away while the part showing scattered translucencies still remained. It is not certain whether the sclerosis is the result of chronic subclinical infection or is entirely due to irradiation. Sclerosis is very rarely seen in the skull as a result of either, but both cause scattered translucencies. Operative findings suggest that most of the translucencies here were the result of irradiation. They lie well beyond the edge of any visible infection

(b)

first examination, cases are encountered from time to time in which the disease has remained localized but has progressed beyond the stage of osteoporosis, so that the area of vault presents as a dense expanded bone containing abnormally thick trabeculae. The appearance in such a localized case superficially resembles fibrous dysplasia, but on close examination the trabeculated texture of the bone is different. (For a systematic study of Paget's disease turn now to page 214.) Trabeculae are not seen within the area affected by fibrous dysplasia; they may be in Paget's disease.

Osteoma (*Figure 127*)

Osteomas of the bones of the vault are very uncommon, though they may be found in the frontal sinuses where they have to be distinguished from ossifying fibromas (*see* Chapter 10 dealing with diseases of the sinuses and nasal bones). They are also found arising in the region of the mastoid process.

It is not uncommon for a hyperostosis due to meningioma to be mistaken for an osteoma, particularly when there is a palpable, hard tumour and the radiograph demonstrates thickening of the outer table of the skull as well as of its deeper layers.

However, a sharply localized, small, prominent exostosis surrounded by bone of normal texture does sometimes occur and may be distinguished from a meningioma because it is confined to the outer table and there is no increase in vascularity of the vault in the neighbourhood. Tangential views show that the thickening does not affect the inner table. Such small, well-defined local exostoses are possibly the end result of local injuries in which a subperiosteal haematoma has organized into bone.

Osteoid osteoma

Osteomas of the skull and mandible are found in Gardener's syndrome, a rare condition in which they coexist with polyps of the colon and sebaceous cysts.

Cephal-haematoma

See the Chapter entitled Head Injury, particularly page 354.

Cerebral atrophy (*Figures 132–134*)

In cerebral hemi-atrophy the affected half of the vault, as well as being smaller than the other side, is usually thicker, while convolutional impressions of the inner table are few and shallow or absent altogether. The unusual thickness of the vault on the atrophic side is presumably due to a lack of the stimulus to bone remoulding which is usually provided by the growth of the underlying cerebrum (*see also* page 126).

Tuberose sclerosis (*Figure 281a*)

In some cases of tuberose sclerosis, small, rather ill-defined areas of increase in density are seen scattered through the vault. They are easily confused with intracranial calcification which may also be visible on the radiograph and is nearly always found in a CT scan.

Radiation necrosis (*Figure 129*)

Most cases in which bone change follows therapeutic irradiation of an intracranial tumour are found to have osteoporosis. However, a sclerotic reaction may occur. The area of dense bone may be extensive. It is thickened and featureless and very hard (*see also* page 75).

Neurofibromatosis

In some cases of neurofibromatosis, dense regions have been described in the vault as a result of involvement. Multiple meningiomas are also occasionally seen in neurofibromatosis and may be the cause of hyperostosis.

4 ABNORMALITIES OF SIZE AND SHAPE OF THE VAULT

The great variety in size and shape of heads is chiefly the result of genetic influence, so that in assessing the significance of a large, small or acromegaloid head it is often helpful to be able to examine the heads of the parents.

Some of the conditions which give rise to abnormalities of shape of the vault are chiefly noticeable because of the alteration to bone texture, for example, in Paget's disease, and these are dealt with fully elsewhere in the book. Details about their appearance will not be repeated here.

A wide head is described as brachycephalic and a long one as dolicocephalic. Bathrocephaly, in which the occipital bone overrides the parietal bones at the lambdoid suture, is important because it is frequently mistaken for the effect of injury.

The classification adopted in this chapter is as follows: (1) asymmetry; (2) overgrowth (other than asymmetry); (3) deficient growth; and (4) miscellaneous conditions.

ASYMMETRY

Postural asymmetry (*Figures 130–131*)

The skull is invariably asymmetrical, and even severe degrees of asymmetry are quite commonplace and are not of any significance if the volume of the two halves of the cranial cavity is approximately equal.

The common form of postural asymmetry is a flattening of one posterior parietal and occipital region with a corresponding bulge of the frontal bone, and the shape is said to result from prolonged recumbency on one side in infancy. It is certainly more often seen to a gross degree in young children than in adult life after the head has remoulded during the period of growth.

Examination of the skull radiographs (in particular of the full axial) shows that in spite of the flattening in the posterior part of the volume of the two halves of the head remains approximately the same. The sutures appear normal.

Another form of postural asymmetry is caused by spinal scoliosis, occurring at an early age and leading to some obliquity of the position in which the head is carried. In these patients the facial asymmetry is more striking than that of the rest of the skull.

Hemiatrophy (*Figures 132–134*)

Cerebral hemiatrophy produces a characteristic deformity of the skull, one half of which is smaller in its total volume than the other. The smaller half is nearly always thicker and lacks convolutional markings. The condition has to be distinguished from postural asymmetry and from plagiocephaly. In hemiatrophy the skull base is usually asymmetrical in a fashion which further diminishes the size of the small half of the cranial cavity, so that the petrous bone on the affected side appears higher than the other. There may also be greater pneumatization of the frontal sinuses on the smaller side. Neither of these findings is present in plagiocephaly, nor is the vault thicker on the affected side. In severe hemiatrophy of the cerebrum the volume of the smaller side may be further diminished by a considerable degree of displacement of the falx (which may be visible on the plain radiograph as a white linear shadow in the postero-anterior view, or its position may also be recognized by the grooves and ridges made by the confluence of sinuses at the torcula).

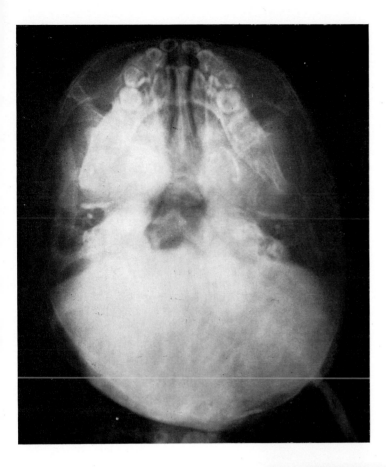

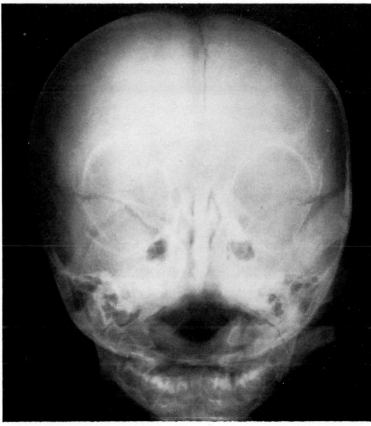

(a)

Figure 130 a and b. Postural asymmetry in an infant. Full axial and antero-posterior views showing that a bulge of the posterior part of the head on the left side is compensated by prominence of the right parietal and frontal regions. The volume of each half of the head is the same. The child is normal

(b)

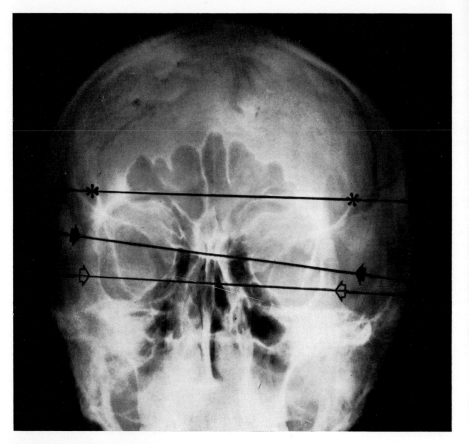

(a)

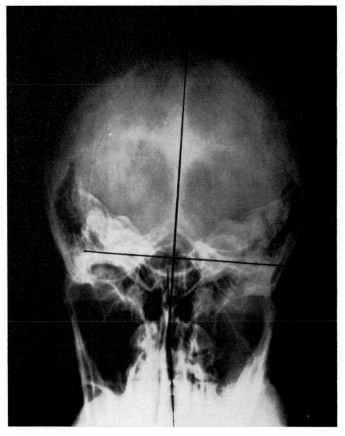

Figure 131. Postural asymmetry in scoliosis. The base of the skull is asymmetrical but in this case the head is carried with the orbits at the same height from the ground. (a) The postero-anterior view. Lines have been drawn through the orbital roofs (asterisk to asterisk), through the planum sphenoidale (closed arrow to closed arrow) and through the floor of the sella (open arrow to open arrow). (b) Half axial view, the axis of the cervical spine and the median plane of the head lie at an angle to each other

(b)

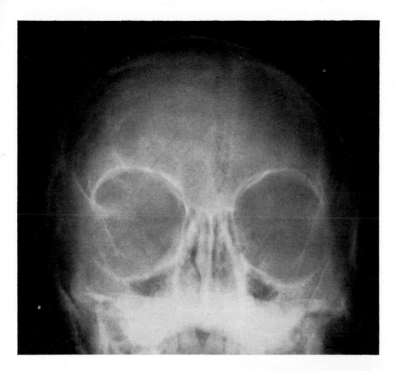

(a)

Figure 132. 'Hemiatrophy' of the cerebrum. The left cerebral hemisphere has failed to grow. As a result, the left half of the cranium is much smaller than the right. (a) In the postero-anterior view some left-sided flattening is evident. (b) The full axial view confirms that there is no left-sided compensatory bulge. The internal occipital protuberance, and therefore the falx, is well over to the left. It is important in doubtful cases to distinguish postural asymmetry from deficient development in this way (cont.)

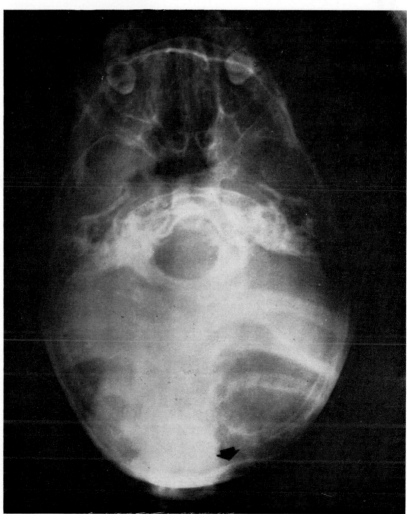

(b)

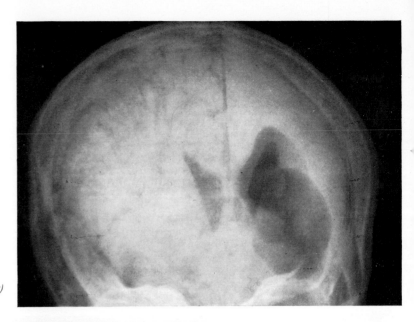

Figure 132 (cont.). (c) Pneumoencephalogram. The division between the hemispheres is to the left of the midline. The left lateral ventricle is dilated. There is no filling of cortical spaces on the left. Note also the absence of convolutional impressions in the vault at this side

(c)

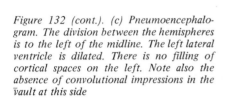

Figure 133. See legend under (c)

(a)

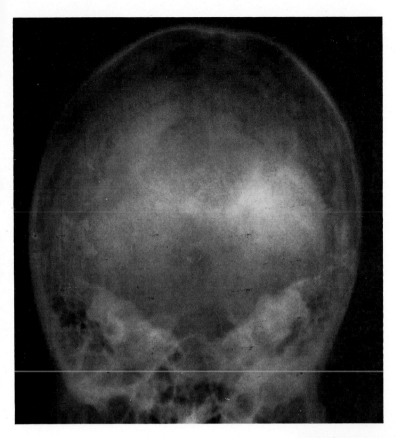

(b)

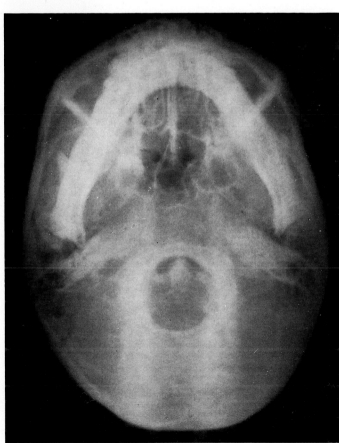

Figure 133 a–c. Cerebral hemiatrophy following 'encephalitis' at the age of 1½ years. The patient had a right hemiparesis. Radiographs at the age of 19 years show the following. In each view there is evidence of a smaller volume to the left side of the head. The left half of the calvaria is also slightly thicker than the right. It is essential with minor degrees of asymmetry to confirm that flattening of the vault in one place is not compensated by a bulge elsewhere before making a diagnosis of atrophy

(c)

132

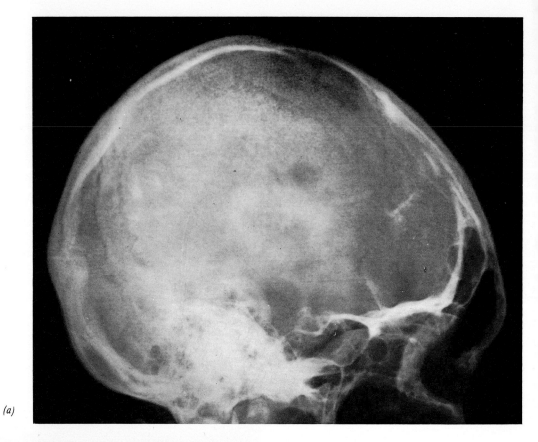

(a)

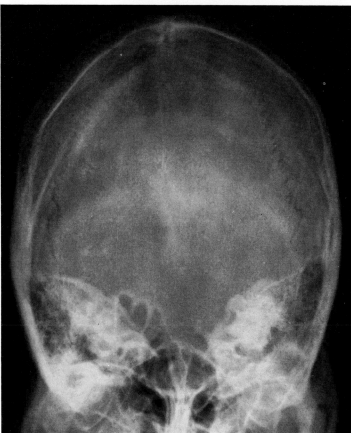

(b)

Figure 134. Hemiatrophy of the cerebrum (Sturge–Weber syndrome) in a young woman with a large cutaneous naevus over the right side of the face. The history was unusual for Sturge–Weber syndrome in that there was a number of episodes possibly explainable as subarachnoid haemorrhages. A diffuse angioma was shown angiographically. (a) Lateral view. There are areas of calcification in the occipital and frontal regions, either cortical or subcortical in position. (b) Towne's view. The right half of the vault is thicker than the left and the right parietal region flatter than the left. Convolutional impressions are less marked on the right (cont.)

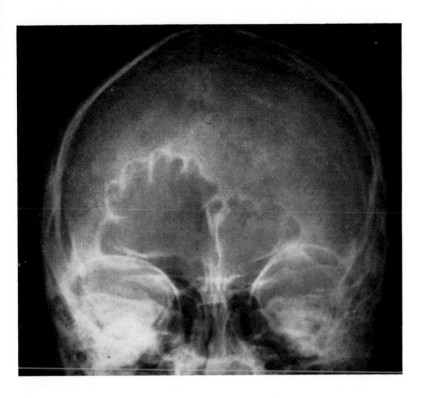

Figure 134 (cont.). (c) Antero-posterior view. The inequality of volume of the two halves of the head is obvious. The right petrous bone is slightly elevated

(c)

Localized atrophy

A localized area of flattening of part of the vault, particularly if the bone is unusually thick, has been taken as evidence in favour of underlying cerebral atrophy, but the point is difficult to prove.

Plagiocephaly

See the section on Craniostenosis on page 142.

On the smaller side the vault is likely to be abnormally thin and to exhibit exaggerated convolutional impressions. There may be an area of compensatory bulging; parts of the sutures will have fused.

Premature unilateral fusion of the coronal suture may cause severe deformity if it occurs before birth. The parietal and frontal bones will be flattened and the orbit enlarged in its vertical diameter. The lesser wing of the sphenoid is elevated, the innominate line pushed outwards (the middle fossa being enlarged) and the lambda is displaced towards the abnormal side. There may be proptosis, and optic atrophy can occur, presumably by pressure on and stretching of the optic nerve (Faure, Bonamy and Rambert–Misset, 1967).

Craniopagus twins (*Figure 12*)

In this very rare abnormality, the head of the children may be joined over a relatively narrow area or the junction may involve the full circumference of the two calvariae. A secondary obliquity and asymmetry, presumably due to the forces produced by growth of the attached twin, is seen at birth and progresses. It may give rise to serious facial distortion.

The normal complement of vault bones usually seems to be present but their relationship to the brains within is often bizarre. The shape of the exterior of the heads gives no indication of the extent to which the cerebrum of one child has encroached upon the territory of the other, though before the end of the first year of life grooves on the inner table along the course of dural sinuses may give some indication of the position of dural shelves and attachments which separate the brains. Normal brain growth produces convolutional impressions chiefly upon the lower parts of the vault as the children tend to lie in a constant posture dictated by the shape of the junction. It is most important to realize when investigating twins of this sort that the lateral ventricles may be of unusual shape and may lie far from their expected positions, so that ventriculography may be impossible and the results of air injection very confusing.

OVERGROWTH

A local bulging of the vault (*Figures 135–140*)

A local bulging of the vault due to an underlying, superficial, space-occupying lesion such as an arachnoid cyst usually causes a considerable degree of thinning of the bones and may appear in *en face* views as an area of translucency. It is therefore considered more fully in Chapter 2.

Expansion of the whole of the middle fossa on one side causes elevation of the lesser wing of the sphenoid (in postero-anterior projections) and forward displacement of the anterior margin of the middle fossa as shown in the lateral view. There is also widening of the curve of this margin in the full axial projection. The commonest cause of such an appearance is the condition usually

134

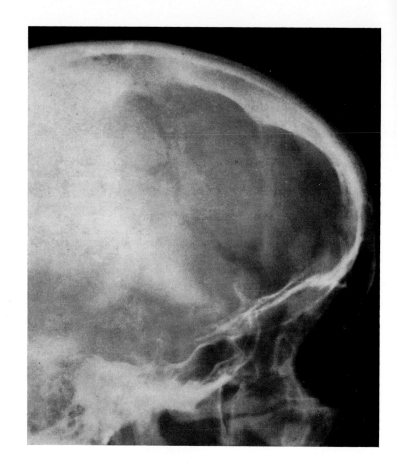

Figure 135. Extradural arachnoid cyst in a woman aged 55 years who had a 'bulge' on the head for an unknown number of years, and then began to develop headaches and papilloedema. (a) The lateral radiograph shows a translucent area in the frontal bone with a somewhat scalloped antero-superior margin

(a)

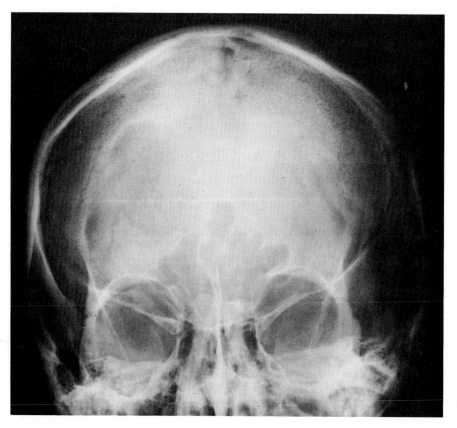

(b) The left side of the frontal bone is much thinner than the right and both it and the temporal bone are slightly bulged. The sphenoid ridge is elevated

(b)

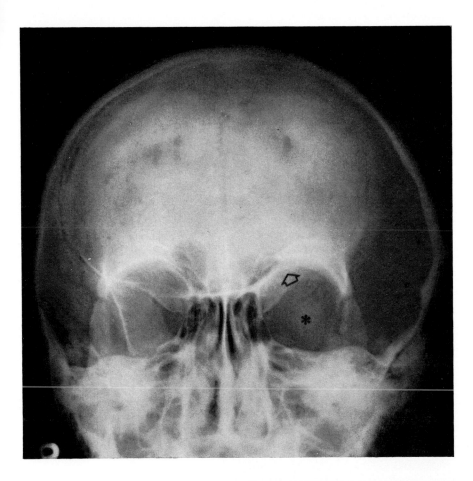

(a)

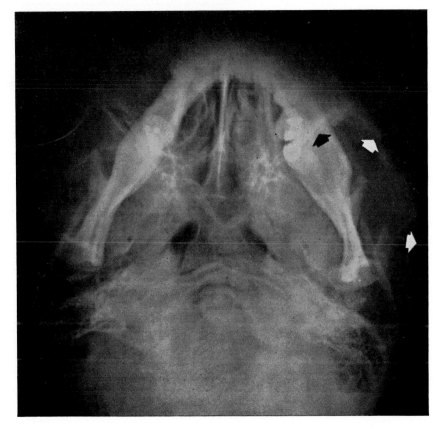

Figure 136. Subdural hygroma in a man aged 53 years who had had a left temporal swelling since childhood. The left half of the middle fossa is expanded as shown in (a), the postero-anterior view, where the greater wing of the sphenoid (asterisk) is thinned and the lesser wing elevated (open arrow). (b) Full axial view, where anterior displacement of the squamous temporal are evident (closed arrows). The time sequence of this condition is still doubtful. Operation and CT scanning show a combination of local bone expansion and underlying cerebral atrophy. It seems likely that many are of the nature of arachnoid cysts

(b)

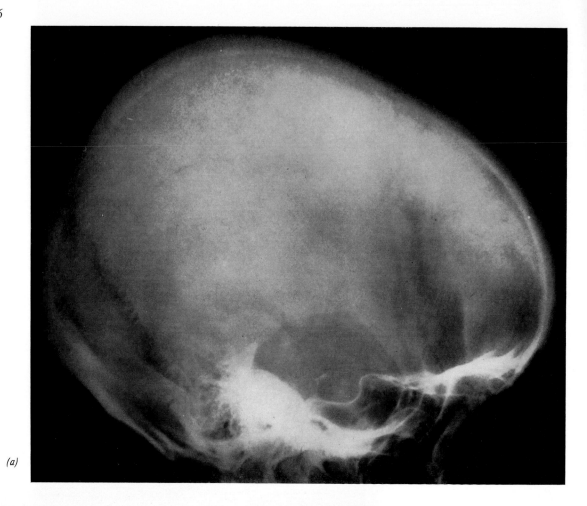

(a)

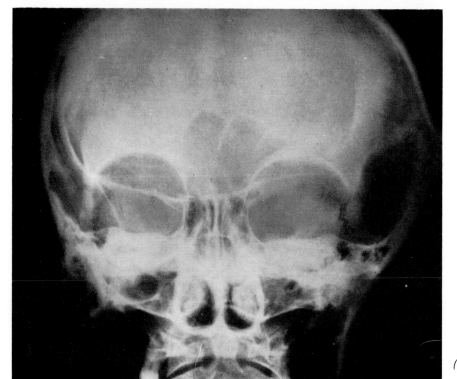

Figure 137 a and b. Localized hydrocephalus, 30 years after a left temporal decompression. The bone has re-formed as a bulging shell. The whole of the left side of the middle fossa is now also expanded. There was gross hydrocephalus confined to the left temporal horn, which was found to be obstructed at its junction with the trigone

(b)

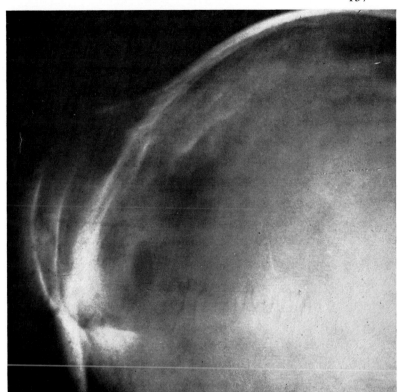

Figure 138. A post-operative bulge. If the dura is left, as in the case of decompression, and the patient survives for a number of years, the vault may re-form in a fresh shape

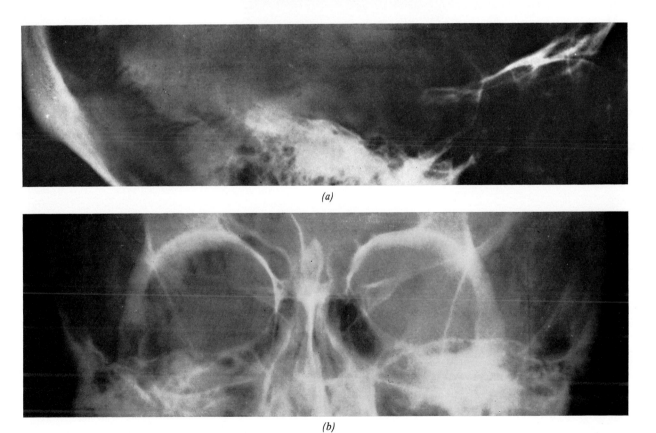

(a)

(b)

Figure 139. A long-standing temporal lobe glioma. There had probably been a recent increase in malignancy which brought about admission to hospital. (a) Postero-anterior view, showing thinning of the sphenoid wings on the right. (b) Full axial view. There is loss of bone detail in the floor and of the anterior margin of the middle fossa on the right side due to the thinning of bone

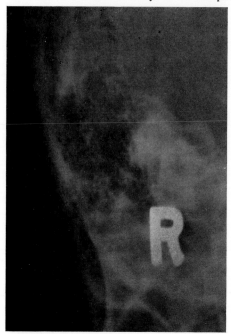

(c)

Figure 139 (cont.). (c) Towne's view. The squamous temporal is thin and bulging. (d) Full axial view. There is a loss of all bone detail in the floor and of the anterior margin of the middle fossa on the right side due to the thinning of bone

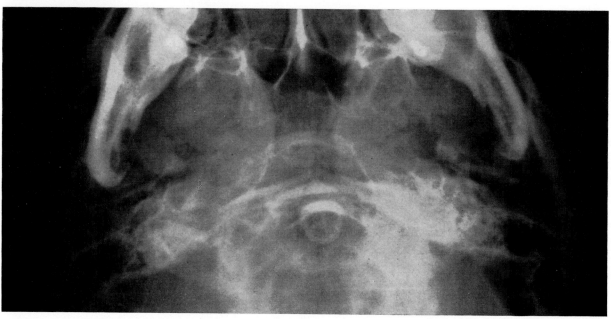

(d)

now known as a subdural hygroma. Some of these may be the result of chronic, overlooked, infantile, subdural haematomas in infancy—they have often been called chronic subdural haematomas. Others, perhaps the majority, may be more in the nature of developmental anomalies in which there is a combination of cystic overgrowth of an extracerebral C.S.F. space with hypoplasia of the underlying temporal lobe, but whether the cerebral or the meningeal abnormality is the primary one has not been decided. In this condition it is not uncommon to see not only a large C.S.F. space, but also some seemingly contradictory evidence of atrophy of the cranial contents such as enlargement of the frontal sinus on the same side as the bulge.

Very slow-growing intracranial tumours of any kind may produce a similar expansion without such evidence of atrophy, as may localized temporal horn hydrocephalus. One special instance of expansion due to tumour affects a portion of the parietal bone superficial to benign masses in the trigone of the lateral ventricle, such as meningiomas and choroid plexus papillomas. In neurofibromatosis there may be a complex asymmetry which includes expansion of one middle fossa.

Hydrocephalus

Enlargement of the whole or part of the head due to hydrocephalus is considered in the chapter devoted to raised intracranial pressure.

Cerebral gigantism (Soto's syndrome)

The large head shows no evidence of raised pressure. There is often an anterior fontanelle bone (Poznanski and Stephenson, 1967).

Gargoylism (Hurler—Hunter syndrome, dysostosis multiplex)

Gargoylism leads to mental deficiency and blindness, followed by death at an early age. In about one-third of the cases there is mild hydrocephalic enlargement of the head due to thickening of the meninges, but the vault is thick rather than thin. Typically the skull is long, with a bulging frontal bone, and abnormalities of the base and mandible have been said to produce a characteristic picture (*see* Chapter 8). There are other members of the group of mucopolysaccharidoses that have less severe cranial deformities; they are described in Chapter 11.

The diagnosis is nearly always made on clinical grounds before radiography.

Dwarfism with a large head

In some cases of achondroplasia (*see* page 237) the head is not only abnormal in shape but actually enlarged by mild hydrocephalus.

There are also a number of other causes of dwarfism with a large head. Thanatophoric dwarfism and achondrogenesis are neonatal lethal conditions presenting somewhat similar clinical appearances, though distinguishable radiologically because of the uniquely retarded skeletal ossification of achondrogenesis (Langer *et al.*, 1969; Saldino, 1971). All these conditions mentioned may involve a skull which shows prominence of the forehead, a depressed bridge of nose and facial bones which are slightly or very small by comparison with the vault.

In the Toulouse-Lautrec Syndrome (pyknodysostosis) the head is also large compared with the face and there is frontal and parietal bossing (*see* Chapter 11).

Ocular hypertelorism

This is dealt with in more detail in Chapters 8 and 10, which are concerned with the skull base and face, and in the chapter on developmental abnormalities. The principal deformities are of the face. The vault will usually be broad and there may, in infancy and childhood, be a midline defect extending forwards from the anterior fontanelle. This is known as cranium bifidum

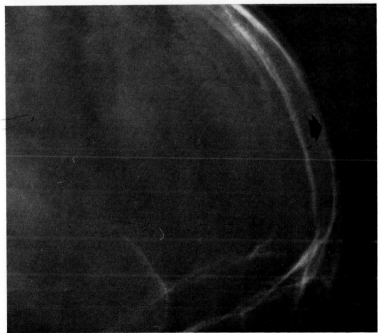

Figure 140. Neurofibromatosis in a boy aged 8 years who has an extensive plexiform neuroma of the face and orbits and neighbouring parts. In addition, there is a right hemiparesis, bilateral optic atrophy and evidence of raised intracranial pressure. He is intelligent and did well after operation for aqueduct stenosis. Several plastic operations have been performed on his face. (a) Localized lateral view of the frontal bone. There is thinning particularly of the outer table (cont.)

(a)

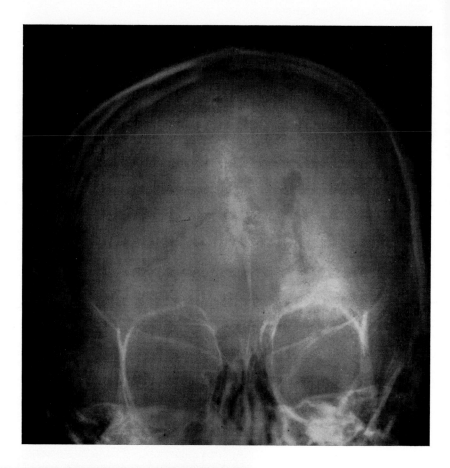

(b)

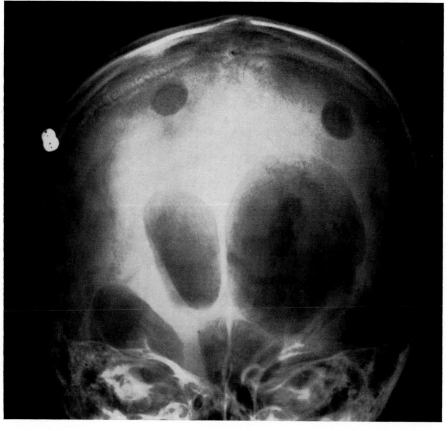

Figure 140 (cont.). (b) The asymmetrical enlargement of the vault and the frontal translucency. (c) The underlying dilatation reveals the same asymmetry (cont.)

(c)

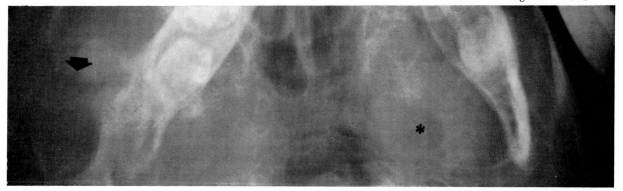

(d)

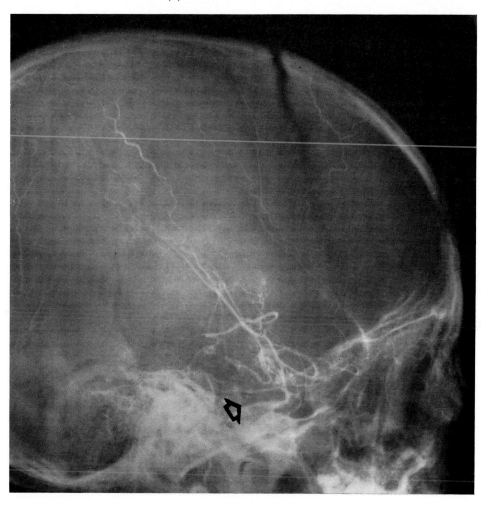

Figure 140 (cont.). (d) Local view of base. Enlargement of foramen ovale (asterisk) and suture diasstasis (arrow). (e) Lateral angiogram showing carotid stenosis, abnormal vessels in the superficial neuroma and, faintly, the enlarged sella (arrow). The internal auditory meatuses were large but not eroded. The orbits were comparatively normal

(e)

occultum frontalis. The defect is bridged by dura and periosteum and tends to ossify in the end.

Osteochondrodystrophia deformans (Morquio's disease)

In most cases the skull is normal; but hydrocephalus occasionally complicates the picture. Morquio's disease is divisible into two or more types, one at least of these is a mucopolysaccharidosis (*see* Chapter 11).

Marfan's syndrome

In the fully developed syndrome the skull is found to be dolicocephalic.

Neurofibromatosis

Cerebral overgrowth and macrocrania are not uncommon. They tend to affect only one region such as the temporal on one side.

DEFICIENT GROWTH

Microcephaly (*Figures 141* and *142*)

The head may be smaller than normal for the patient's age as a result of endocrine dwarfism, in which case the vault will be of normal thickness for the size of the head and will show normal convolutional impressions.

Moderate deficiencies in cranial size at birth should not necessarily be taken as of poor prognosis. Only those measurements which are particularly small in neonates tend still to lag at school age (Schmidt and Holthusen, 1972).

The head may be small as a result of failure of normal development of the brain, and in these cases the skull bones are usually thicker; sometimes the paranasal air sinuses, particularly the frontal sinuses, are unusually large.

The head may be small as a result of generalized craniostenosis.

A number of syndromes associated with microcephaly are described in Chapter 11.

Craniostenosis (*Figures 2, 4, 26, 111, 143–145*)

The coronal, sagittal and lambdoid sutures, the sutures around the squamous temporal and the pterion normally remain open into adult life, and in some individuals synostosis never occurs. Craniostenosis consists in the fusion of one or more of these sutures at an age earlier than normal; but the extent and the age at which this occurs vary widely from case to case. It may even begin *in utero*. When craniostenosis is widespread, and when it begins in the first few years of life, its clinical effects may be severe since, in addition to the deformity, it may lead to severe headache, mental retardation and blindness.

The condition may be hereditary and other congenital abnormalities may be present.

Craniostenosis (craniosynostosis means the same) may be part of Crouzon's syndrome (craniofacial dysostosis) in which it is associated with hypoplasia of the facial bones. It is one of the features of Apert's syndrome (acrocephalosyndactylism) and of Carpenter's syndrome (acrocephalopolysyndactyly). It is the essential feature of Kleeblattschädel (clover-leaf skull) in which the deformity is due to intra-uterine closure of the coronal and lambdoid sutures with concomitant hydrocephalus.

There is premature closure of the metopic, coronal and sagittal sutures in craniotelencephalic dysplasia in which it is clinically associated with ear deformities, mental retardation and some degree of hypotelorism. Orbital hypotelorism itself is sometimes used as a name to include not only those mild cases in which early fusion of the metopic suture was the principal abnormality, but a whole spectrum of much more severe abnormalities including trigonocephaly with, in the worst cases, cyclopia or arrhinencephaly.

Craniostenosis is occasionally associated with Treacher–Collin's syndrome (mandibulo-facial dysostosis). There is a separate chapter (11) devoted to such congenital malformations.

In addition, craniostenosis may appear in some cases of vitamin D resistant rickets under treatment, in idiopathic hypercalcaemia, in vitamin D poisoning, in hypophosphatasia and after the relief of raised intracranial pressure in hydrocephalic children. It is occasionally seen following treatment for hyperthyroidism in children. Duggan, Keener and Gay (1970) list other rare causes such as the Hurler type of gargoylism and certain equivocal associations.

There are three main radiological features in most cases of craniostenosis. These are: (1) the absence of part or the whole of one or more sutures of the vault; (2) the deformity of the skull; and (3) the exaggeration of convolutional impressions.

Severe cases are often diagnosed clinically before radiography is undertaken because of the abnormal shape of the head and the presence of palpable bony ridges along the closing suture lines. However, confirmation is required and detailed examination is of importance before surgical treatment is attempted.

The radiological recognition of the closure of sutures may be difficult in infancy and in young children unless particular attention is paid to the problem. In the early stages of craniostenosis the shape of the head is not altered, and in the lateral radiographs the coronal sutures are, in any case, often difficult to see. In postero-anterior and antero-posterior views, however, portions of the sagittal suture can be seen and, when viewed tangentially with a bright light, the more opaque region of the radiograph may reveal some heaping up of the bone on either side of the narrow or obliterated suture line.

In the full axial projection (most useful in recognizing suture diastasis in childhood) the sagittal or coronal suture will not be seen, but because of superimposed basal shadows it would be unwise to make the absence of the visible suture line in this view the only basis for the diagnosis.

Confirmation of the closure of any suture is probably best obtained by a radiograph made with the beam tangential to the vault and firing along the line of the suture.

In cases of craniostenosis where closure of sutures took place in childhood some months or years before the radiological examination, there will be a deformity, the nature of which depends upon the distribution of the stenosis. The literature on this subject is confused by too many classifications. Much early work was done in Germany and the German names for the various deformities have entered general medical usage alongside their English translations in addition to names of Greek derivation for substantially the same conditions.

Most authors use the term 'brachycephaly' to describe the short, wide head which results from fusion of coronal and/or lambdoid sutures. They apply the terms scaphocephaly and dolicocephaly to the long, narrow head of premature fusion of the sagittal suture. Brachycephaly and dolicocephaly also describe the broad or long and narrow heads of normal people and it is confusing to use the same words for abnormal features. In practice, fusion of the coronal suture is usually accompanied by early fusion of some part (usually posterior) of the sagittal suture. The skull grows upwards in the region of the anterior fontanelle and is broad in inverse proportion to the degree of sagittal suture synostosis. Tall heads of various shapes are described by the terms turricephaly and acrocephaly (pointed head). Oxycephaly (*oxus* = sharp, Greek) really means the same thing. In

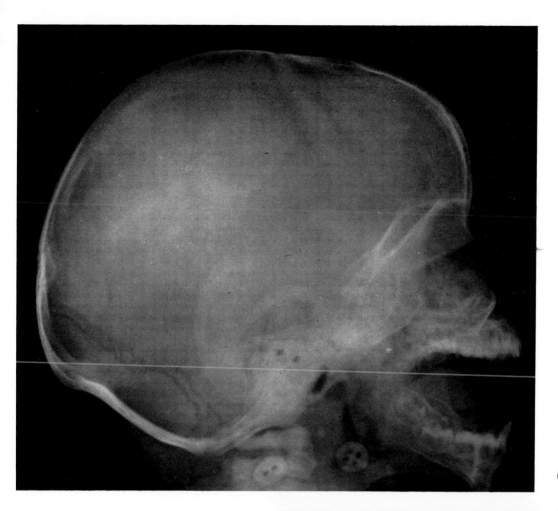

(a)

Figure 141 a and b. Microcephaly of unknown cause in a girl aged 5 months. Compare with microcephaly due to craniostenosis. The head is symmetrical. The sutures are open and the bones show few convolutional impressions

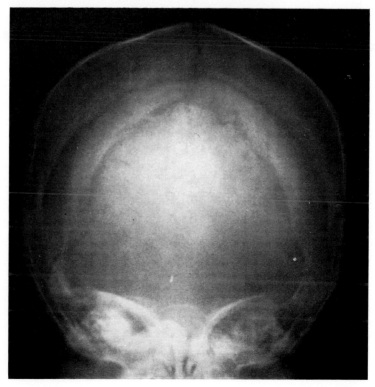

(b)

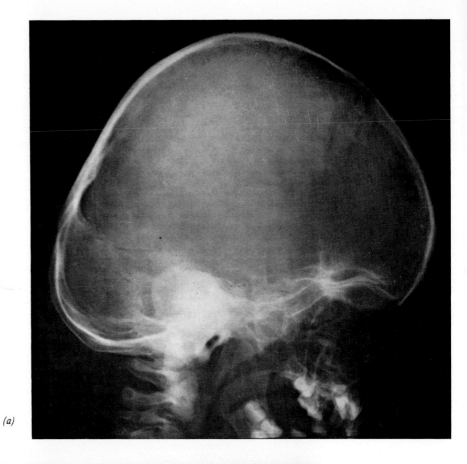

(a)

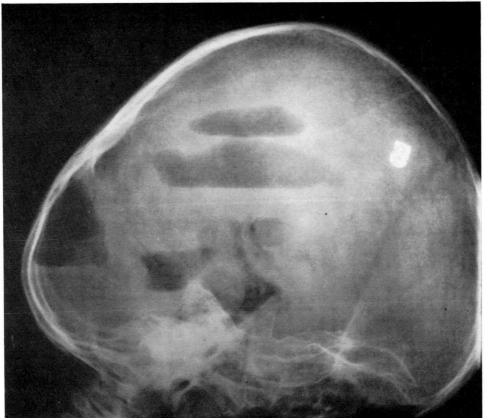

(b)

Figure 142. Failure of development in a child aged 3 years who is grossly retarded and has evidence of a cerebellar defect. She was born with an abnormally shaped head. (a) There is flattening of the posterior parietal regions together with expansion of the posterior fossa. (b) Pneumoencephalography shows dilatation of the lateral ventricles most marked posteriorly – presumable due to failure of brain growth – as well as an enormous cisterna magna (of unknown significance but associated with a small cerebellum)

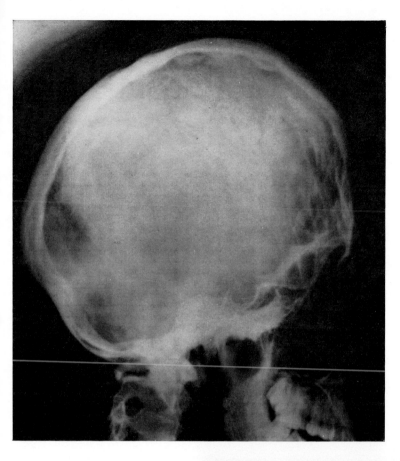

(a)

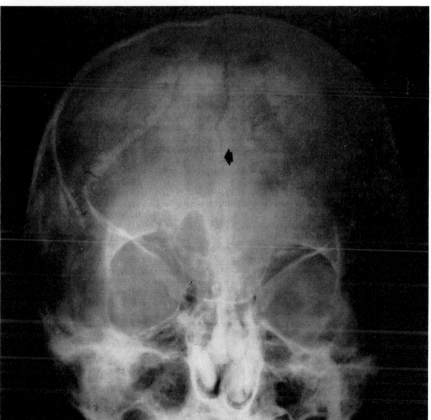

Figure 143. Craniostenosis (oxycephaly) in a woman aged 23 years. (a) The head is tall and wide but its antero-posterior diameter is short. There are pronounced convolutional impressions on the frontal bone. There is no coronal suture. (b) The postero-anterior view shows a metopic suture (cont.)

(b)

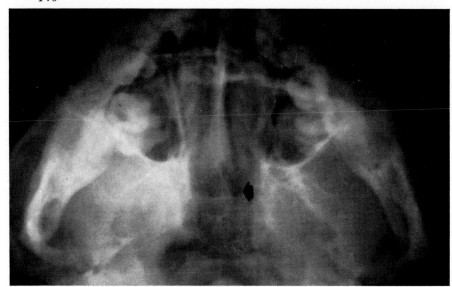

Figure 143 (cont.). (c) The full axial view demonstrates that the sagittal suture is still unfused. There may also be partial fusion of the right lambdoid suture

(c)

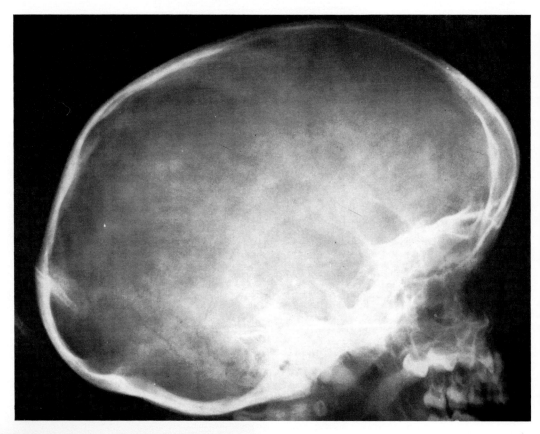

(a)

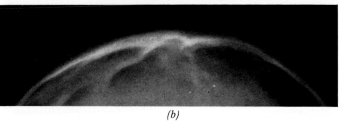

(b)

Figure 144. Craniostenosis (scaphocephaly) in a boy aged 2 years 9 months. The head is too narrow for its length. (a) This slightly oblique lateral view shows the coronal, lambdoid and parieto-temporal sutures. (b) A portion of the half axial view confirms that the sagittal suture is completely fused. Tangential views of this kind are the most reliable for confirmation of synostosis of any particular suture

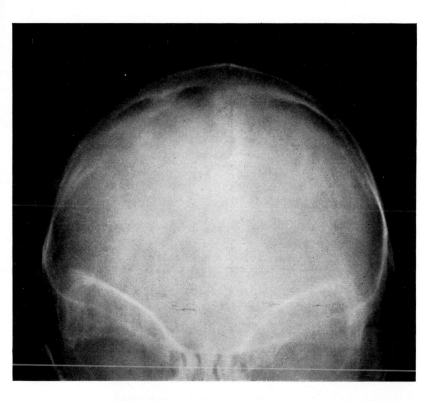

(a)

Figure 145. Craniostenosis (predominantly scaphocephalic in type). (a) Antero-posterior view. The sagittal suture is nearly closed (the coronal suture also). (b) Lateral view, 2 months later. Closure of the coronal and sagittal sutures still spares the region of the anterior fontanelle, and a bulge is appearing here due to growth. The head is long and narrow, the lambdoid suture still remaining open

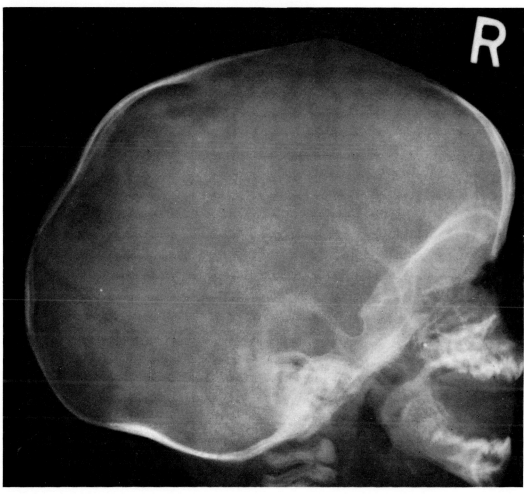

(b)

oxycephaly, where stenosis took place at an early age and also involved the metopic suture, the middle fossae may be expanded, the child showing exophthalmos.

Most of the brachycephalic types of craniostenosis are tower-shaped or pointed and may be described as turricephaly or oxycephaly (or acrocephaly), and it is rarely necessary to confuse the issue by using the name 'brachycephaly' without qualification in the group of craniostenoses.

Trigonocephaly (narrow in front, broad behind) results from premature closure of the metopic suture. Plagiocephaly is an asymmetrical head after unilateral craniosynostosis and has to be distinguished from postural asymmetry and from hemiatrophy.

Convolutional impressions in many of these cases become very deep and obvious due to the exaggerated process of bone remoulding which takes place in an attempt to accommodate the growth of the child's brain.

Grundy, Goree and Jimenez (1970) have pointed out a diagnostic pitfall in oxycephaly when patients in adult life complain of bitemporal visual field defects due to the skull deformity. Because the pituitary fossa is so low and obscured by other basal structures they may at first be thought to have pituitary tumours.

MISCELLANEOUS

Rickets

In children and adults a four-cornered appearance to the head due to 'bossing' of the frontal and parietal bones may be the result of healed rickets. The vault may become very thick over the frontal and parietal 'bosses'.

In infants with active rickets the bones of the vault may be extremely thin, but the abnormality of shape is less evident.

Trauma

A local flattening of any part of the vault may be due to a depressed fracture. The subject of skull trauma is dealt with in a separate chapter (page 334).

In neonates, who have lain *in utero* with the feet pressed to the head, local depressions may be found on inspection and are sometimes shown radiographically.

Tam-o-shanter skull

The combination of great thickening of the vault with basilar invagination in Paget's disease produces an appearance described as tam-o-shanter skull.

5 THE SELLA TURCICA

First-class radiographs of the sella may reveal minor abnormalities which are easily overlooked at a cursory examination, but since they may precede definite clinical evidence of serious disease it is most important that a careful study of the region should be made. If a magnifying glass aids memory or concentration on this, it should be used routinely.

The abnormalities may be classified: (1) osteoporosis and erosion; (2) enlargement; (3) flattening; or (4) calcification in the neighbourhood.

These may be found alone or in combination in a variety of diseases, sometimes making interpretation of the radiograph very difficult.

Consideration of the sella is probably the most complex part of the skull radiology, and this chapter is the most difficult one in the book. The reader is encouraged to remember the overall classification and observe the broad differences between the groups of illustrations.

In the most general terms the usual causes of sellar abnormalities are: raised intracranial pressure; pituitary tumours; suprasellar space-occupying lesions; parasellar space-occupying lesions; bone diseases.

The size of the sella is related to the size of its contents. Not only can it enlarge, even in adult life, but it can also shrink if the pituitary gland diminishes in size. An extreme example is provided by the unusually small sellas sometimes seen after post-partum pituitary necrosis (Meador and Worrell, 1966).

(1) OSTEOPOROSIS AND EROSION

The shadow of the sella in the lateral view may appear at a glance indefinite, 'rubbed out', obviously eroded with-out being enlarged, or sometimes careful study of a sella of more normal appearances will reveal minor erosions. The causes of these abnormalities are analysed in the first section of the chapter, where it will be found that raised intracranial pressure and the earlier stages of intrasellar, suprasellar and parasellar erosions are described.

(2) ENLARGEMENT

Definite enlargement of the pituitary fossa may occur at a later stage of the diseases which begin with erosion. Enlargement is also sometimes found without any defect or loss of definition. The second section of the chapter is concerned with the causes of this sellar expansion with and without erosion, often due to intrasellar tumours.

Parasellar expanding lesions also fall, strictly speaking, into this category; but since a few of them may appear to erode the sella without causing obvious enlargement, they are divided between Sections 1 and 2.

(3) FLATTENING

Suprasellar tumours often present by flattening the sella from above with erosion or forward displacement of the dorsum. They and their differential diagnosis form the basis for Section 3.

(4) CALCIFICATION

Calcification may be an additional sign or may complicate the picture, and requires separate analysis.

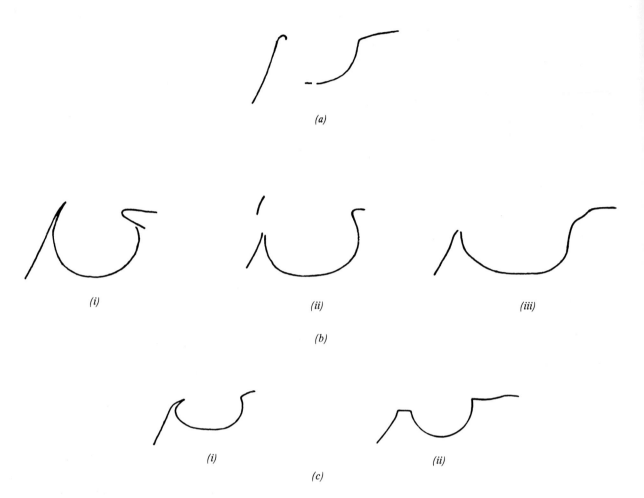

Figure 146. Typical profiles. (a) Erosion (due to raised intracranial pressure). (b) (i and ii) Ballooning (due to pituitary adenoma), (iii) non-specific enlargement. (c) (i and ii) Flattening, (due to suprasellar masses)

(1) OSTEOPOROSIS AND EROSION WITHOUT EXPANSION OF THE SELLA TURCICA

The term 'osteoporosis' is often used to describe changes in the sella which, on analysis, include or are entirely due to definite small erosions. In this context the distinction on radiographs between osteoporosis and erosion is really one of size of defect, and depends partly on overlying shadows (*Figure 147*). The word 'osteoporosis' should mean here detectable diminution in density on the radiograph but without measurable gaps in the bone, and very little further mention will be made of it because of the difficulties which surround its recognition.

Erosion is usually first observed in the lamina dura (cortex) of the sella, which may be indistinct or obviously interrupted by small holes. The diploë of the dorsum sellae may also have pathological defects which are masked by the remaining trabeculae. In severe cases the individual areas of destruction are greater and erosions are recognized as such.

From a practical point of view the important criterion is interruption or disappearance of the lamina dura. With advancing age the cancellous structure may become more translucent and overlying arterial calcification confuses the picture; but though the cortex may be thin, and careful inspection is required to see it, it is preserved in the aged, so that *absence of this thin white line on a correctly centred radiograph made with high definition screens, standard film and a reasonably fine-grain development, should be regarded as a most suspicious sign.*

Causes

RAISED INTRACRANIAL PRESSURE (*Figures 5–7, 13–19, 148* and *149*)

This is the commonest cause of erosion of the sella without enlargement. The author believes that the abnormality is recognizable at any age, and need not be confused with the general translucency of senile bones.

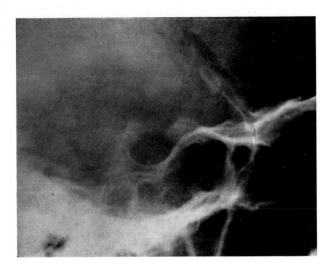

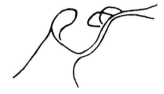

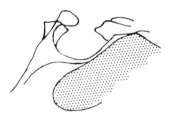

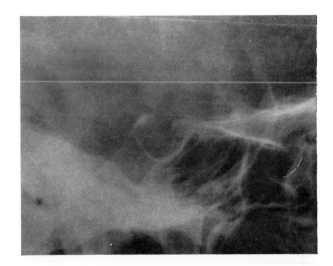

Figure 147. The normal sella in old age. In spite of some osteoporosis the floor of the sella and the anterior surface of the dorsum are perfectly intact

Figure 148. Raised intracranial pressure in a patient aged 34 years. There is a 6-month history of headache, vomiting and unsteadiness of gait. The patient had bilateral papilloedema. A cerebellar hae-mangioblastoma was removed. The radiograph shows the very earliest detectable loss of cortex of the anterior part of the base of the dorsum sellae. The relationship of the moderately dilated third ventricle is shown

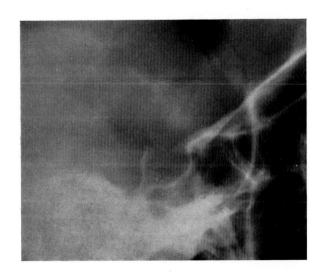

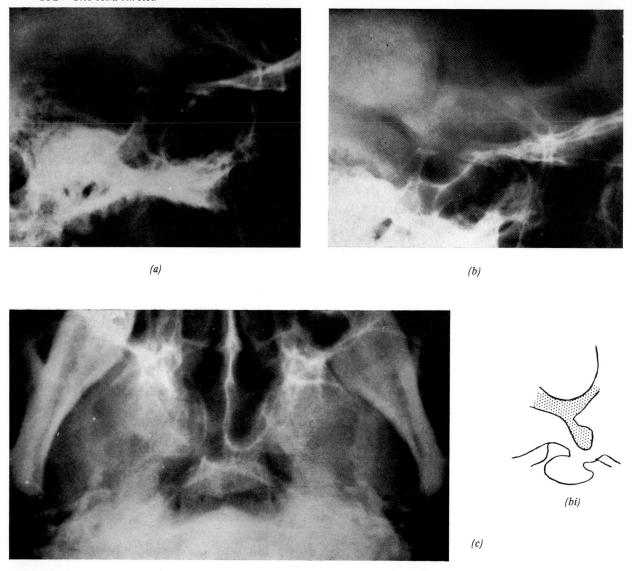

Figure 149. A paraphyseal cyst of the third ventricle in a woman aged 39 years with a 2½ year history of headaches. She has severe bilateral papilloedema. (a) Lateral radiograph. There may be a few erosions of the lamina dura, but the dorsum is, as often with colloid cysts, otherwise undamaged in spite of gross hydrocephalus. (b) The lateral ventriculogram shows why. The anterior end of the third ventricle is quite small. (c) The full axial view shows 'pseudo-erosions' of the floor of the middle fossa. In reality they are exaggerated convolutional impressions on the base due to long-standing raised intracranial pressure which has thinned the skull

It occurs in about one-third of all patients with raised intracranial pressure of more than a few weeks' duration, whether or not they have papilloedema.

Any part of the floor of the pituitary fossa may be affected, but the most common situation for the loss of clearly defined lamina dura is the anterior surface of the dorsum sellae near its base. A general haziness of outline may be apparent at first glance or there may be more severe destruction of the dorsum. The changes are said to be delayed when, due to well-developed pneumatization, a double thickness of dense cortex is all that separates the floor of the sella turcica from the sphenoid air sinus (Mahmoud, 1958).

In advanced cases, the degree of erosion may render the walls of the sella turcica almost invisible.

The mechanism responsible for these erosions is not understood, but the association of destruction of the walls of the pituitary fossa and raised intracranial pressure is common at necropsy. Because, however, a certain amount of time is required for pitting of the surface of the bone, the change is not always recognizable on radiographs, and certainly never before 5 or 6 weeks have elapsed since the beginning of the process.

Twenty per cent of patients with sellar changes due to pressure, who are subsequently found to have intracranial tumours, do not have papilloedema and some

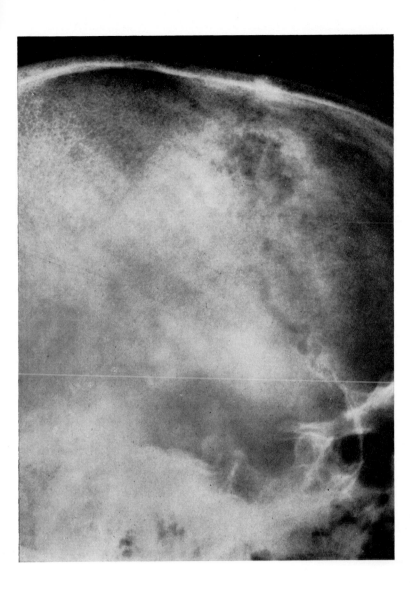

Figure 150. Meningioma (pressure erosion of top of dorsum) in a man aged 37 years who had a two year history of headaches and more recent visual deterioration. He had a mild right hemiparesis and sensory inattention on the left. The skull radiographs show hyperostosis and erosion near the coronal suture on the right side due to meningioma. There is a hypertrophied middle meningeal groove. The tumour was extremely large and had caused severe tentorial herniation (the pineal is depressed). It may be that the direct downward displacement of the hypothalamus has been responsible for the erosion of the top of the dorsum sellae. The floor of the sella is ill-defined as a result of the raised intracranial pressure

Figure 151. Olfactory groove meningioma in a man aged 33 years in whom the clinical findings pointed strongly to the correct diagnosis. The lateral skull radiograph shows destruction of the top of the dorsum sellae without any expansion of the sella but with complete loss of its cortical bone lining. In spite of the loss of lamina dura, the subjacent sphenoid bone is remarkably dense. Bone in the region of the olfactory groove shows no definite radiological abnormality but at operation the cribriform plate was 'spongy and thickened' where the tumour attachment lay. The meningioma was large, extending backwards to overlay both optic nerves and the sella. The shape of the dorsum sellae suggests a suprasellar lesion. The

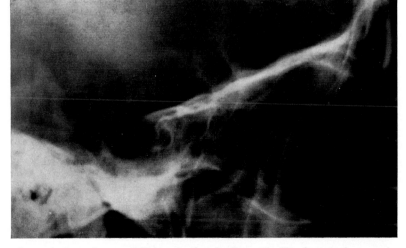

dense nature of the remaining bone is in favour of a meningioma, but not definite enough to be diagnostic. The absence of a recognizable hyperostosis in the olfactory groove is most unusual (sclerosis of bone at some distance from the point of attachment of a meningioma is, of course, common)

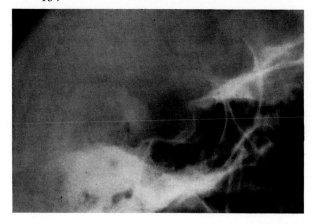

Figure 152. Chromophobe adenoma. The dorsum sellae has been completely destroyed but the rest of the sella may be normal. There are several possible causes for such an appearance, of which pituitary tumour is the least likely. However, this patient had a chromophobe adenoma. There was calcium in its capsule (see Figure 268 on page 263)

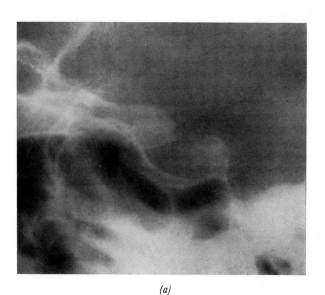

(a)

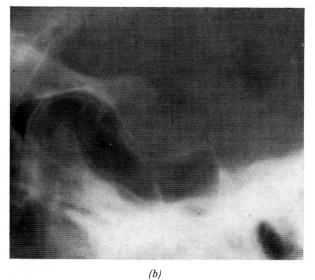

(b)

Figure 153. Craniopharyngioma. (a) The sella appears normal. (b) Three years later, there is severe destruction of the dorsum sellae with little alteration in the remainder. The appearance suggests an expanding lesion immediately above the dorsum. (A flake of calcium probably lies in the carotid siphon.) There was also some very fine suprasellar calcification which is not visible on reproduction

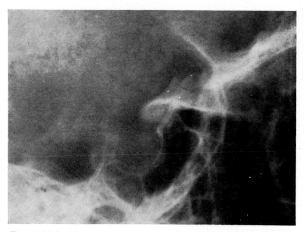

Figure 154. Glioma of the optic chiasm in a boy aged 11 years with a history of headaches, vomiting and loss of vision for 12 months. The top of the dorsum sellae is eroded. The floor of the sella is a little ill-defined. At operation a glioma of the optic chiasm was removed. This had invaded the third ventricle and obstructed the foramen of Monro. The appearance is that of any suprasellar mass

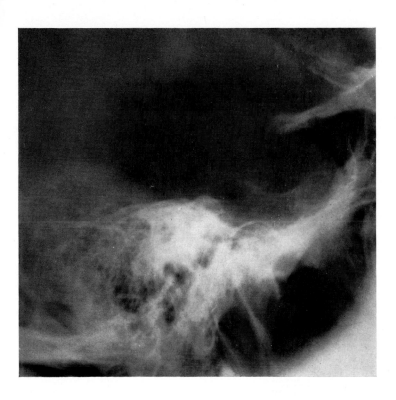

Figure 155. Secondary carcinoma in the sphenoid bone. The floor of the sella is eroded and there is also a soft-tissue mass protruding into the sphenoid sinus. The primary growth was believed to be in the prostate

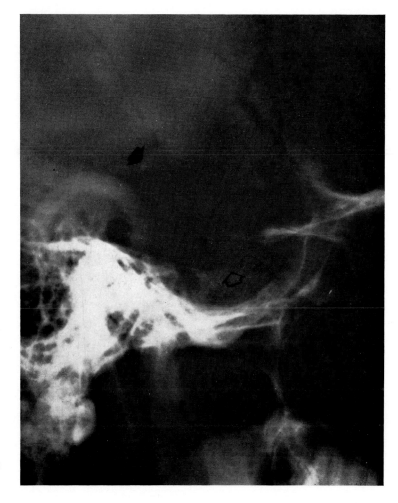

Figure 156. Chromophobe adenoma (parasellar extension) in a man aged 44 years who complained of slight blurring of vision and unsteadiness of gait for 8 months. On examination he had a little left facial weakness and a left lower quadrantic homonymous field defect. (a) The lateral radiograph shows a 'ghost' of the sella, without the dorsum in its normal position (open arrow) and with only one anterior clinoid. A curved flake of bone or calcium (closed arrow) suggesting that the dorsum has been pushed upwards and backwards. There are thus features of a suprasellar, intrasellar and parasellar expanding lesion (cont.)

(a)

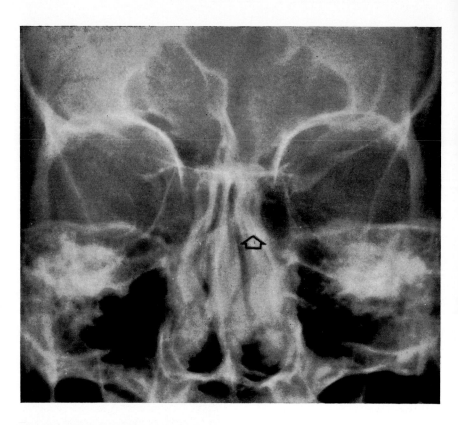

(b)

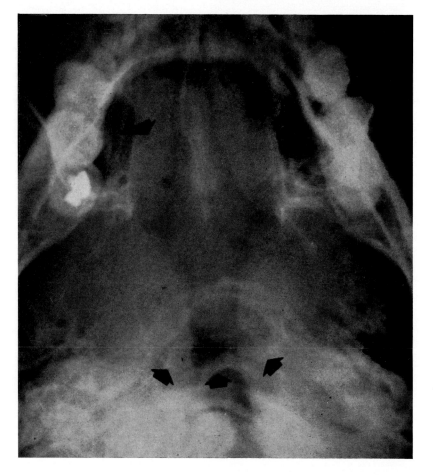

Figure 156 (cont.). (b) The postero-anterior view confirms the parasellar position of part of the mass. Half of the floor of the pituitary fossa (open arrow) is absent (which is why only a 'ghost' is seen in lateral projection). The right lesser wing of sphenoid is much thinned and therefore very translucent. The right ethmoid air cells are opaque. (c) The full axial radiograph demonstrates an extensive mass in the ethmoid and nasal cavity (in the lateral view this post-nasal soft-tissue shadow is difficult to see). The medial part of the right middle fossa is featureless due to erosion. The shell of bone or calcium which partly surrounds the mass is clearly visible (closed arrow). Contrast studies excluded an aneurysm and demonstrated a lobulated mass with a vascular capsule, thus also tending to exclude the possibility of a craniopharyngioma. The absence of any hyperostosis and the shell of calcium were points against the diagnosis of meningioma. A presumptive diagnosis of chromophobe adenoma proved correct, but its temporal extension was far larger than the radiographs suggest

(c)

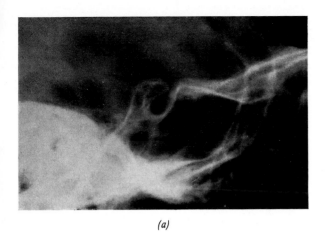

(a)

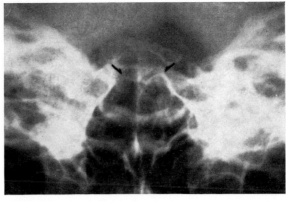

(b)

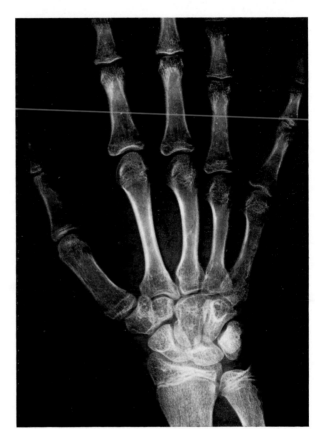

Figure 157. An unusually small sella turcica. It is often considered, but wrongly, that a small-sized sella is of no significance. This girl, aged 17½ years, showed evidence of hypopituitarism. (a) and (b) The sella: lateral and antero-posterior views. (c) The hand and wrist of the same patient showing retarded development

(c)

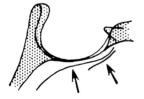

(a)

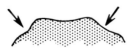

(b)

Figure 158. The carotid sulcus. (a) Lateral view. (b) Antero-posterior view

of them do not complain of headache. Of this particular group a high proportion are found to have slow-growing, benign or treatable tumours, which makes the recognition of pressure changes in the sellar region a matter of importance in the preliminary screening of neurological patients. Any serious suspicion of sellar abnormality is an indication for further investigation, perhaps by C.T. scanning.

It should also be noted that the changes in these occult cases of slow-growing tumours are often severe.

The author, with the help of El Gammal (1966), divided sellar pressure changes into three categories, the aim being to provide help in choice of contrast investigations. Category I erosion was as described above, a loss of the lamina dura of the dorsum sellae. Category II was erosion, often with forward tipping, of the remainder of the top of the dorsum sellae, with or without erosions of the lamina dura.

Category III consisted of those sellas in which there was not only erosion of the top of the dorsum but from which erosion of the lamina dura had extended to the planum sphenoidale.

It was found that Category I erosion provided no clear pointer to the cause in either children or adults, and could also be due to severe vascular hypertension (Fry and du Boulay, 1965).

Category II erosion was due to dilatation of the 3rd ventricle resulting from obstruction of the ventricular pathway behind it. It could be confused with the direct pressure of a local tumour such as a craniopharyngioma. When the whole of the dorsum sellae is invisible, a distinction between raised intracranial pressure, pituitary tumour and suprasellar tumour may be impossible. The great majority of patients with a Category III sella had slow-growing frontal tumours which had pushed the hypothalamus and inferior surface of the frontal lobes downwards onto the bone: most were gliomas.

GENERALIZED BONE DISEASE (*Figure 49, 50, 111* and *112*)

A diminution of bone density may be the result of widespread bone disease such as the osteoporosis of Cushing's syndrome. The cortex of the bone may also be lost, for example, in hyperparathyroidism. The abnormality will not be confined to the sella and the clinical findings should prevent misinterpretation of the radiograph.

SUPRASELLAR MASSES (*Figures 150–154*)

Although suprasellar masses often produce a characteristic shape to the pituitary fossa (*see* Flattening of the Sella on page 167), they may also sometimes present with only osteoporosis or erosion of the sella turcica. When this occurs (in contra-distinction to the change in raised intracranial pressure and in pituitary adenoma) the effect is usually erosion of the posterior clinoid processes and tip of the dorsum sellae with less severe change at the base of the dorsum and in the sellar floor.

PARASELLAR MASSES (*Figures 156, 182, 186, 217–219*)

Lateral parasellar masses (aneurysm, meningioma, rarely chordoma, pituitary adenoma and craniopharyngioma)

may cause erosion of one side of the sella without expanding the portion which remains, thus giving the superficial appearance of a mere loss of bone density in lateral projections. The distinction between them may be attempted from the criteria described in the section on Enlargement other than Ballooning in this Chapter, the presence or absence of hyperostosis being a most important point to observe. (For systematic reading on meningiomas turn to page 167.)

METASTATIC DEPOSITS (*Figures 155, 227, 331*)

Metastatic deposits of carcinoma in the pituitary itself and in the surrounding bone are not particularly uncommon. They give rise to osteoporosis and erosion, which is less localized than the usual effects of pressure or suprasellar tumours. They extend through the basisphenoid.

Carcinoma spreading from the nasopharynx may produce a similar ill-defined, but widespread erosion, with or without a soft-tissue mass in the nasopharynx on the lateral radiograph. Occasionally, a mixture of erosion and sclerosis is provoked by metastatic carcinoma, and then the distinction from meningioma may be difficult. (For systematic reading on malignant disease of the skull turn to page 213.)

(2) ENLARGEMENT OF THE SELLA

Enlargement of the sella turcica is very often, but not invariably, accompanied by some erosion or loss of definition of its borders. Numerous papers deal with the dimensions of the pituitary fossa, its area or its size relative to the rest of the skull in the lateral view – The Sella Index (Riach, 1966).

A sella which seems long or deep in lateral projection may be narrow and not truly enlarged. On the other hand, a slight enlargement in the lateral view may be thought more significant when in the postero-anterior projection the sella is seen to be very wide.

Normal antero-posterior and transverse measurements have been published and the volume predicted, notably by di Chiro and Nelson (1962) and by Oon (1963); but the figures are to some degree contradictory, and in any case the limits of the normal are bound to overlap with the measurements in some abnormal cases. On the borderline, where doubt is felt by an experienced observer, and if there is no erosion or other direct contributory evidence, an opinion based purely on the size of the sella is not of much value.

Israel (1970) has demonstrated the interesting fact that the area of the pituitary fossa in the lateral view increases with advancing age. In men the mean increase between 40 and 59 years is 15 per cent. In women it is rather less.

THE BALLOONED SELLA

Enlargement of the sella (*Figure 159*) may have no particular recognizable abnormal shape, or it may be enlarged in the particular fashion described aptly as 'ballooning'. Some authors have described other characteristic shapes (notably a cup-shaped enlargement, the

'J', and the 'omega' or 'cottage-loaf' sella), but this seems to add confusion to an already difficult subject.

The ballooned sella is the commonest manifestation of the presence of a pituitary tumour. As seen in the lateral view the sella has a shape suggesting expansion of its contents. The dorsum may be unusually curved, tipped or even dislocated backwards. The floor may be

cisterns. Ballooning of the sella may occasionally reach such proportions that the sphenoid or ethmoid sinuses are not merely encroached upon but perforation of their walls takes place. Tumours of this order of size usually extend laterally as well.

Destruction of the lateral part of the dorsum, a laterally sloping floor, and erosion of the undersur-

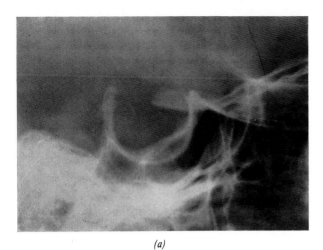

(a)

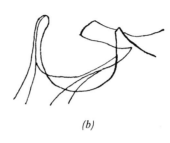

(b)

Figure 159 a and b. Ballooning of the pituitary fossa due to a chromophobe adenoma. The top of the dorsum is intact. Only an intra-sellar expanding lesion could produce such a picture

Figure 160. Chromophobe adenoma in a man aged 42 years with headache, exhaustion, gain in weight and loss of libido. The sella is slightly enlarged. The contour of the dorsum is a little suggestive of expansion from within the sella; that is, ballooning. The top of the dorsum is intact. Chronic raised intracranial pressure without hydrocephalus would be likely to cause more destruction of the sella, but a dogmatic diagnosis from a picture like this would be dangerous

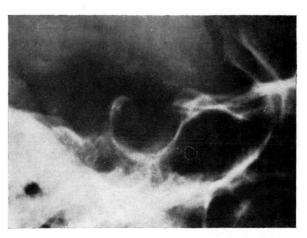

depressed in whole or in part (but a prominent carotid groove on the side of the body of the sphenoid may look very like a depression of one part of the sella floor if only the lateral projection is studied, and lead to an erroneous diagnosis of an asymmetrical deepening; (*see Figure 158*). The anterior border of the sella may be difficult to see because it is pressed forwards, giving the anterior clinoids the appearance of being undercut, or, rarely, the anterior clinoids themselves may be abnormally flattened by pressure from below and medially.

In postero-anterior projection, the floor of the sella will be concave and may be very deeply depressed.

If in addition to general enlargement of the sella the dorsum is dislocated backwards and lifted, it may be assumed that the tumour has encroached on the basal

face of an anterior clinoid process are evidence of asymmetrical enlargement which is not uncommon, particularly with chromophobe adenomas. More severe asymmetrical enlargement of the tumour may result in parasellar extension, and this may be suggested by widening of the sphenoid fissure in addition to the evidence of asymmetry within the sella itself. Occasionally, one or both anterior clinoid processes may be severely eroded from above and suprasellar extension of the mass can press downwards in the region of the planum sphenoidale, causing deformity here also.

In addition to expansion, there may be loss of the normal thin layer of dense bone over some part of the sellar floor, particularly in its posterior part; or there may be irregular destruction which eats into the structure of the sellar floor or dorsum.

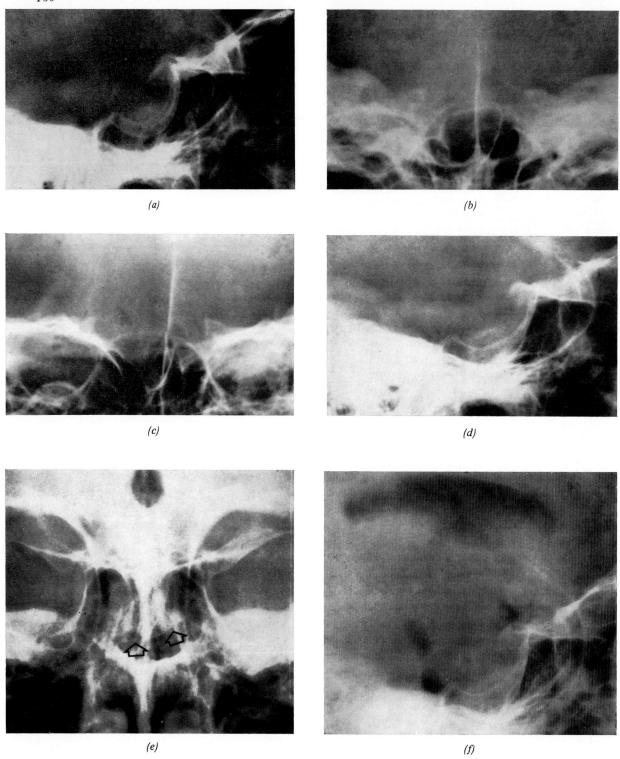

Figure 161. Progress of a chromophobe adenoma. (a) Lateral view at the age of 48 years. The sella shows expansion of the 'ballooning' type; with thinning and backward dislocation of the dorsum. (d) There is elevation of a flake of calcium or bone on the tumour sur-face—perhaps an interclinoid ligament. (c) Eleven years later, at the age of 59 years, she had begun to have minor visual disturbance. The anterior clinoids are a little shortened and the flake of calcium has disappeared. (It was still present at the age of 49 years.) (d) One year later the patient had bitemporal hemianopia. Her lateral skull view shows much depression of the central part of the sella floor with total destruction of the dorsum, so that the appearance now resembles the later stages of hydrocephalic erosion. The anterior clinoids are also eroded from below. (e) Antero-posterior view at encephalography shows the sella floor. (f) Lateral view shows the tumour, which has broken out of the confines of the sella, outlined by air

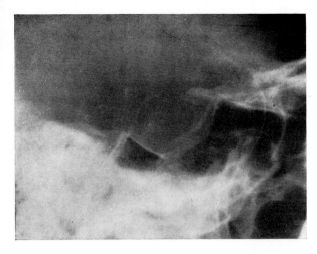

Figure 162. Chromophobe adenoma. Note that the only part of the dorsum sellae shows backward displacement

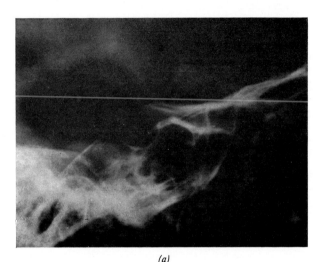

(a)

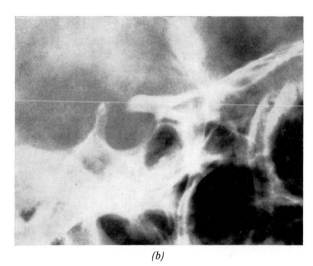

(b)

Figure 163. Pituitary tumour, perhaps malignant. (a) At the age of 16 years this girl was investigated for dwarfism and failure of secondary sexual development. The skull is small and the sella is in proportion to it. (b) At the age of 20 years (after some success with hormone therapy) she began to have headaches and visual deterioration. The sella had enlarged considerably, but its floor remained reasonably well defined. A large suprasellar extension of the pituitary tumour was partially removed. It surrounded the carotid and anterior cerebral arteries and invaded the brain. She regained her vision but developed diabetes insipidus. Subsequent progress has been satisfactory. It is now 3 years since she received radiotherapy. The tumour was a locally invasive, pleomorphic, poorly differentiated, chromophobe adenoma

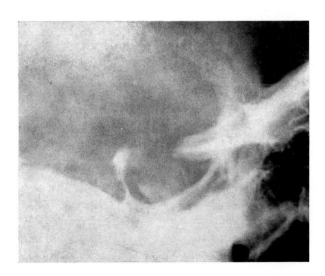

Figure 164. Acromegalic giant aged 24 years. An eosinophil adenoma often causes a striking increase in the depth of the sella. In this case the enlargement is chiefly in the antero-posterior direction. The shape of the dorsum suggests ballooning

Just as the distinction of erosion from osteoporosis is largely a matter of degree, the differences between expansion and erosion are difficult to define in logical terms. The size of tumour alone may be responsible for the disappearance of part of the sellar wall, but the factors which influence osteoclasts are not well enough understood to explain fully why, for instance, one chromophobe adenoma should give rise to a large, smooth sella, while another not only causes some expansion but also a visible fine pock-mark of the floor or the anterior surface of the dorsum.

In recent years endocrinologists and radiologists working with them, have recognized changes in the sella accompanying very small adenomas (McLachlan, Wright and Doyle, 1970). These local bulges of the pituitary fossa may be present long before there is any suprasellar extension and therefore before any eye-signs have developed. Small adenomas are also much more common than had been generally appreciated. Unfortunately, a catch-word has become associated with the early radiological signs sometimes found in such cases. The catch-word is 'double-floor'. Radiologists and clinicians, having picked up this term and ignoring anatomical considerations, some of which are outlined in this chapter, jump to the conclusion that when two or more lines contribute to the shadow of the floor of the sella in the lateral view a pituitary tumour is likely to be present. This is quite wrong when applied to the general run of skull radiographs for headache, head injury and neurological disease. Anatomical asymmetry, radiographic inexactitude and the superimposition of other irrelevant lines are much more commonly the cause of a 'double-floor' to an otherwise normal sella than pituitary adenomas (Swanson and du Boulay, 1975).

Causes

PITUITARY ADENOMA (*Figures 100, 159–165*)

By far the commonest cause of 'ballooning' of the sella is a pituitary adenoma, whether predominantly chromophobe or eosinophil, the radiological change in the pituitary fossa is the same.

Distinction between the usual benign and the rare malignant pituitary adenoma is not possible on the evidence of plain radiographic studies, since either may show expansion with or without erosion. Occasionally, a pituitary tumour may first manifest itself by sellar enlargement after adrenalectomy. Often, of course, there is enlargement of the sella in Cushing's syndrome before adrenalectomy.

CRANIOPHARYNGIOMA (*Figure 166*)

A few examples of primarily intrasellar craniopharyngiomas are seen in which there is enlargement of the sella and erosion of its floor or dorsum. When calcification is absent from the tumour, no distinction from pituitary adenoma can be made, but the presence of amorphous calcification makes the diagnosis of craniopharyngioma very likely.

RAISED INTRACRANIAL PRESSURE (*Figure 167*)

Very rarely a mild degree of ballooning appears to be the result of long-standing raised intracranial pressure. The dorsum sellae in such cases is never dislocated backwards.

THE EMPTY SELLA

A moderately ballooned sella, particularly if it is deep rather than long, may be largely occupied by a C.S.F. space in continuity with the chiasmatic cistern.

There are several causes; spontaneous or post-irradiation shrinkage of a pituitary tumour, or an exaggeration of the normal diverticulum with or without a history to suggest raised intracranial pressure. The appearance is very difficult to distinguish from pituitary tumour, but CT scanning may obviate the necessity for air-study.

ENLARGEMENT OTHER THAN BALLOONING

Sometimes the sella turcica is enlarged, but its shape remains approximately normal. Scrutiny of the postero-anterior and submento-vertical views is a most important part of the assessment. Measurements are not very valuable in borderline cases. Distinct forms of enlargement are seen in some cases of hydrocephalus, with parasellar and with suprasellar masses (and particularly with optic chiasm gliomas). They are arranged here to bring out their similarities and contrasts.

Causes

PITUITARY ADENOMA

Uncommonly, patients are seen in whom a pituitary adenoma has caused an enlargement of the sella which cannot be described as 'ballooning'! Osteoporosis and erosion may be very mild or sometimes extreme. In such cases the differential diagnosis from raised intracranial pressure depends largely on the clinical picture.

RAISED INTRACRANIAL PRESSURE

Long-standing raised intracranial pressure without excessive dilatation of the anterior end of the third ventricle may eventually cause sufficient erosion at the base of the dorsum sellae to give an appearance of slight sellar enlargement. Much more dramatic enlargement may be seen when, usually in Category III sellar erosion, the lamina dura becomes so weak that the whole sellar floor, together with parts of the planum sphenoidale, herniates downwards into the sphenoid sinus.

CHORDOMA (*Figure 181*)

Slight expansion of the sella, accompanying erosion which, though small in degree may be widespread through the basisphenoid, is sometimes due to a chordoma in this situation. The erosion is often very difficult to localize and cannot be interpreted as the

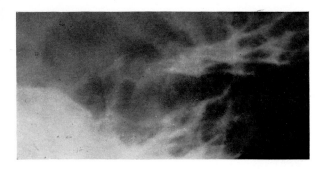

Figure 165. Acromegaly in a woman aged 50 years with a 10-year history of enlarging hands, feet and face. The sella is ballooned

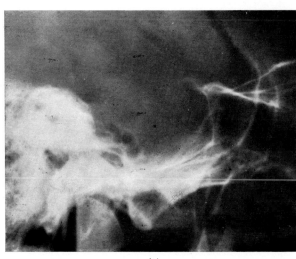

(a)

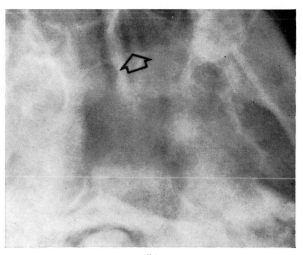

(b)

Figure 166. Parasellar tumour (craniopharyngioma). The patient, a man aged 58 years, presented with increasing headaches for 4 years. There was a right homonymous hemianopia and a partial left third nerve palsy. (a) The lateral radiograph shows an enormously expanded sella with a thin shell of calcium somewhat behind the normal position for the dorsum. The anterior clinoid processes appear to be lifted up. The floor of the sella is less affected on one side. At operation the anterior part of the sella was empty, but a large partly cystic tumour attached to the diaphragm projected into the left temporal lobe as well as upwards on the left side and backwards into the posterior fossa. (b) Full axial view showing anterior wall of the sella. The asymmetrical sella enlargement does not, of course, prove the existence of a parasellar extension of the tumour. In this case localization was only possibly by contrast examination. CT would have been helpful

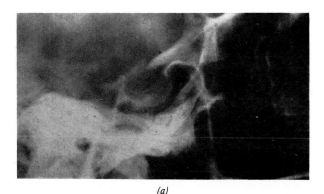

(a)

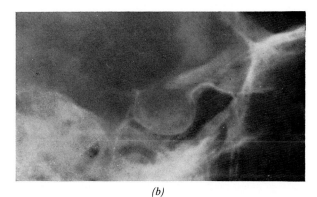

(b)

Figure 167. Raised intracranial pressure in a woman aged 49 years with a history of failing vision for 6 months. She had had papilloedema for at least 2 weeks. There was a left frontal meningioma, the posterior surface of which lay well away from the region of the sella. The pituitary fossa is a little expanded as by a pituitary tumour, and its floor and the anterior surface of the dorsum show erosions and loss of definition. However, the expansion is of the anterior rather than the posterior part. Had the dorsum sellae been dislocated backwards the diagnosis of pituitary tumour would be unavoidable. As it is, distinction between the effect of raised intracranial pressure and a pituitary tumour in this case has to rest on the presence of a frontal hyperostosis (see Chapter 2). Ballooning, as distinct from less well-defined forms of enlargement with erosion is a very uncommon manifestation of raised intracranial pressure (but remember that when chronic hydrocephalus is present, complete destruction of the dorsum sellae may make a picture indistinguishable from that due to a pituitary tumour). (a) Lateral radiograph of the sella. (b) Six months after the removal of the tumour, the sella floor has re-ossified

effect on an extra-osseous mass encroaching from any particular situation. Sometimes the bone appears unusually dense. There may also be a soft-tissue mass in the nasopharynx, and occasionally scattered, coarse calcification in the tumour may show behind the clivus or alongside the sella.

The diagnosis from meningioma is particularly difficult and may be impossible.

PARASELLAR MENINGIOMA

The 'intrasellar' meningioma is usually an extension from a tumour alongside and is then likely to show widespread bone changes, particularly sclerosis. In some cases, however, the osteoclasts are much more active and expansion is accompanied by erosion rather than hyperostosis. If the tumour has reached into the sella, it may also enlarge the

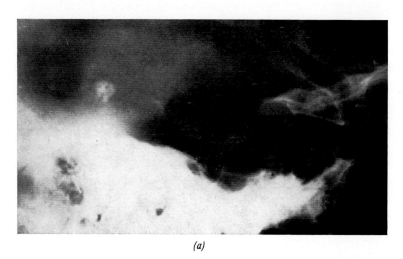
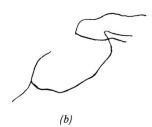

(a)

(b)

Figure 168. Aqueduct stenosis in a woman aged 37 years with long-standing raised intracranial pressure due to aqueduct stenosis. The sella is enlarged (elongated) with a steeply sloping floor, but the dorsum which is very thin is not bent backwards. If anything, displacement is in the forward direction. The appearance is typical of hydrocephalus with ballooning of the front of the third ventricle, and should be distinguished from a pituitary tumour by the position of the dorsum. Note also the depressed pineal due to tentorial herniation

Figure 169. Two effects of the anterior end of the third ventricle in chronic hydrocephalus, particularly in childhood

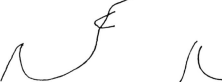
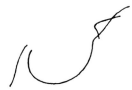

HYDROCEPHALUS (*Figures 8, 11, 22, 23 168–171*)

When, as a result of an obstruction in the aqueduct or fourth ventricle, there is severe hydrocephalus of long duration, beginning in infancy or early childhood, the region of the sella may be altered in shape in a characteristic fashion. By a slow process of absorption the top of the dorsum sellae tends to disappear and the sulcus chiasmaticus to elongate, while the pituitary fossa itself is driven downwards, often without enlarging. The whole tentorium may be pressed downwards. The anterior clinoids are often blunt and massive. This is the appearance which must originally have given rise to the name 'J' sella. It is seen most commonly in aqueduct stenosis and, rarely, with midbrain tumours or very long-standing masses within the fourth ventricle.

sphenoid fissure and cause destruction of bone over the medial surface of the floor of the middle fossa. Erosion is apt to be gross while the expansion of the pituitary fossa is small. Poor definition of the bones makes them difficult to see, but the Towne's view, lateral stereoscopic pictures and tomography may show that one half of the sella is destroyed much more than the other.

ANEURYSM

An aneurysm of the internal carotid may sometimes so enlarge medially in the cavernous sinus that it destroys the lateral part of the sella turcica and may cause some expansion of the rest. Here, as in meningioma in the same situation, erosion overshadows expansion and there may be enlargement of the sphenoid fissure. However, the bone that is not destroyed tends to preserve a crisp outline (unlike the bone alongside a meningioma), and there may be flaky or curvilinear calcification.

An aneurysm may very occasionally reach such a size that, having destroyed the floor of the middle fossa, it encroaches on the nasopharynx.

CRANIOPHARYNGIOMA

A craniopharyngioma may lie partly within and partly above the sella. Commonly the sella is flattened, but cases are sometimes seen with enlarged sellas of a variety of shapes. There is usually erosion of the upper part of the dorsum.

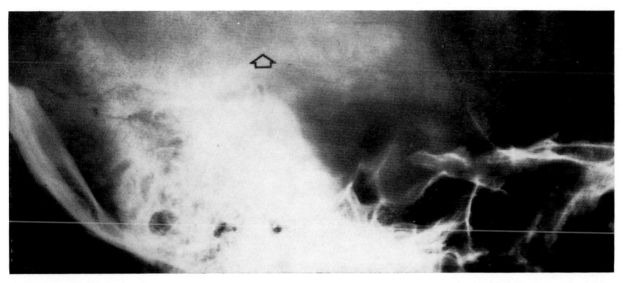

(a)

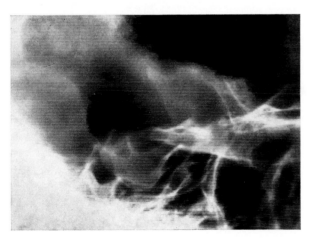

(b)

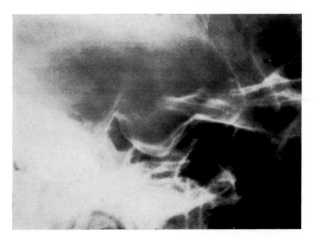

(c)

Figure 170. Sella—chronic hydrocephalus and relief. At the age of 40 years this man had had a history of occipital headaches for 1 year. He had bilateral papilloedema but no other signs. (a) The lateral radiograph shows disappearance of the top of the dorsum sellae. The pituitary fossa is a little deeper than it should be, and the floor is very indistinct in places in spite of full development of the sphenoid sinus. The presumptive diagnosis is of ballooning of the front of the third ventricle (obstructive hydrocephalus) or some other supra-sellar expanding lesion. Raised intracranial pressure without established hydrocephalus is unlikely to cause such severe destruction of the top of the dorsum sellae and a pituitary tumour will usually cause more obvious expansion before the dorsum disappears. The diagnosis may be taken a stage further since a small speck of calcification is present in the pineal (arrow), and this is not displaced downwards. Hydrocephalus without downward tentorial herniation is usually due to a posterior fossa tumour. Rarely it may be caused by obstruction to the exits from the fourth ventricle. It is most unlikely in aqueduct stenosis and somewhat improbable with a supra-sellar tumour. (b) The ventriculogram demonstrates the relationship of the third ventricle and the sella. (c) 3½ years after subtotal removal of a posterior fossa haemangioblastoma. The patient has no clinical evidence of raised intracranial pressure. Considerable re-ossification of the sella floor is shown and there is now a clearly defined lamina dura. There has even been some re-appearance of one posterior clinoid process

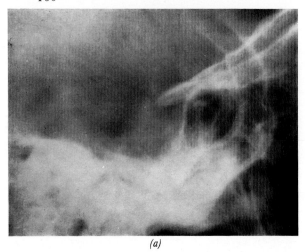

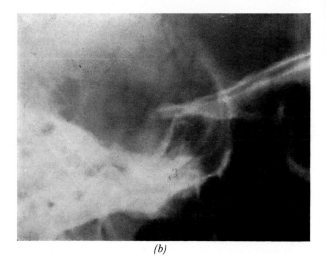

(a)   (b)

Figure 171. Gross ballooning of the third ventricle. Hydrocephalus plus raised intracranial pressure. The patient had clinical evidence of raised intracranial pressure. Ventriculography showed an obstruction of the aqueduct with gross ballooning of the third ventricle, the anterior end of which intruded into the sellar cavity. (a) At this stage differentiation between hydrocephalus, a suprasellar tumour, an intrasellar tumour and raised intracranial pressure would be very difficult, but close inspection reveals the ghost of the dorsum sellae not displaced backwards, so an intrasellar tumour is unlikely. (b) Eighteen months after a Torkildsen's operation the ventricles had returned almost to normal size, although the brain-stem tumour had enlarged. The sella margins have become much better defined with re-ossification and even the top of the dorsum has re-appeared. There is calcification in an interclinoid ligament. The sella is still large

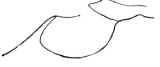

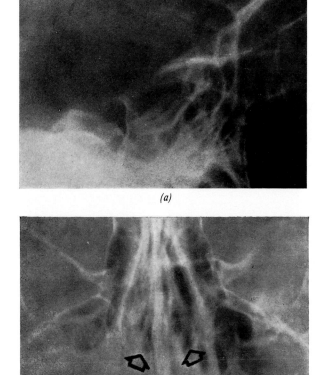

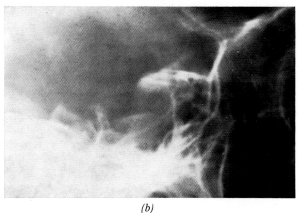

(a)   (b)

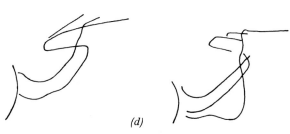

(d)

(c)

Figure 172. Glioma of the optic chiasm in a girl aged 12 years presenting with a history of severe disturbance of vision in the right eye for 2 years. She had a little vision in the upper temporal quadrant on this side and a left temporal hemianopia. (a) Lateral view of the sella. There is erosion of the top of the dorsum indicating a suprasellar space-occupying lesion. (b) Ten months later there is a deep excavation of the anterior part of the sella and early erosion of the undersurfaces of one or both anterior clinoids. There is also suture diastasis. (c) Postero-anterior view to show the deep concavity of the sella floor. A large glioma of the optic chiasm was found in this situation extending into the third ventricle and causing obstruction of the foramen of Munro

SUPRASELLAR MENINGIOMA

So-called suprasellar meningiomas usually arise in front of the sella and have a small hyperostosis at their origin, which will be seen on scrutiny of the radiographs — if only in retrospect. Enlargement of the sella in such cases is nearly always very slight and it may also show the characteristics of pressure by a suprasellar mass, erosion of the top of the dorsum or of the anterior clinoids and lesser wings of the sphenoid. Herein lies a difficulty, for erosion of the top of the dorsum sellae, often with only minimal change in the lamina dura but with some

by the term 'omega' or sometimes 'cottage-loaf' sella. Not all cases of optic chiasm glioma present in this way (6 out of 25 in the series of Schuster and Westberg, 1967), since some merely show erosion of the top of the dorsum, and in a few no definite abnormality is demonstrated. In neurofibromatosis, enlargement of the sella is not proof of the presence of an optic chiasm glioma. Because erosion or enlargement of the sulcus chiasmaticus is associated in this way with optic chiasm glioma, and elongation of the sulcus is one of the features of the 'J' sella, unnecessary confusion has occurred between the 'omega' and the 'J'.

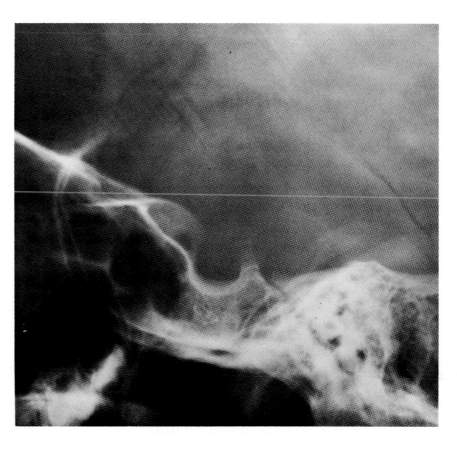

Figure 173. A child with aqueduct stenosis. Note the long, rather vertical sulcus chiasmaticus, the large anterior clinoid, the short dorsum and the normal-sized bowl of the sella itself. These changes are produced by the expanded anterior end of the third ventricle and the abnormally low position of the tentorium. They constitute a 'J' sella. In this particular child one half of the dorsum sellae has been shortened more than the other

enlargement of the pituitary fossa, is also seen in a fair number of patients suffering from parasagittal meningiomas. This kind of abnormality, caused not by the usual suprasellar tumour but by one at a great distance, seems to be peculiar to long-standing masses capable of pressing into the brainstem downwards towards the mass. (For systematic reading on meningiomas turn to page 172.)

GLIOMA OF THE OPTIC CHIASM (*Figure 172*)

A particular form of erosion of the bones around the sella turcica is sometimes exhibited by cases of glioma of the optic chiasm in which, in the lateral view, a cavity is shown extending forwards through the anterior wall of the sella turcica underneath the anterior clinoids and the planum sphenoidale. The appearance of the sella may be that of a double fossa (*Figure 174*) and has been described

(3) FLATTENING OF THE SELLA

A long, shallow, boat-shaped sella is a normal form, and is always wide in a postero-anterior view. Abnormal flattening of the sella is caused by very long-standing suprasellar tumours and is distinguished from the normal flat forms by the presence of erosion, usually of the tip of the dorsum sellae.

If the dorsum is eroded to the shape of a spike and seems to be tipped forwards, or is truncated, with or without definite elongation of the pituitary fossa, a suprasellar tumour mass is probably present.

Causes

In the great majority of cases, flattening of the sella is due to pressure from a mass immediately above and in front, or above and behind. Many are *craniopharyngiomas* and some of these will show calcification (*Figures 17.5, 176, c.f. Figure 21*).

Much more rarely, *glioma of the optic chiasm* or in the region of the hypothalamus will give the same effect, usually without calcification.

Meningiomas arising from the region just in front of the sella often produce a small enostosis at their point of origin. For some reason enlargement of the sella is very much more common than 'flattening' with suprasellar meningiomas. Erosion of the top of the dorsum in cases of parasagittal meningiomas and long-standing intracerebral tumour have already been discussed (page 167).

Another rare cause of such a shape of sella may be *aneurysm* in the midline, arising on the first part of the anterior communicating artery.

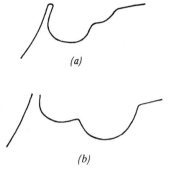

(a)

(b)

Figure 174. (a) A deep sulcus chiasmaticus. (b) The sella eroded by a glioma of the optic chiasm

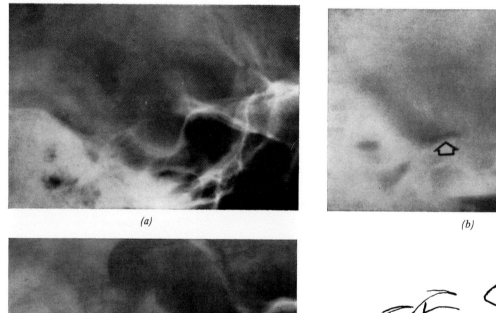

(a)

(b)

(c)

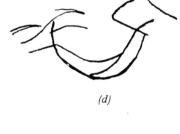

(d)

Figure 175. Craniopharyngioma in a woman aged 37 years. (a) Lateral radiograph. The dorsum sellae is very thin and is bent forwards. The pituitary fossa is of normal size. There is some fine spotty calcification above and behind. (b) A lateral brow-up tomogram during encephalography. A little of the air was introduced by chance in the subdural space and has come to lie on the posterior surface of the dorsum (arrow) sellae, demonstrating that in spite of its appearance the tumour is separated from the dorsum by a narrow space. The anterior end of the third ventricle was completely obliterated. (c) Four months after the partial removal, some re-ossification has taken place in the posterior clinoids. The dorsum is the same shape as before. The re-appearance of the posterior clinoids makes the sella appear much less flattened

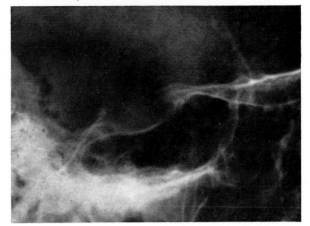

Figure 176. Suprasellar tumour (glioma) in a man aged 54 years who had suffered drop attacks with headache and slowing up of his intellect for 2 months. There was a right inferior quadrantanopia, but no other signs. The lateral radiograph shows erosion of the top of the dorsum sellae. He had an astrocytoma which filled the third ventricle and had invaded the interpeduncular and pontine cisterns. It involved the optic chiasm and surrounded the carotid arteries

(4) CALCIFICATION IN AND AROUND THE SELLA

Calcification in the region of the sella will always be seen more clearly in a lateral view than any other, but the Towne's and the postero-anterior views may give useful information confirming the site of the lesion.

The most common difficulty in recognition is due to small areas of thicker bone in the pterion region or in the squamous temporal, casting ill-defined superimposed shadows. These are particularly clearly visible if the remainder of the squamous temporal is thin. When in doubt, a stereoscopic pair or any two lateral views with different centring will clearly demonstrate whether the opacities are near the midline or more peripheral. Small fugitive shadows of this kind, even if they represent abnormal

Classification

Calcification in this region may be classified according to exact situation or type. The possible causes may be: (1) atheroma of the internal carotid (common); (2) calcification in an aneurysm of any artery of the circle of Willis (quite unusual); (3) craniopharyngioma (relatively common); (4) meningioma (the calcification in a meningioma is often not recognized in this region); (5) chordoma (a rare tumour which does not often calcify); (6) healed tuberculous meningitis (common after streptomycin); (7) pituitary adenoma (between 1 and 6 per cent of chromophobe adenomas show some calcification); (8) angioma (unlikely because of the situation, though angiomas are relatively common); and (9) glioma of the optic chiasm (very rare).

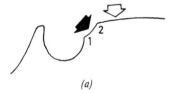

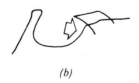

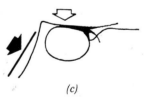

(a) (b) (c)

Figure 177. The normal sella. (a) Common form—the sulcus chiasmaticus (closed arrow); the planum sphenoidale (open arrow); the tuberculum sellae (1); the limbus chiasmaticus (2). (b) Unusual form—the middle clinoid process (open arrow). (c) The same, with calcified ligaments—the interclinoid ligaments (open arrow); the petroclinoid ligament (closed arrow)

calcification, are often very difficult to pick up in axial views. The ability to use stereoscopic radiography is therefore important.

Calcification in the interclinoid and petroclinoid ligaments provides a second cause of difficulty, but no pathological structure ever takes quite the same form as these. Calcification may sometimes appear in ligaments around the sella at an early age (*Figure 177*).

All other causes of calcification in and around the sella are abnormal.

Conditions in and around the pituitary fossa may also be subdivided according to their exact situation, as follows: (1) intrasellar; (2) suprasellar (including the area immediately above and in front, and above and behind); (3) parasellar; and (4) retrosellar (clivus).

Localization is sometimes of help in deciding the cause of the calcification and is of importance in planning treatment, but many cases show calcification spreading from one area to another, making a topographical approach to the differential diagnosis difficult.

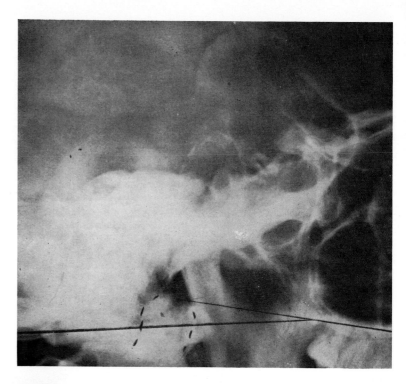

Figure 178. Suprasellar and intrasellar cranio-pharyngioma (cystic type of calcification) in a man aged 24 years complaining of headaches and visual deterioration. He was known to have had an intracranial tumour for at least 6 years. The lateral radiograph shows a mixture of 'cystic' calcification and dense nodules in, above and behind the region of the sella. The sella is deformed and very much enlarged. There is deformity of the whole skull base (basilar invagination and platybasia) presumably due to the presence of the tumour during childhood. At operation a cystic craniopharyngioma was removed. Note: Bull's angle has been drawn. The posterior limb of the angle in this case corresponds closely with the modified Chamberlain's line

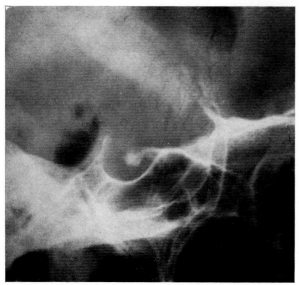

Figure 179. Intrasellar and suprasellar craniopharyngioma in a girl aged 16 years who for 6 months had had headaches and vomiting and had a bitemporal hemianopia. She showed the Lorain type of dwarfism. A largely cystic craniopharyngioma was removed from above and from within the sella. The plain radiograph shows a single nodule of calcium within the sella. The sella itself is not definitely abnormal. (The radiograph was made at pneumoencephalography)

The form taken by calcification may be subdivided into a number of types as follows: (1) flakes and specks; (2) dense masses; and (3) monogeneous faint calcification, but one disease process may produce a variety of forms.

Calcification which may be found in any position

Calcification which may be found in any position within or around the sella, and may have a variety of forms, may be caused by the following: (1) craniopharyngioma; (2) meningioma; (3) chordoma; or (4) chromophobe adenoma.

CRANIOPHARYNGIOMA (*Figures 178–180, 276*)

The commonest cause of calcification in the midline above and behind, directly above, or above and in front of the pituitary fossa is a craniopharyngioma. When these tumours present in childhood, some 80–90 per cent exhibit calcification. In adults, calcification is only seen in about 30 per cent. It may or may not extend downwards into the pituitary fossa itself, and it is only rarely that it spreads much more to one side than the other. Very rarely, however, a craniopharyngioma is parasellar or lies only to one side of the midline above the sella. In such cases the type of calcification may help to make the diagnosis.

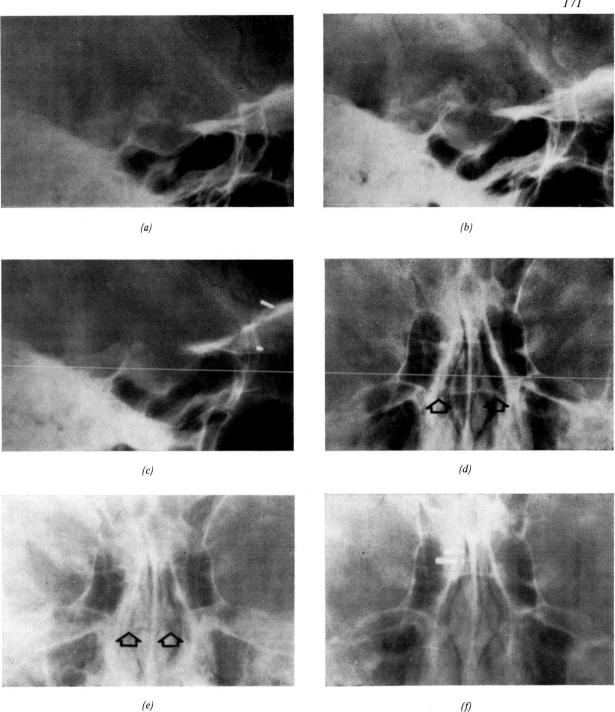

(a)

(b)

(c)

(d)

(e)

(f)

Figure 180. Craniopharyngioma in a girl aged 20 years complaining of amenorrhoea for 2 years, remittant visual deterioration for 1 year and recent occipital headaches. She had early bilateral papilloedema, and a partial right third nerve palsy and a small right central scotoma. (a) The lateral radiograph shows calcification (proved to lie above the sella by other views). The calcification consists of fine dots, distributed irregularly in a tumour whose main outline seems well defined. The sella is long and flat, as it often is with a cranio-pharyngioma. It shows no erosion, even at the top of the dorsum. Pneumoencephalography revealed a tumour, much larger than the calcification, causing partial obstruction to the foramen of Monro and lateral ventricular dilatation. Six months later her scotoma had increased in size and she began to complain of a continuous heavy sensation in the frontal region. (b) The lateral radiograph shows an increase in density of the calcification, slight expansion of the sella and destruction of parts of its floor. At operation a week later a large cyst (9 cc) as well as the whole of the hard calcified suprasellar mass and all the intrasellar extension of the tumour were removed, leaving the sella empty, relieving pressure on the optic chiasm and the right third nerve. (c) A lateral view 17 days after operation shows the bone erosion well. The anterior part of the sella is slightly fuller in outline than before, perhaps due to weakness. The calcified mass has gone. (d) Postero-anterior view at first admission. Normal sella floor. (e) Postero-anterior view before operation. Sella floor indistinct due to erosion and change of position of the floor. (f) Postero-anterior view after operation. Sella floor completely invisible (cont.)

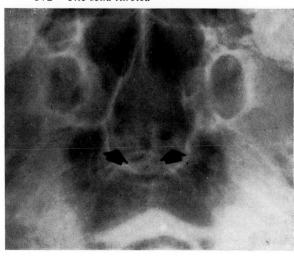
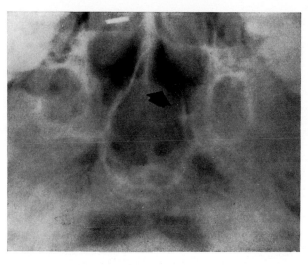

(g)   *(h)*

Figure 180 (cont.). (g) Full axial view at first admission. Anterior margin of sella invisible because of the direction in which it runs. Posterior margin of the sella just visible. (h) Full axial view after operation showing the anterior margin of the sella clearly because of its change of direction

Two types of calcification are commonly seen in craniopharyngiomas. There are usually a number of shapeless specks at least 2 mm in diameter and of considerable density. They may be scattered or packed closely together. Sometimes curved flakes are also visible suggesting the walls of a cyst, but on histological examination flakes are also found enclosing solid nodules of tumour. The size of the tumour is not necessarily to be judged by the area covered by the calcification. Although enormous areas of dense calcification are occasionally found, some of these tumours extend well into the frontal region or through the tentorium and show calcification scantily only near their bases.

Details of the bone of the sella turcica may be difficult to see through the investing dense calcification, but when it is visible it will usually be found abnormal. This abnormality is usually in the nature of 'flattening'.

MENINGIOMA

Meningiomas arising from the clivus or extending around the sides of the sella may show calcified shadows of one or other type. The diagnosis may be made if there is a characteristic hyperostosis of the neighbouring bone, but this is not invariably present or may be obscured by the density of calcification, and confusion with chordoma may easily arise, particularly in those cases where the bone involved in the chordoma is abnormally dense.

Purely suprasellar meningiomas seem to show dense calcification much less commonly. A meningioma is less likely to lie symmetrically in the midline than a craniopharyngioma. (For systematic reading on meningiomas turn to page 180.)

CHORDOMA (*Figures 181, 182*)

Chordomas are encountered in which very dense calcification has been laid down. It is unlikely to be confined to the suprasellar region and may extend on both sides of the sella. Such calcification has been known to appear very rapidly in tumours which have been present for some time. If the bones of the pituitary fossa are visible through the calcification they may show very little alteration of structure or they may be dense rather than eroded.

CHROMOPHOBE ADENOMA (*Figures 183* and *268*)

A very few cases of adenoma have been described in which heavy calcification is seen within the tumour. The sella may be ballooned and contain a mass of solid-looking calcification which may or may not protrude upwards. It has a clear-cut edge.

Rather more commonly, flakes of calcification are seen on the surface of chromophobe adenomas where they show as curved lines or even complete shells, suggesting the presence of a cyst. Differentiation from a craniopharyngioma or from an aneurysm may not always be possible on the plain radiograph, but if the sella is ballooned the changes are in favour of an adenoma.

Calcification not extending into the sella

Calcification not extending into the sella, but which may be above, behind or at the side may have the following additional causes: (1) atherosclerosis; (2) aneurysm; (3) glioma; (4) tuberculous meningitis (after treatment); or (5) angioma.

ATHEROSCLEROSIS (*Figures 184, 185*)

Calcification in atheromatous plaques is common in the carotid siphon. It usually forms a shadow which is recognized as having the shape and position of one wall of the carotid artery, or of both walls showing as parallel

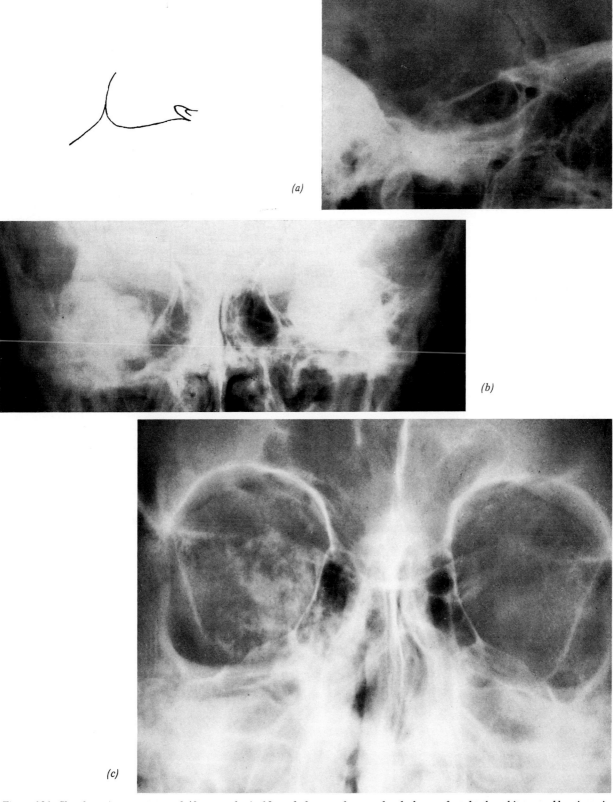

Figure 181. Chordoma in a woman aged 40 years who in 12 weeks became demented and who was found to have bitemporal hemianopia, bilateral sixth nerve palsies and some impairment of sensation over the distribution of the right fifth nerve. (a) Lateral view. The floor of the sella is flat, the dorsum extremely thin and eroded. The texture of the basi-sphenoid is probably normal. There is widespread calcification above and behind the clivus and within the pituitary fossa. (b) The right sphenoid fissure is enlarged. (c) A similarly placed tumour with extensive parasellar calcification

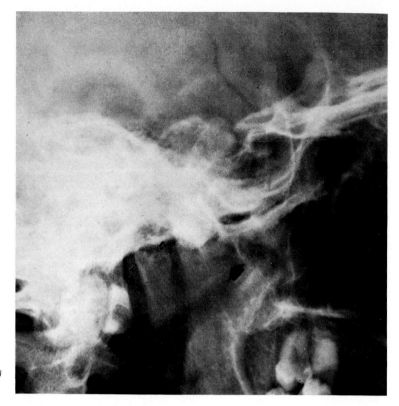

(a)

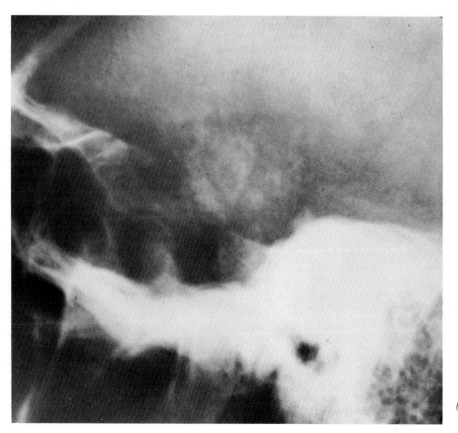

Figure 182. Chordoma in a woman aged 27 years with an 8-year history of steadily increasing cranial nerve palsies. (a) The lateral view shows a calcified mass behind and partly overlapping the sella. There is a soft-tissue shadow in the naso-pharynx (arrow). (b) A very similar case with the additional feature of increased density of the remains of the clivus

(b)

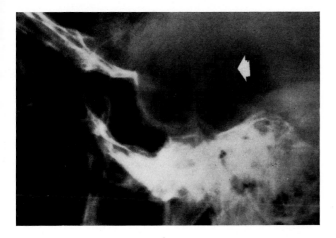

Figure 183. Chromophobe adenoma. The sella is enlarged and the walls are ill-defined. The dorsum sellae has been almost completely destroyed. The shape of the sella is of no help in this case in distinguishing between a pituitary tumour and the effect of raised intracranial pressure, but there is a fleck of calcium (arrow) above and behind the normal position of the dorsum sellae, and this strongly suggests, by its shape, the presence of a mass growing out of the sella. The calcium lay on the capsule of a chromophobe adenoma

(Reproduced by courtesy of the Editor of *Br. J. Radiol.*)

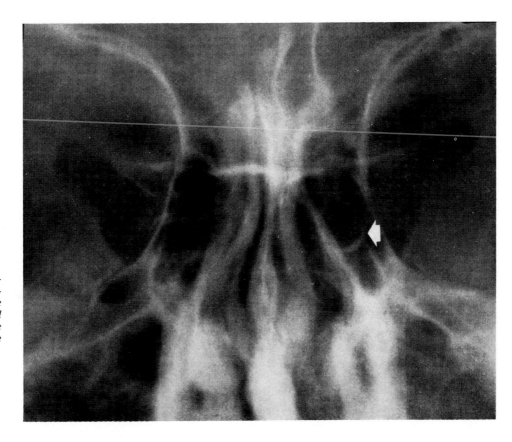

Figure 184. Carotid calcification. Rings and semicircles of calcium may be seen through the ethmoid sinuses in cases where there is atheroma of the carotid syphon

lines. In the lateral view it is usually a little below the interclinoid ligament and has a slightly curved course.

The calcification can often be seen as a crescent or circle on the postero-anterior views on one or both sides in or just medial to the superior orbital fissure where the artery is projected end-on, and rarely it is also recognizable in the Towne's projection and full axial view.

It is to be distinguished from calcification in aneurysms.

Calcification in the basilar artery is much less common than that in the carotid siphon but is occasionally seen. Distinction between calcification in atheroma of this

artery and in an aneurysm may only be made if the calcification is extensive.

CALCIFICATION IN AN ANEURYSM (*Figure 186*)

Calcification is rarely seen in an aneurysm of the main cerebral arteries as a ring or a crescent shadow, but it is much more common in those aneurysms which arise from the intracavernous part of the carotid artery and reach large proportions.

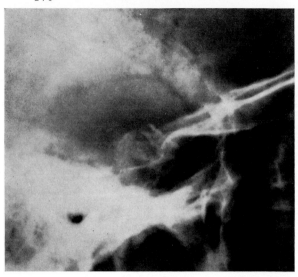

Figure 185. Calcification in the carotid syphon. There is an extreme degree of calcification in this old lady's carotid syphon

Figure 186. Parasellar aneurysm in a woman aged 71 years with a history of gradual loss of sight in the right eye over the course of 1 year. There was also a left lower quadrantic temporal field defect. (a) The lateral view reveals an area of irregular calcification. Below and partly overlapped by it, the pale ghost of an outline of the floor and dorsum of the sella can just be seen. They are more or less normal in position, but very faint because severely eroded from the right-hand-side. There is a large soft-tissue shadow in the nasopharynx. (b) Posteror-anterior view. The right sphenoid fissure is expanded and the remains of the lesser wing of the sphenoid elevated (cont.)

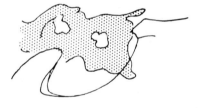

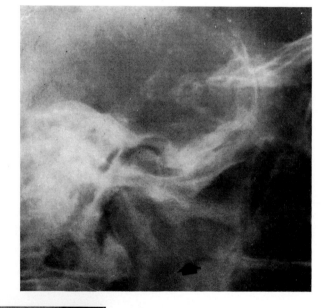

(a)

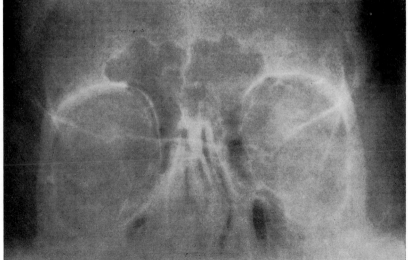

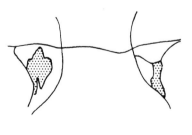

(b)

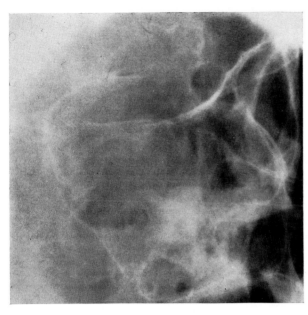

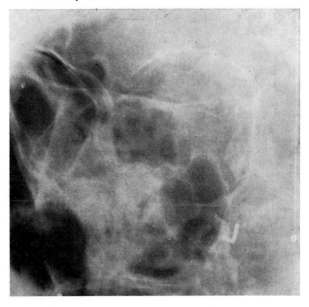

(c)   (d)

Figure 186 (cont.). Oblique ethmoid view shows a large erosion extending downwards and forwards from the sphenoid fissure. (d) Left side for comparison. The mass was an aneurysm of the intracavernous portion of the carotid

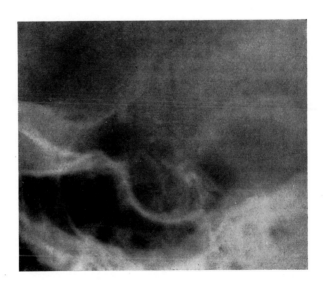

Figure 187. Calcified tuberculous exudate. The patient had been successfully trated for tuberculous meningitis. The nodular and amorphous calcification lies, as it usually does, around the optic chiasm and in the medial parts of the Sylvian fissures

Depending upon the relationship between the beam of x-rays and the calcification, it may be shown as a curved line or a flat plaque. It is only occasionally that the whole circumference of the aneurysm is outlined with uninterrupted calcium, but the general size and shape of the aneurysm can quite frequently be made out when it extends beyond the confines of the cavernous sinus and the obscuring sphenoid bone.

When the aneurysm is not large enough to have caused bone erosion, the distinction from atheroma in an undilated carotid must rest upon the position of the calcification beyond the normal situation of the carotid siphon.

If there is bone erosion the conditions with which the appearance is most likely to be confused are craniopharyngioma (which is rarely purely parasellar) and chordoma or meningioma (if the ring-like shape of the calcification is not obvious).

The diagnosis is usually settled by angiography, though in a few patients such aneurysms are found to have become filled with clot.

GLIOMA

Calcification in gliomas may take almost any form, but is rare in the suprasellar region. Speckled calcification is, however, seen in some cases of glioma of the optic chiasm. Schuster and Westberg (1967) found it in 20 per cent of optic chiasm gliomas, but all were large tumours. If the sella turcica has an omega-shaped enlargement, the diagnosis is probable; but other cases are indistinguishable from craniopharyngiomas.

TUBERCULOUS MENINGITIS (*Figure 187*)

Calcification commonly takes place in the exudate after tuberculous meningitis has been treated with streptomycin, and may then be seen in the suprasellar region and the Sylvian fissures as well as in the interpeduncular cistern. It consists of collections of small, not very dense, amorphous nodules.

ANGIOMA (ARTERIOVENOUS MALFORMATION)

Calcification occurs in about 20 per cent of angiomas and is then seen to consist of a mixture of small faint dots and curvilinear streaks. It might, therefore, be mistaken for the appearance of a faintly calcified craniopharyngioma, but angiomas in the suprasellar region are exceedingly uncommon so that this differential diagnosis is usually dismissed if the lesion can be shown to be in the midline close to the sella.

Calcification chiefly above the sella, or above and in front which is homogenous and faint with a clear-cut edge

Calcification of this type is characteristic of a meningioma. Meningiomas frequently contain widespread areas of calcification but it is only on rare occasions that this is sufficiently dense to cast a recognizable shadow through the bones of the skull.

However, tumours are seen from time to time in which the calcification, consisting of very large numbers of microscopic dots, forms a homogeneous shadow with a sharp edge corresponding to the edge of the tumour.

6 EROSIONS OF THE BASE

INTRODUCTION

It is particularly difficult to see the bones of the base of the skull clearly because they cannot, for the most part, be placed in a position near the x-ray film. The single exception to this difficulty is the sphenoid wing whose greater and lesser wings may be observed through the appropriate orbit. The other bones of the base of the skull are demonstrated best in the lateral and the full axial projections with various degrees of angulation; their shadows will be enlarged with consequent loss of detail, and confused by the markings of the vault bones through which they must be viewed.

In the lateral projection, only the largest erosions are recognizable as such (*Figures 331, 332*) (although tomography may provide rather more information, it is not usually attempted unless other evidence of erosion has already been discovered), but an important feature to be looked for is the presence of a soft tissue mass encroaching upon the nasopharynx or occasionally on the oropharynx. The upper cervical canal will be included upon the view, and since some tumours which affect the base of the skull also affect the upper cervical vertebrae, they should always be examined for erosions, for expansion of the cervical canal and for abnormalities of position of the bones (*Figure 248*).

The full axial projection provides more information about the presence and situation of erosions. The translucency of the pharynx should not cause confusion. It has a more or less symmetrical distribution, sharp margins and through the translucency all the normal bone detail may be clearly recognized.

In the normal full axial projection, with the beam of x-rays at right-angles to the base-line of the skull, the foramina ovale, spinosum and lacerum with the carotid canal are grouped fairly close together to one side of the sella in the middle fossa. Erosions in this region may

cause loss of definition of the margins of any or all of these foramina.

Midline erosions are rarely complete and are particularly difficult to recognize.

Erosions of the tips of the petrous bones are usually easy to see, and enlargement of the internal auditory meatuses or erosions at their mouths may also be visible, particularly if coned views are used. The exact relationship of the meatus to the posterior surface of the petrous bone makes a great deal of difference to its visibility, and it is therefore advisable when making a special examination of the region to have views taken with slight alterations in the angulation of the x-ray beam to the patient's head in order to see the internal auditory meatus to the greatest advantage. Valuable special techniques are in use for this area.

Unless they are particularly large, erosions around the jugular foramina are difficult to demonstrate in the routine projections. The axis of the jugular foramen lies at an angle of about 60 degrees to the base-line in the average adult skull and the margins of the jugular foramen will be obscured by the superimposed petrous bone. In order to demonstrate the jugular foramen to the best advantage, a submento-vertical view should be obtained in which the angle of the x-ray beam to the base-line is considerably less than 90 degrees. Oblique views and tomography are also of value. It is easy to confuse the appearance of the foramina transversaria of the cervical vertebrae with the medial part of the jugular foramen unless this possibility is remembered. The jugular foramina are frequently asymmetrical. Enlargement is usually accompanied by a loss of the normal cortex of the margin and there will probably also be some erosion of the adjacent petrous bone.

There is little difference in the appearance of erosions due to many causes, but some assistance towards a differential diagnosis may be obtained by consideration

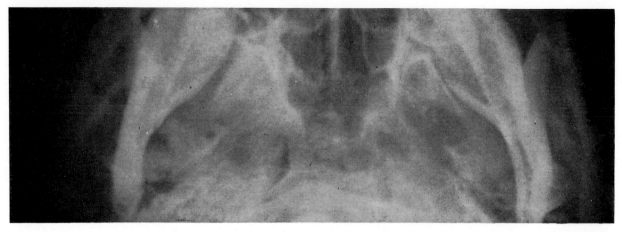

Figure 188. Extradural sarcoma in a girl aged 17 years with progressive left cranial nerve lesions for 5 months, beginning with numbness of the left cheek. Later she developed cerebellar and long tract signs and recently papilloedema. The full axial view shows enlargement of the foramen ovale. No other plain radiographic changes were visible, but angiography demonstrated a mass. The isolated enlargement of a single foramen was thought to indicate that the tumour had been present for some considerable time in the region and that perhaps it began in association with the fifth nerve. At operation a tumour was found occupying and expanding Meckel's cave, invading the cavernous sinus and extending into the posterior fossa. It was a sarcoma

of the situation and the associated clinical signs. Erosions of the base will, therefore, be discussed in relation to their position and will be grouped as erosions of the middle fossa, of the temporal bone and around the jugular foramen, with a further section devoted to erosions of the sphenoid bone as seen in postero-anterior projections.

At first this may confuse the reader; the same diseases appear again and again with rearrangement and additions; but the broad outline of the chapter should be appreciated before the individual paragraphs are studied.

The purpose here is to discuss a series of localized areas of the base in turn without much reference to the topographical overlap which must occur, and to consider all the likely diagnoses in each area.

This method is based on a diagnostic line of thought rather than a pathological classification and is intended to help the radiologist who has a radiograph in front of him.

The actual topographical subdivisions have been chosen for clinical as well as radiological reasons.

EROSION OF THE FLOOR OF THE MIDDLE FOSSA

An erosion of the floor of the middle fossa may amount to no more than the enlargement of one of the natural foramina as, for instance, the foramen ovale in rare cases of neuroma of the fifth nerve, either benign or malignant, or occasionally from the invasion of a foramen by some other tumour in the neighbourhood, such as a cylindroma.

The area of destruction may be confined to one half of the middle fossa or it may extend to and involve the structures in the midline as well, showing bone change in the basisphenoid, basi-occiput and perhaps the sella turcica (*Figures 188–191*).

INVASION BY MALIGNANT NASOPHARYNGEAL TUMOURS AND METASTATIC DEPOSITS (*Figure 192*)

Typically, such an erosion has an ill-defined margin and is not accompanied by any sign of sclerotic bone reaction. In lateral views a soft-tissue mass is not invariably found intruding into the air space of the nasopharynx.

MENINGIOMA

Generally speaking, there is also evidence of hyperostosis when a meningioma is attached to the floor of the middle fossa. The hyperostosis may affect the sella as seen in the lateral view, or the sphenoid wings, demonstrated by a postero-anterior radiograph; but hyperostosis is not quite invariable and the full axial view may show a more or less ill-defined area of bone destruction, closely resembling the appearance due to invasion by a malignant neoplasm. Other projections will be required to demonstrate the full extent of the lesion. It is particularly difficult from plain x-rays to determine the extent of meningiomatous attachment to bone and dura. Meningiomas within the cavernous sinus may, however, expand into the sphenoid air sinus and cause a soft-tissue bulge into the air shadow. Tomography is particularly valuable in such cases. (For systematic reading on meningioma, turn to page 201.)

CHORDOMA (*Figures 181, 182*)

All degrees of erosion take place and sometimes there is, in addition, either some sclerosis of uneroded bone or calcification in the tumour, or both. The differential diagnosis from meningiomas may therefore be difficult or impossible. A large erosion accompanied, however, by evidence of a soft-tissue mass in the nasopharynx is far

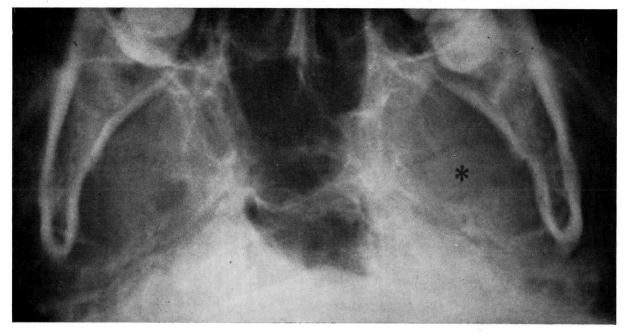

(a)

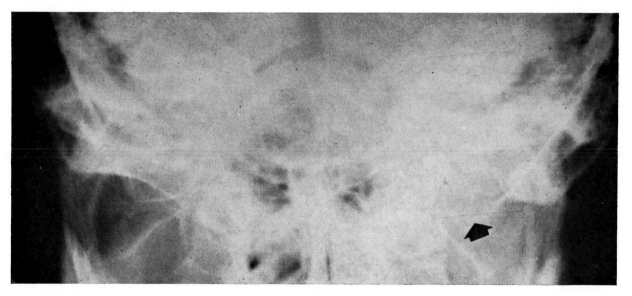

(b)

Figure 189. Neuroblastoma deposit in a boy aged 10 years with a history of 6 weeks' illness. For the last month he had had left temporal pain and numbness in the seond and third divisions of the trigeminal nerve. A neuroblastoma was found. (a) Full axial view showing erosion of the floor of the middle fossa on the left; the foramen ovale is missing. (b) A half axial view also demonstrates this erosion

more common with a chordoma than a meningioma. Chordomas are very rare in early childhood. Less than a dozen pre-pubertal cases had been described up to 1967 (Sassin and Chutorian, 1967). Malignant nasopharyngeal tumours show a more rapid advance of symptoms. Huge aneurysms may be recognized by angiography.

ANEURYSM (*Figure 186*)

Very large aneurysms of the internal carotid (originating usually in its intracavernous course) may cause erosion not only of the lateral wall of the sella and the sphenoid wings around the fissure, but of the whole of the medial

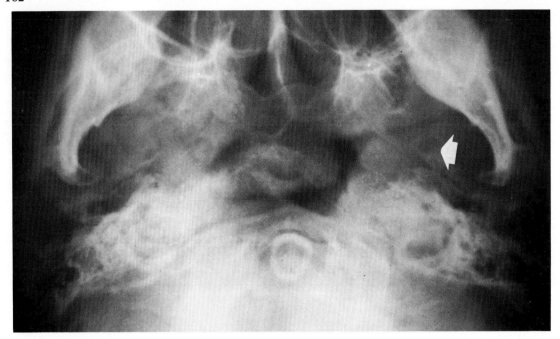

(a)

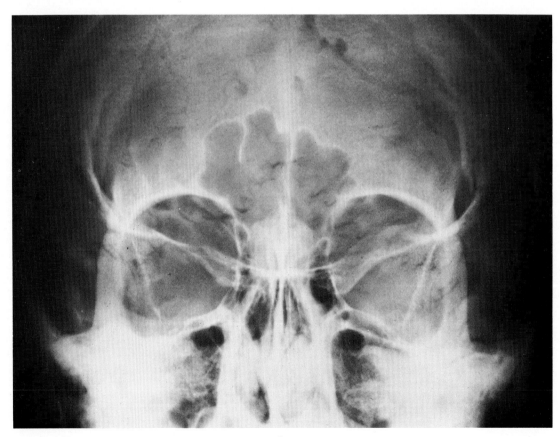

(b)

Figure 190. Enlargement of foramen spinosum. (a) The patient had a very vascular meningioma in the middle fossa. The left foramen spinosum (arrow) is greatly enlarged by hypertrophy of the middle meningeal artery. However, inequality of the foramina spinosa is a most unreliable sign, and should be interpreted with the greatest caution. (b) There is slight increase in density of the left sphenoid wings

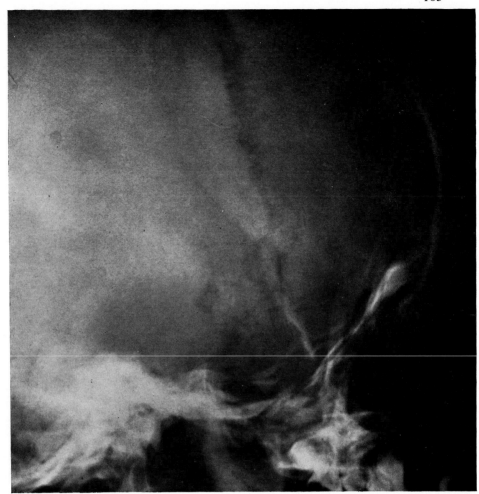

Figure 191. Xanthomatosis in a girl aged 8 years. There is almost total destruction of the floor of the anterior fossa as well as erosion of the sphenoid around the sella. The large size of the intracranial mass is responsible for the suture diastasis

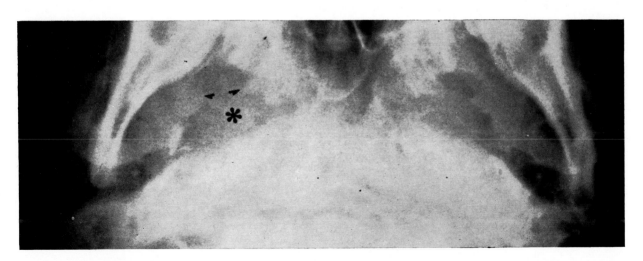

Figure 192. Nasopharyngeal carcinoma spreading to the ear. At this time there was no clinical evidence of involvement of cranial nerves. The patient was a little deaf in the right ear. A large soft-tissue mass in the nasopharynx had been removed and reported as a cylindroma. It recurred and at biopsy the histological picture was of an anaplastic carcinoma. The full axial view shows erosion (asterisk) of the sphenoid bone on the right-hand side, invading the foramen ovale (arrows) and spreading along the path of the pharyngo-tympanic tube. The left side is also suspect

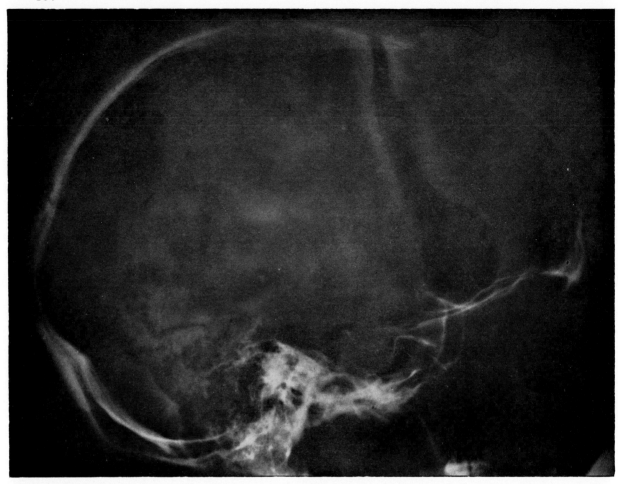

(a)

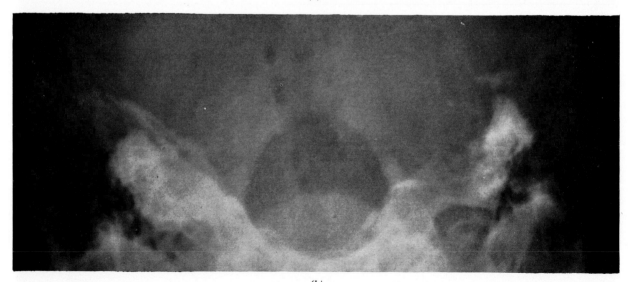

(b)

Figure 193. An acoustic neuroma in a girl aged 16 years. She had complained of progressive deafness in the left ear for 2 years and then developed signs of intracranial pressure, ataxia, nystagmus, left-sided hypotonia and left sixth and seventh nerve weakness. A massive acoustic neuroma was removed. On radiological evidence alone the differential diagnosis was thought to include acoustic neuroma and a developmental type of epidermoid. (a) Lateral view. The sutures are spread, convolutional markings are prominent and the cortex of the sella is eroded (as seen with a magnifying glass). The sella is slightly enlarged. There is therefore long-standing raised intracranial pressure. (b) Half axial view. There is an enormous erosion of the left petrous bone (cont.)

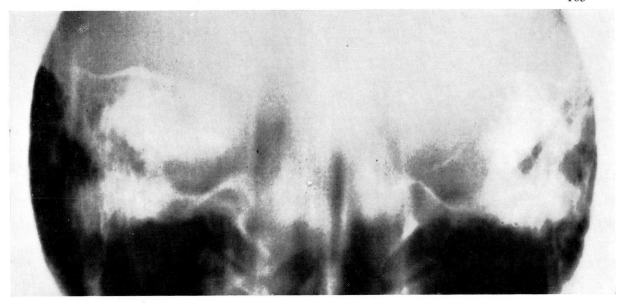

(c)

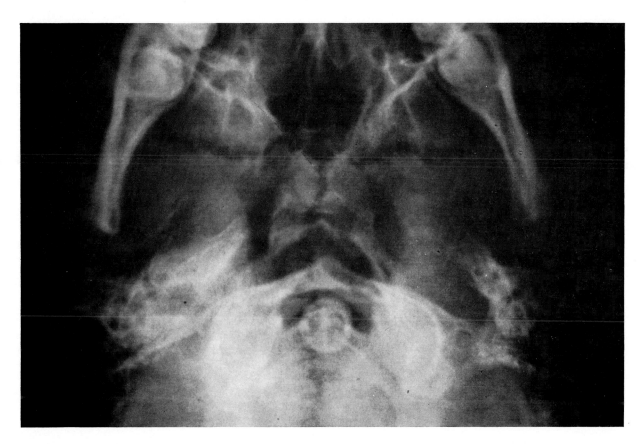

(d)

Figure 193 (cont.). (c) Antero-posterior tomogram of the petrous bones shows an expanded shell of bone around the lower margin of the mass. There was also a flake of bone over the upper surface. (d) Full axial view demonstrates the erosion and the suture diastasis (cont.)

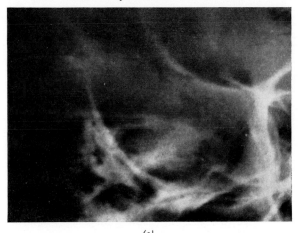
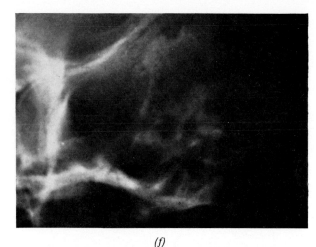

(e)   *(f)*

Figure 193 (cont.). (e) Stenver's view of the normal side. (f) Stenver's view of the left side showing erosion up to, but not into, the cochlea

part of the floor of the middle fossa. They may even enlarge to such a degree as to produce a nasopharyngeal soft tissue mass. Calcification will frequently be present in some part of the aneurysm wall. Angiography is essential to confirm the diagnosis and to distinguish the cause of the erosion from meningioma and from chordoma.

EPIDERMOID (CHOLESTEATOMA)

Any part of the floor of the middle fossa may occasionally be destroyed by an intracranial or intra-osseous epidermoid. By the time that bone destruction is demonstrated, the tumour will have expanded beyond its original confines so that the term 'intracranial' or 'intra-osseous' refers to the presumed site of origin of the tumour. The erosion has a well-defined margin, and destruction of bone over the centre of the area is likely to be complete. There may be an incomplete ring of calcification or ossification around the edge of the mass, derived either from calcification in the capsule of the tumour itself, from remoulded bone or produced by the displaced periosteum.

GLOMUS TUMOUR (*Figure 213*)

The erosion extends from elsewhere (the petrous bone or behind it) and is considered under the heading Erosions around the Jugular Foramen.

HISTIOCYTOSIS X

The lesions have similar characteristics whenever they occur. There is rarely any evidence of reactive sclerosis. The erosion is complete but may have an irregular margin. Erosion can be very extensive.

RAISED INTRACRANIAL PRESSURE (*Figure 23*)

In some cases of long-standing raised intracranial pressure, the floor of the middle fossa may be so thinned as to present the appearance of an erosion or erosions of one or both sides. Characteristically, these have ill-defined edges and there is often enlargement of one or both foramina ovale. Other radiological signs of raised intracranial pressure are invariably present.

TEMPORAL LOBE GLIOMA (*Figure 139*)

Very slow-growing temporal gliomas may occasionally, after a number of years, produce a certain degree of erosion and thinning of the overlying bone, and this may show as a loss of definition of the structures on one side of the base of the skull in the temporal fossa. Such cases are extremely rare.

EROSIONS OF THE TEMPORAL BONE

Large areas of destruction in the petrous bones are easy to see in the full axial, the Towne's and the postero-anterior projections, but small erosions are easily overlooked because of the density of the bone, its complicated anatomy, and the shadows of other overlying areas. It is therefore often necessary to use additional radiographic views where a lesion is suspected in the region of the petrous bone, even though routine radiographs appear normal. There are a number of possible additional projections and techniques which are described in the chapter devoted to radiographic technique.

In order to gain some knowledge of the nature of the cause of the erosion, it is essential to try to discover the area most severely affected and to judge, if possible, from where the erosion began. The temporal bone will, therefore, be discussed under several headings: The Internal Auditory Meatus; The Petrous Apex; and The Tympanic Part and its Surroundings.

The internal auditory meatus

The internal auditory meatus is visible in the full axial and Towne's projections but may be much more clearly seen in the antero-posterior projection through the orbit, in

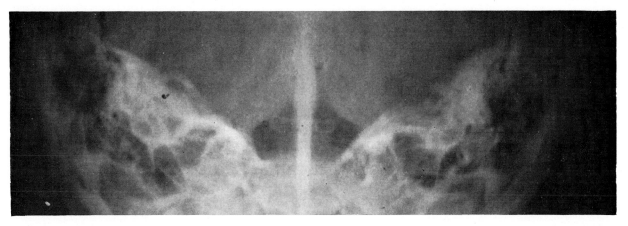

(a)

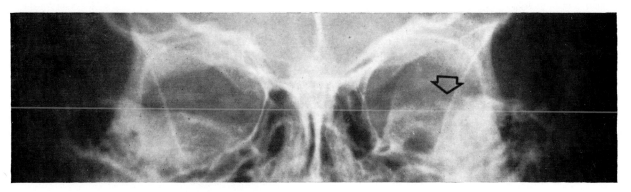

(b)

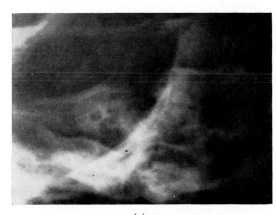

(c)

Figure 194. Bilateral acoustic neuroma in a girl who at the age of 18 years had the typical signs and symptoms of a left acoustic neuroma. There was also some right-sided tinnitus and loss of hearing. (a) Half axial view. There is a rather ragged erosion around the left internal auditory meatus. (b) Per-orbital view showing elevation of a thin section of bone (arrow) by the expanding tumour. The right internal auditory meatus was considered normal. (c) Stenver's view. Erosion has destroyed the normal outline of the internal auditory meatus. The cochlear wall is still visible. (d) Four years later the patient developed unequivocal signs of a right acoustic neuroma. The half axial view shows an erosion on the right very like the original one on the left, with elevation of a flake of bone. Note evidence of previous left-sided operation. The right-sided tumour was also removed with success

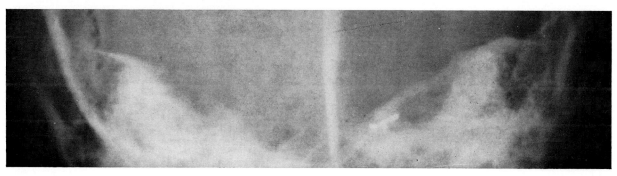

(d)

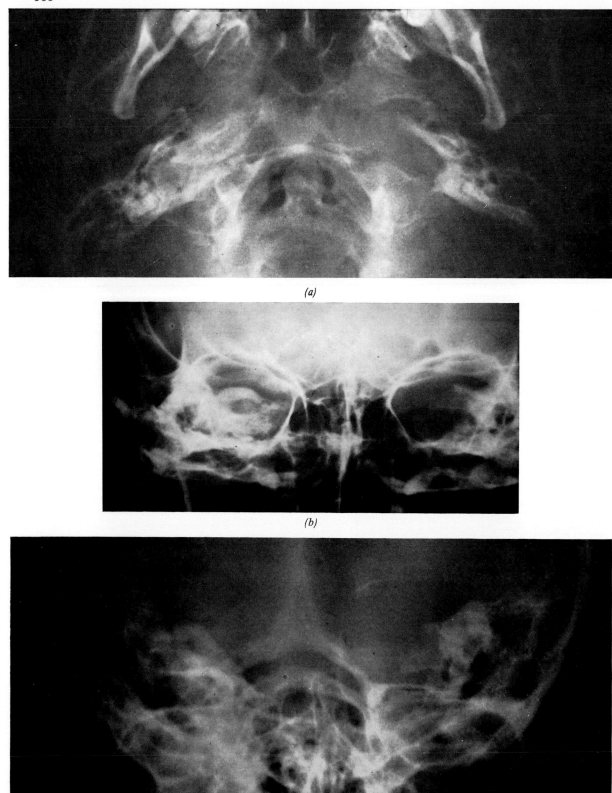

(a)

(b)

(c)

Figure 195. Acoustic neuroma. (a) Full axial view. There is severe erosion of the tip of the petrous bone and, apparently, of the lateral part of the basiphenoid, but the erosion is centred on the internal auditory meatus. (b) Per-orbital view. The erosion is clear, but the details of its margins are difficult to interpret. (c) Half axial view. A shell of bone has been lifted on the surface of the tumour

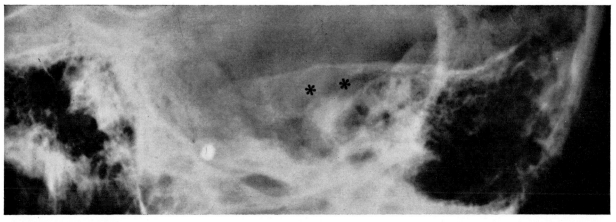

(a)

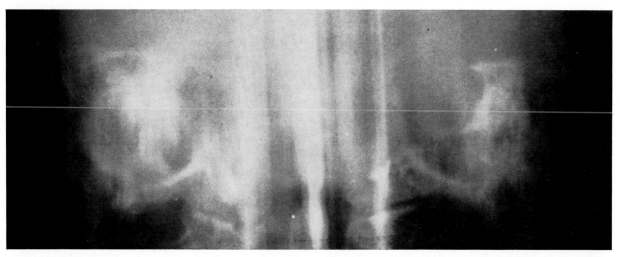

(b)

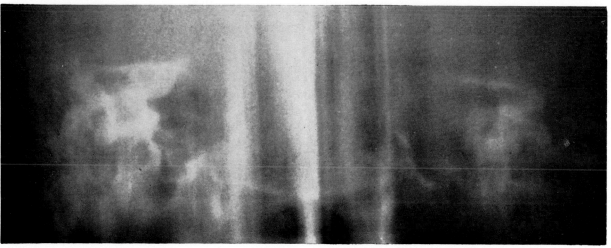

(c)

Figure 196. Acoustic neuromas in a woman aged 45 years who presented with evidence of raised intracranial pressure after an 11-month history of failing vision. There was a minimal left facial weakness, complete loss of taste over the anterior two-thirds of the tongue and some depression of hearing on the left. Ataxia and nystagmus were present. There was no response to caloric tests. (a) Stenver's view shows much enlargement of the internal auditory meatus (asterisks). There is still a thin shell of bone representing the roof of the canal. (b) Antero-posterior tomogram cut at 7 cm. A large scooped out erosion on the posterior surface of the petrous bone. (c) Antero-posterior tomogram cut at 8 cm showing the roof of the (anterior) part of the expanded meatus. A large acoustic neuroma was removed. It has burrowed deeply into the cerebellum but also crossed the midline

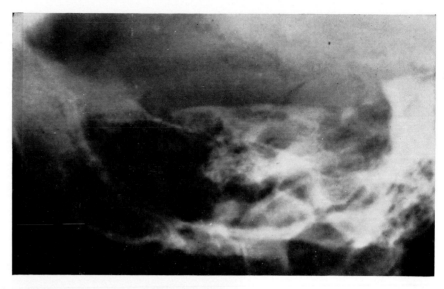

(a)

(b)

Figure 197. Acoustic neuroma in a woman aged 50 years complaining of deafness and a history typical of a right acoustic neuroma. (a) The right Stenver's view shows an internal auditory meatus apparently of normal size, but the neighbouring bone is much less dense than on the left side. This is because of erosion of the posterior surface, leaving the upper and lower margins of the meatus more or less unchanged, but diminishing the depth of bone through which the rays have to pass. The tumour was a substantial one and protruded well into the meatus. (b) The left side for comparison

Stenver's views and in tomograms. The meatuses of the two sides are not necessarily symmetrical in their shape. The maximal diameter may be at the medial or the lateral end of the meatus and the normal canal therefore either bottle-shaped or trumpet-shaped. This makes small degrees of enlargement of part of the canal particularly difficult to recognize. Valvassori (1966), after examining the radiographs of 100 normal subjects, stated that in 90 per cent the meatuses were the same shape. In the remaining 10 per cent differences of diameter were no more than 2 mm. He went on to say that it was abnormal to find the medial end of the canal 1 mm or more wider than the lateral, and abnormal to find more than 3 mm of difference between the length of the posterior walls of the canals on the same side. The

posterior wall should be from 4 to 11 mm in length. The diameter of the canal should be between 2 and 9 mm. (A diameter as small as 2 mm presumably implies that the 7th and 8th nerves are passing through individual canals.)

In good pictures, including tomograms, the crista falciformis is always visible and is usually a linear density between 1 and 7 mm in length. When the 7th and 8th nerve canals are separate, the crista falciformis, prolonged, forms the division between them.

Pathological enlargement of the canal may involve its whole length. More commonly, the enlargement is confined to the medial end and is accompanied by an erosion on the postero-medial face of the petrous bone. In such cases, the meatus appears trumpet-shaped to a degree greater than normal. However, a shallow erosion

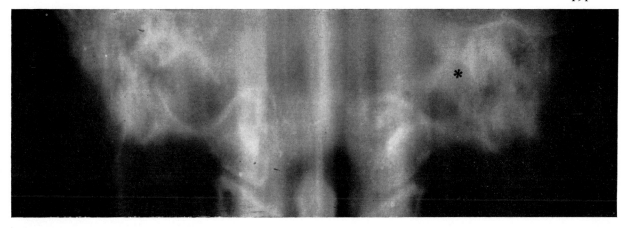

(a)

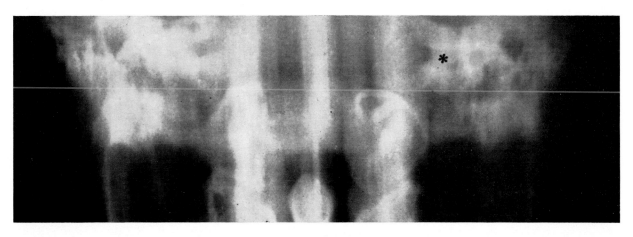

(b)

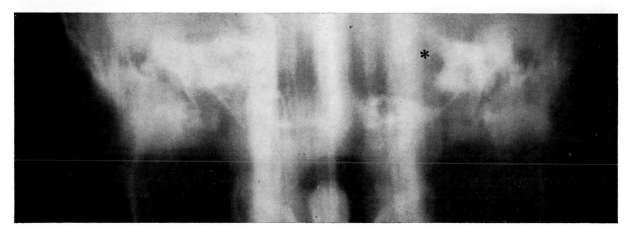

(c)

Figure 198. Erosion of the tip of the left petrous bone. Plain radiographs revealed an isolated erosion of the petrous bone. Antero-posterior tomograms at 0·5 cm intervals show the following. (a) A normal jugular foramen. (b) A normal internal auditory meatus. (c) The erosion lying medially in front of the internal auditory meatus. The tumour was shown to be slightly indenting the carotid artery in its vertical intra-osseous course. No operation yet. Differential diagnoses include epidermoid and chordoma or, less probably because the jugular foramen look normal, 9th or 10th nerve neuroma

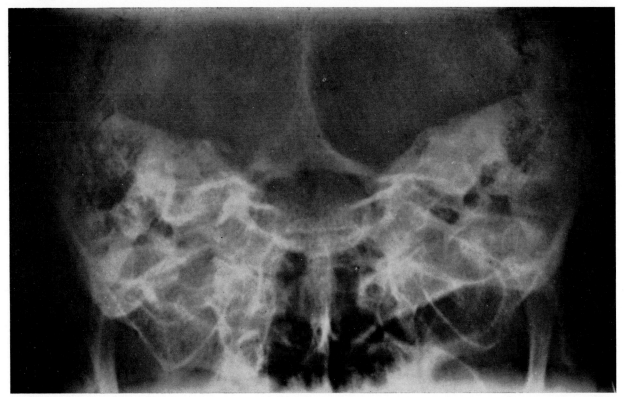

(a)

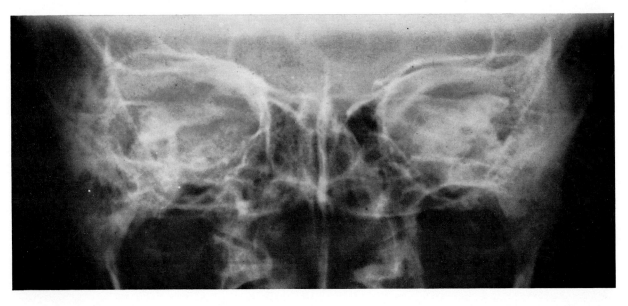

(b)

Figure 199. A woman aged 56 years who had had chronic mastoiditis. In the 7 years before these investigations she had suffered from frequent spasms of the right side of her face, and now recently pain in the right cheek. There was diminution of pain and light touch perception over the right side of her face, an absent corneal reflex and bilateral incomplete deafness. At operation a large meningioma was removed. Its attachment covered an area from the posterior margin of the jugular foramen up to and just through the tentorial hiatus, and from the lateral margin of the foramen magnum to the tentorial attachment. (a) The half axial radiograph shows an ill-defined erosion, which together with some calcification or hyperostosis has obscured the internal auditory meatus. (b) The per-orbital view demonstrates the intact deep part of the meatus and the irregular specks of calcium over the eroded tip (cont.)

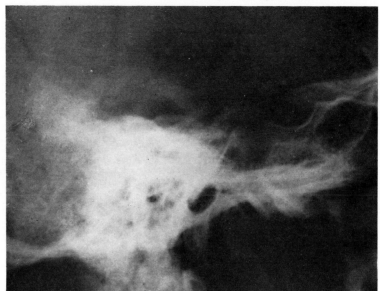

Figure 199 (cont.). (c) Lateral view shows that much of the calcium must lie in the lower antero-medial part of the tentorium (petroclinoid ligaments). Such heavy calcification in the presence of definite evidence of a tumour in the region is strongly suggestive of a meningioma

(c)

around the mouth of the meatus may affect neither the upper nor the lower wall of the canal. Thus, the width of the shadow of the porus acousticus will remain unaltered in antero-posterior and Stenver's views. They will show hypertranslucency and a diminution of contrast range on the affected side (*Figure 197*).

Much more rarely, enlargement of the canal is confined to its distal deep end in which case an exaggerated form of the normal bottle-shape is demonstrated on the radiographs.

In time, erosions of the meatus may enlarge to such a degree that little of the normal anatomy remains, but a large depression is easily visible on the posterior surfaces of the petrous bone. Sometimes a flake of bone may become detached from its normal position and be lifted away on the edge of the eroding tumour.

ACOUSTIC NEUROMA (*Figures 193–197*)

Almost invariably the cause of pathological widening of the internal auditory meatus and erosions near its mouth is an acoustic neuroma. In a few cases, patients suffering from neurofibromatosis, these are bilateral, making it unwise to rely too much upon comparison of the two sides in distinguishing the normal from the abnormal.

MENINGIOMA (*Figure 199*)

Meningiomas of the cerebello-pontine angle are uncommon but they too may, on very rare occasions, produce erosions difficult to distinguish from those due to acoustic neuromas. A certain amount of surrounding hyperostosis or increased density of bone can sometimes be detected, and there is often calcification in the near parts of the tentorium which is striking in its density.

Meningiomas of the petrous apex are not radiologically distinguishable from those in the cerebello-pontine angle.

OTHER CEREBELLO–PONTINE ANGLE TUMOURS

Other long-standing cerebello-pontine angle masses may be encountered from time to time as cases for widening of the internal auditory meatus. The author has seen a seventh nerve neuroma, an arteriovenous malformation, and a brain-stem glioma present in this way.

Fifth nerve neuromas may occasionally destroy the upper surface of the petrous bone and when they make a large erosion it will be difficult to distinguish from any other.

A fourth ventricular choroid plexus papilloma, expanding out of the foramen of Luschka — a very rare entity — may also cause bone erosion in the region.

METASTATIC CARCINOMA

The second or third commonest cerebello-pontine angle tumour is a metastasis from carcinoma. Bone erosion may be detectable, though it is usually slight. The internal auditory meatus is not widened in the smooth, well-defined way sometimes seen with neuromas.

The petrous apex

If the destruction predominates in the apex of the petrous bone (although it may spread to some extent to neighbouring areas of the temporal, occipital and sphenoid bones) (*Figure 198*), the following causes should be considered.

CHORDOMA (*Figure 200*)

The destruction is not commonly confined to the petrous apex and may be very widespread, even crossing the midline and involving the apices of both petrous

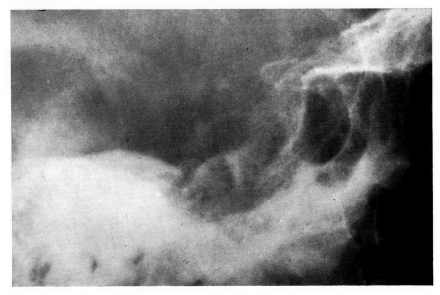

(a)

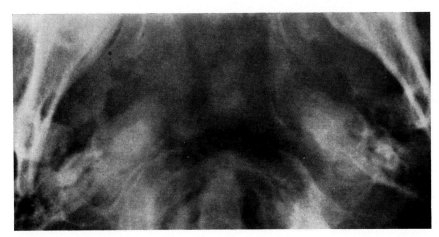

(b)

Figure 200. Chordoma in an adult who had suffered from double vision for 3 years. He had had pain in the right eye for 6 months and a drooping right eyelid and unequal pupils for 3 months. At operation a tumour was found filling the right cavernous sinus and elevating the bone and dura in the region of the posterior clinoid. (a) Lateral view shows erosion of the posterior part of the sella, and a basisphenoid of normal or more than normal density. (b) Full axial view shows that the apex of the petrous bone is much denser than that on the left

bones. Some increase in density of bone and some calcification may also be seen. The differential diagnosis from meningioma may not be resolved without angiography.

EPIDERMOID (CHOLESTEATOMA)

Epidermoids very occasionally occur in the medial part of the petrous bone and may be separated from the cavities of the middle ear by intact and normal structures. They may grow to a large size and involve neighbouring bones to a greater or lesser degree. Surrounding bone reaction is minimal, although there may be a curvilinear flake of bone or calcification on the capsule of the tumour. The limited surrounding reaction and the complete bone destruction produced by the tumour make erosions due to epidermoids appear particularly translucent.

GLOMAS JUGULAR TUMOURS

Due to the difficulty of demonstrating the jugular foramen in the routine views, erosion due to these tumours when severe may be thought at first examination to affect predominantly the petrous apex. Bone destruction in the region of the tumour is complete and there is little or no surrounding sclerosis. Special views will almost always demonstrate that the erosion is continuous with the translucency of the jugular foramen, and in the majority of cases the jugular foramen itself will be grossly enlarged and have lost its clear-cut margins.

OSTEOMYELITIS

Osteomyelitis of the petrous apex is an extremely uncommon cause of erosion and is usually accompanied by a certain amount of sclerosis. Unlike most of the destructive lesions described above, the edge of the erosion is

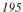

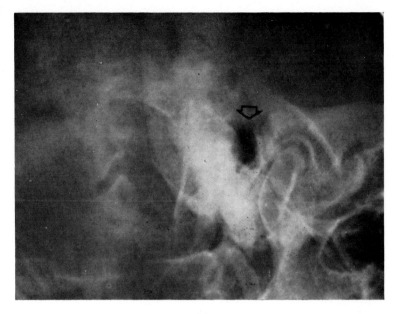

(a)

Figure 201. Post-infective cholesteatoma. The patient had a chronic discharge from the ear. There had been no previous operation. (a) The lateral oblique view shows erosion (arrow) above the middle ear and sclerosis of bone around the antrum and in the mastoid process. (b) Stenver's view shows expansion of the tympanic antrum (asterisk) which contained cholesteatoma. The tegment tympani is intact

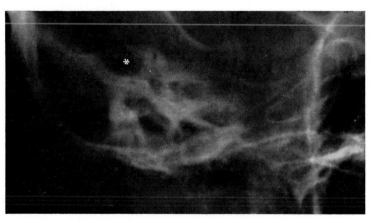

(b)

indefinite and probably extends laterally towards the region of the middle ear. Neighbouring bones are not affected. The most difficult differential diagnosis on radiological grounds will be from a meningioma. The author has never seen a case.

HAEMANGIOMA OF BONE

Haemangioma may affect any bone. A few cases have been described and the author has seen one in which the petrous apex showed irregular destruction with coarse trabeculae of spicular bone. The diagnosis, although unlikely, is important because of the difficulties which may be encountered at operation.

The tympanic part and its surroundings

Small areas of destruction in the lateral part of the petrous bone are easily confused with the mastoid air cells and the normal cavities of the middle ear. The four routine radiographs of the skull may show only a proportion of the destructive lesions which are found at operation or may be demonstrated by special techniques, particularly tomography. The differential diagnosis of areas of erosion includes some of the causes already mentioned but there are other more likely ones.

CHOLESTEATOMA (POST−INFECTIVE) (*Figures 201−207*)

The cavity of the middle ear or the antrum, or both, and the mastoid air cells may be occupied by products of chronic infection and desquamated epithelium. The detection of such a cholesteatoma is not always easy.

If the middle ear on the affected side (seen in the full axial view) shows hypertranslucency and particularly if the ossicles are not visible; if the translucency of the middle ear is enlarged, or if there is a neighbouring translucent cavity in the generally dense bone, the

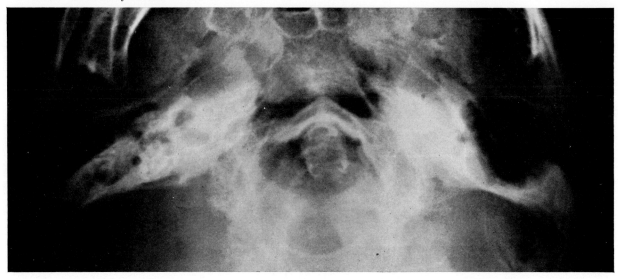

Figure 202. A very large cholesteatoma with a classical appearance. The area of destruction is completely translucent, and there is a shell of eburnated bone around the mass. The destructive process has extended into the labyrinth

presence of a cholesteatoma as a complication of chronic infection may be suspected.

Sclerosis of the surrounding bone may tend to obscure the translucent area occupied by the cholesteatoma. An additional difficulty, not generally appreciated, is the fact that cholesteatomatous material may contain specks of calcium which will render it partially opaque. Nevertheless, observation of the trabeculae of the bone between air cells is important. If in spite of moderate translucency the walls intervening between cells are invisible, a cholesteatoma is probably present. If the cells are less translucent than normal, but intact bony walls are visible, the cause is swollen mucosa, retained secretions, pus or long-standing fibrosis.

Tomography of the petrous bone is particularly useful in demonstrating the presence and extent of abnormal translucencies in this region. Tomography and special projections may also show perforation of the upper cortical surface of the petrous bone over an erosion, indicating the route through which infection may reach the extradural space, or they may reveal destruction spreading to the labyrinth (*Figure 203*). It is also sometimes possible to recognize a fistula between the midde-ear cavity and the labyrinth (usually between the antrum and the lateral semi-circular canal). This may be a useful diagnostic finding in a patient complaining of vertigo, but both in the author's experience and in that of Rovsing and Jensen (1968) false positive radiological diagnoses are not uncommon.

Very careful radiography with special apparatus is necessary to show details of disruption of the auditory ossicle (*see* page 224). In the routine submento-vertical view the rather ill-defined shadow thrown by the combination of the malleus and the incus is nearly always visible (*Figure 208b*) and absence or diminution of the ossicle shadow may be discovered in chronic otitis media, particularly with cholesteatoma formation.

Cholesteatomas may reach a very large size and when, for instance, destruction extends into the squamous temporal, the distinction between the post-infective and the neoplastic type of cholesteatoma (epidermoid) becomes impossible on radiographic evidence alone.

ACUTE MASTOIDITIS

Bone destruction may sometimes be visible after 2 weeks. The thin air-cell walls are usually first affected, but they tend to be obscured by pus which fills the cells.

Osteomyelitis thus produces little evidence of erosion in a very opaque mastoid.

CHRONIC MASTOIDITIS (*Figures 206–210*)

Chronic osteomyelitis usually presents the appearance of considerable sclerosis around a localized erosion. The presence of a cholesteatoma is difficult to exclude. Osteomyelotis due to tuberculosis is sometimes seen and may produce a strikingly irregular area of translucency spreading from the region of the middle ear (*see also* Acute and Chronic Mastoiditis on page 223).

KERATOSIS OBTURANS

In this rare condition progressive enlargement of the external auditory meatus may be demonstrated. The external auditory meatus is filled with desquamated epithelial debris.

DERMOIDS AND EPIDERMOIDS

Epidermoids are very much more common in this situation than dermoid cysts. The distinction between inflammatory and neoplastic types may be difficult or impossible (*see* above). Generally speaking, the very large erosions which spread to involve other bones are believed to be neoplastic.

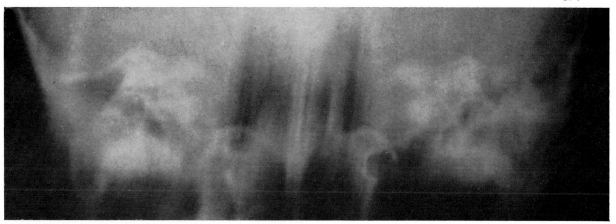

Figure 203. Cholesteatoma. A tomogram showing, on the left side, expansion of the tympanic antrum and a fistula between antrum and horizontal and semi-circular canal. On the right side an operation has been performed

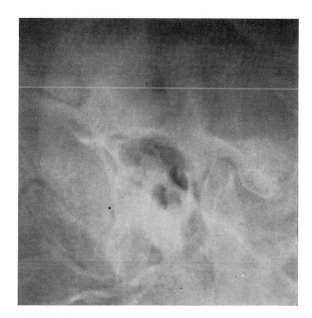

Figure 204. Cholesteatoma, in a man aged 63 years who had had pain in the ear for 1 month and a right facial palsy for 1 week. Cholesteatoma was protruding into the external auditory meatus. The lateral oblique view shows an erosion with a smooth wall. The translucency consists of the expanded middle ear, tympanic antrum and external auditory meatus. There was erosion of the tegman tympani

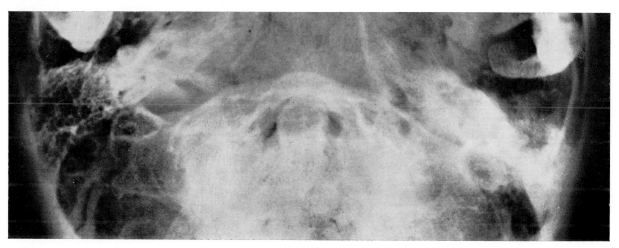

Figure 205. Cholesteatoma. The patient had had a discharging left ear for 40 years. Cholesteatomatous material was seen in the external meatus. Full axial view reveals expansion of the left middle ear cavity and the external auditory meatus with an ill-defined extension in the antral region. The ossicles have entirely disappeared

198

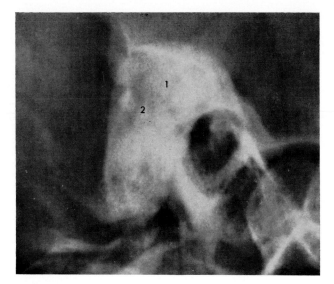

Figure 206. Chronic mastoiditis. The mastoid is diploetic. The tympanic antrum (asterisk) is very large and was filled with cholesteatomatous material. The superior (1), posterior (2), and lateral (3) semi-circular canals show up clearly through the dense bone. (a) Lateral oblique view. (b) Modified Stenver's view

(a)

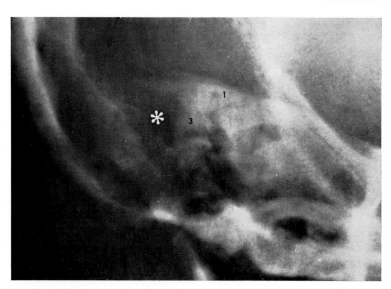

(b)

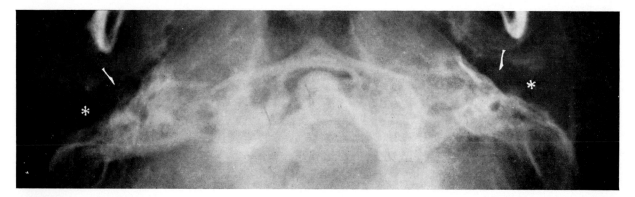

Figure 207. Chronic mastoiditis. Cholesteatoma. On both sides there is only very limited pneumatization of the petrous bones. The external auditory meatuses (asterisks) are wide and the middle ears fully translucent. The shadow of the ossicles (arrow) on the left is small and faint. On the right the shadow is large (arrow) but not of normal dimensions. The patient had had a recurrent otorrhoea, and pain and was deaf. Both drums showed old perforations and granulation tissue. At operation large amounts of cholesteatoma were removed from the attic regions of both ears. The ossicles have been partly destroyed in the chronic inflammatory process

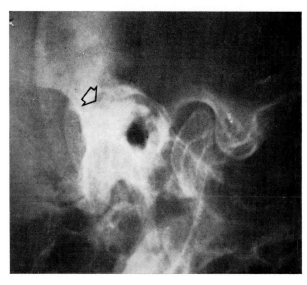
(a)

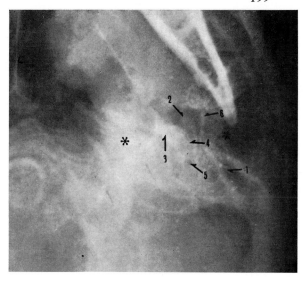
(b)

Figure 208. Chronic mastoiditis. (a) Lateral oblique view. The mastoid is acellular and the bone sclerosed. Around the tympanic antrum (arrow) (which is opaque) there is a suggestion that trabeculae are eroded. (b) The opposite side of the same patient. Normal full axial view. Note: (1) A few cells in the mastoid process; (2) the head of the malleus with the incus; (3) vestibule; (4) semi-circular canal; (5) facial nerve canal; (6) the middle ear bounded laterally and above by the shadow of the tympanic ring. The external and internal auditory meatuses (asterisk)

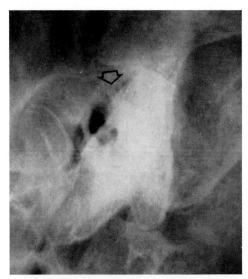
(a)

Figure 209. Chronic infection in a man aged 49 years who has been deaf since childhood and who has had a discharging ear for several years. At operation the antrum contained pus and the tympanum granulation tissue. The dura was visible in the region of the tegmen. There was cholesteatomatous material on the inside of the drum. The ossicles were intact. (a) Lateral oblique view shows a diploetic mastoid. The peri-antral region is translucent due to erosion (arrow). (b) Full axial view. The left middle ear is opaque by comparison with the right, but the ossicle shadows are distinctly seen on both sides (arrows)

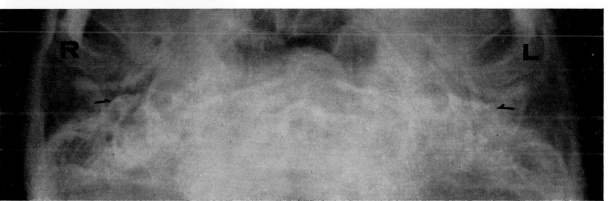
(b)

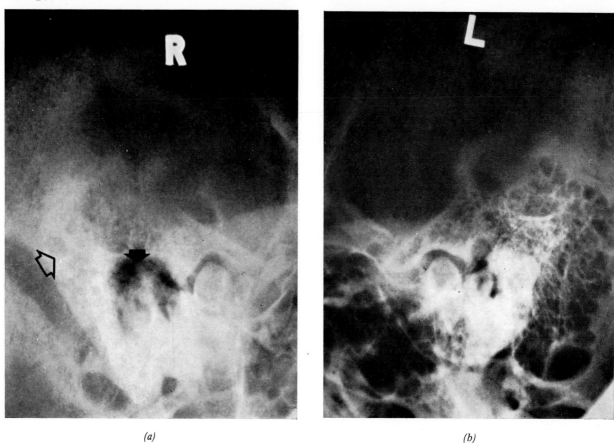

(a) (b)

Figure 210. Chronic mastoiditis in a cellular mastoid. The patient, a woman aged 25 years, had had many years of recurrent discharge from the right ear through a small perforation in the drum. Tympanoplasty after a cortical mastoidectomy had been only a partial success. (a) The lateral oblique view shows a number of pre-antral cells (open arrow) all abnormally opaque but with intact bony walls. The area of bone removal (closed arrow) is shown. (b) The normal side (in which at one time the patient also had acute mastoiditis)

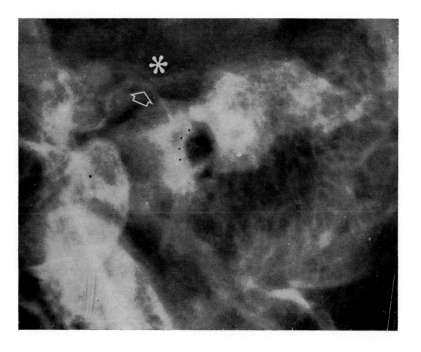

Figure 211. Carcinoma of the external auditory meatus. The anterior margin of the external auditory meatus has disappeared (outlined with dots). There is an extensive erosion spreading in the squamous temporal (asterisk) and probably invading the condylar fossa (arrow). In the radiograph slight clouding of the mastoid air cells is apparent

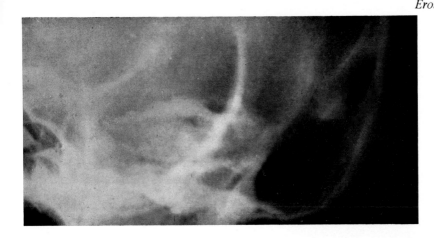

(a)

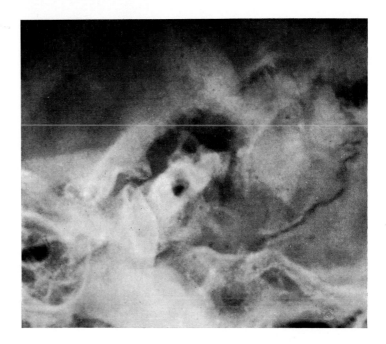

Figure 212. Squamous carcinoma of mastoid. The area of erosion is a little more lateral than that produced by a glomus jugulare tumour and has extended to the squamous temporal. (a) Stenver's view. (b) Lateral oblique view

(b)

MENINGIOMA

Meningiomas arising in the posterior fossa may involve the posterior surface of the lateral part of the petrous bone as well as the occipital bone in the region of the groove for the transverse sinus. Erosion is usually very slight and extremely difficult to see. A certain amount of hyperostosis is likely which will also be masked by the density of the overlying bone, and there may be evidence of hypertrophied vascular channels in the neighbourhood. (For systematic reading on meningiomas, turn to page 203.)

PRIMARY CARCINOMA (*Figures 211, 212*)

The early radiographic features are those of the chronic infection which often precedes it. The particular feature of carcinoma is an erosion which increases rapidly in size.

MALIGNANT INVASION BY NASOPHARYNGEAL TUMOURS

Secondary invasion of the petrous bone may take place around the middle ear and Eustachian tube from nasopharyngeal carcinoma. Bone erosion when demonstrated is usually part of a larger area of destruction involving the floor of the middle fossa.

GLOMUS JUGULARE TUMOUR

An erosion with little or no surrounding sclerosis which invades the lateral part of the petrous bone from below may well be the result of a glomus jugulare tumour. A very few cases are encountered in which the tumour appears to arise from the region of the promontary, and these may be indistinguishable radiologically from cholesteatoma.

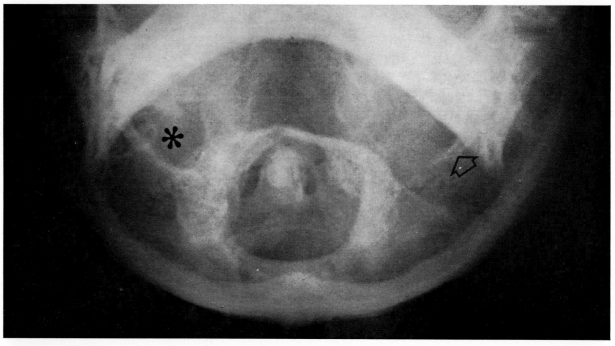

(a)

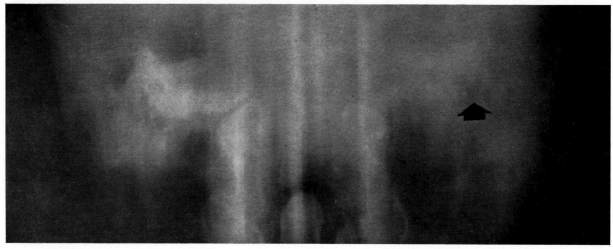

(b)

Figure 213. Glomas jugulare tumour. (a) In the subaxial projection the right jugular foramen is clearly seen (asterisk). It has a well-defined edge and is normal. On the left most of this margin has disappeared due to an erosion, exact limits of which are impossible to define. Note the styloid process superimposed upon the erosion (open arrow). (b) Antero-posterior tomogram showing the typical destruction of the undersurface of the petrous bone (closed arrow)

HAEMANGIOMA OF BONE

This uncommon tumour has similar features wherever it occurs (*see* page 195).

OTHER MALIGNANT TUMOURS IN THE REGION

When a carcinoma or rodent ulcer of the pinna is present, radiological examination is required to determine the extent of the underlying erosion of bone.

Rarely, other primary or metastatic tumours are found, as they are in all bones.

PAGET'S DISEASE

Though thickened, bone affected by Paget's disease may be hypertranslucent. Demineralization often affects the cochlear and other parts of the optic capsule. It also sometimes affects the ossicular chain, though this is much more difficult to recognize radiologically.

Erosions around the jugular foramen

The jugular foramina are obscured in the four routine radiographic projections, but may be shown clearly in a full axial view taken with considerably less than the usual 90 degrees of angulation, and in mento-occipital views. The foramina are frequently of unequal size on the two sides.

GLOMAS JUGULARE TUMOUR (*Figures 213, 214*)

Erosion when it occurs around the borders of the jugular foramen is generally the result of a glomus jugulare tumour, which will almost inevitably be accompanied by cranial nerve palsies. The glomus tumour is vascular and relatively slow-growing. The erosion produced usually extends forward and upward into the petrous bone and medially, and the edges of the erosion do not show any sclerosis. In the postero-anterior projection, in antero-posterior views, and in the Stenver's projection, a considerable amount of destruction of the undersurface of the petrous bone may be demonstrated in most cases.

9th AND 10th NERVE NEUROMAS

Both are very rare and either may cause moderate enlargement of the jugular foramen, especially of its medial part and of the petrous apex.

EROSION OF THE SPHENOID WINGS AND EXPANSION OF THE SPHENOID FISSURE

In postero-anterior projections of the skull in which the x-ray beam is angled cephalad (20–25 degrees) the greater and lesser wings of the sphenoid, with the sphenoid fissure between them, are visible through the orbits, unimpeded by superimposed shadows except those of the posterior part of the vault.

The major difficulty in the radiology of this region lies in the recognition of normal from abnormal degrees of asymmetry.

LESSER WINGS OF THE SPHENOID

Recognition of abnormality

The lesser wings of the sphenoid are more often than not asymmetrical in shape and, to some extent, in position. Asymmetry of shape and of position may lead to an apparent asymmetry of density of the bones on the two sides. Unless, therefore, there is definite erosion as detailed below, or alteration in bone texture, inequality between the lesser wings is better ignored.

It is essential to start with a clear idea of the clinical lateralization of the lesion.

If the lesser wing of the sphenoid on the clinically abnormal side is denser than that on the opposite side, an attempt must first be made to decide whether the dense sphenoid wing shows bone of normal or abnormal texture. Increased density with obvious abnormality of texture indicates the presence of a meningioma or sometimes fibrous dysplasia (*see* page 115) but lesser degrees of density in which the texture of the bone is normal are rarely of any significance.

If the sphenoid wing on the clinically abnormal side is the more translucent, difficulties of interpretation are greater. When (1) the asymmetry is severe and not part of a generalized obliquity of the base; and (2) there is loss of corticated edge to the lesser wing, some significance may be attached to the translucency.

The lesser wing of the sphenoid may be eroded from above or below. (Erosion from below will widen the sphenoid fissure.)

Causes of erosion of upper surface of lesser wing (*Figure 216*)

When the shape of the lesser wing of the sphenoid has been altered by the presence of a long-standing space-occupying lesion above it, the anterior clinoid process and the planum sphenoidale on this side are very likely to show a similar alteration. To be of significance, depression of the upper surface of the lesser wing of the sphenoid and neighbouring areas must be severe and fairly obvious, or there must be other evidence (such as calcification) of a tumour in the region.

Any sufficiently long-standing space-occupying lesion in the subfrontal region may produce this type of abnormality. The commoner causes are as follows.

MENINGIOMA

Meningiomas arising from the anterior clinoid process or planum sphenoidale or the lesser wing of the sphenoid may produce depression and erosion of the upper surface of the lesser wing, but with very few exceptions they also cause a recognizable hyperostosis at some point. Both erosion and hyperostosis may extend across the midline but the change is rarely of equal severity on the two sides. (For systematic reading on meningiomas, turn to page 209.)

GLIOMA

From time to time slow-growing gliomas are encountered which have caused a definite deformity of the upper surface of one or both sphenoid wings. The flattening is usually unilateral and no hyperostosis is present.

CRANIOPHARYNGIOMA

Rarely, craniopharyngiomas lie above and in front of the sella turcica and in such cases they may cause depression of the medial parts of the lesser wings of the sphenoid as well as of the planum sphenoidale and sometimes of the anterior clinoid processes. The abnormality is more often symmetrical than asymmetrical. Calcification is present only in a proportion of cases and may be confused with calcification in slow-growing gliomas of the region.

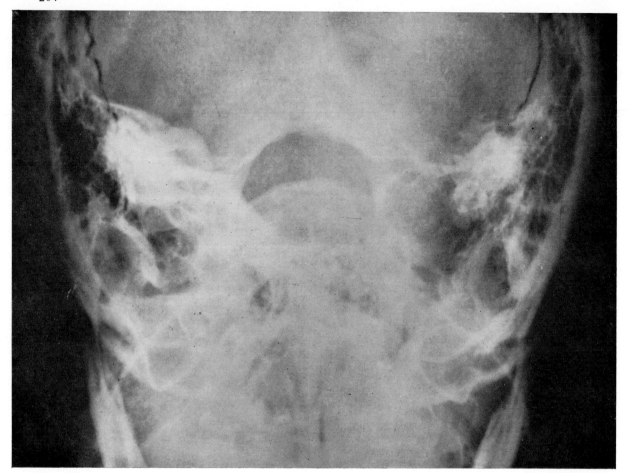

(a)

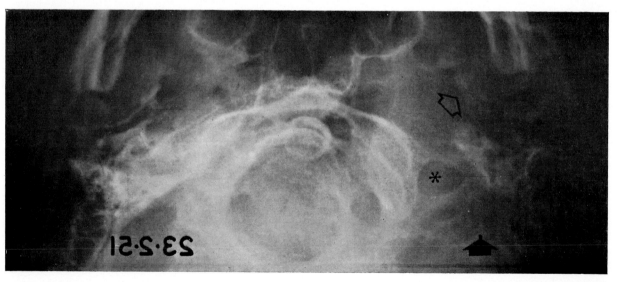

(b)

Figure 214. Glomus jugulare tumour in a girl aged 21 years who gave 4 years' history indicating steadily increasing left cranial nerve palsies. The lateral skull radiograph was normal. (a) Half axial view showing a large erosion which has destroyed much of the left petrous temporal bone and the squamous occipital below and behind it. (b) Full axial view showing that the erosion extends into the floor of the middle fossa, stopping short of the foramen spinosum but damaging the sphenopetrosal fissure (open arrow). The foramen transversarium (asterisk) of the atlas stands out against the general loss of detail in the bone of the skull (cont.)

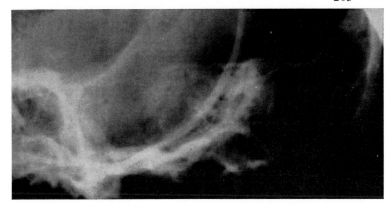

(c)

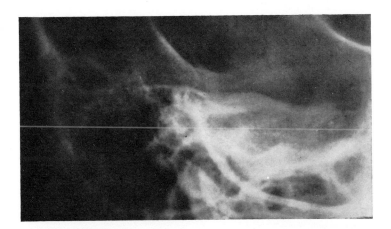

(d)

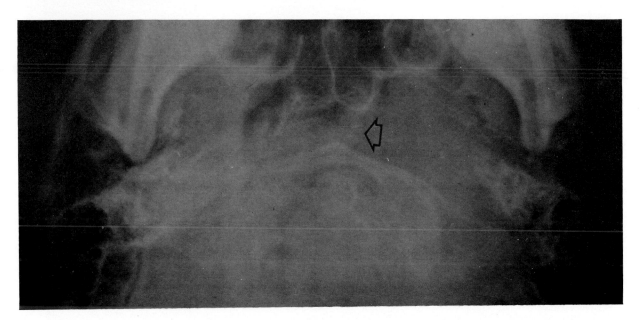

(e)

Figure 214 (cont.). (c) Stenver's view. Erosion of the petrous bone is rather patchy and, although it extends for a long way, is more complete at the tip and inferiorly than above. (d) The normal side for comparison. (e) A sub-axial view 2 years later shows the erosion much more clearly. It has probably altered only slightly; but less head tilt demonstrates the destructive process entering the basisphenoid and basi-occiput (open arrow) as well as showing more detail behind the petrous bone. The situation of the erosion below the petrous bone should raise a strong suspicion of a glomas jugular tumour, but it can only be confirmed by direct inspection

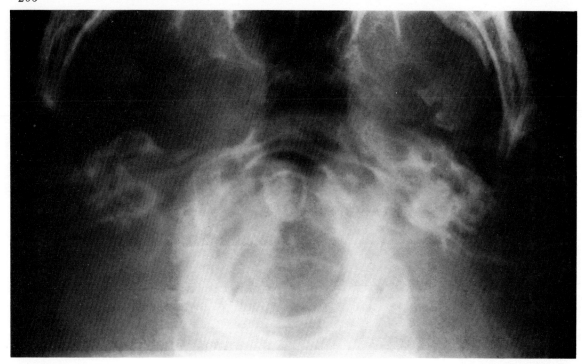

(a)

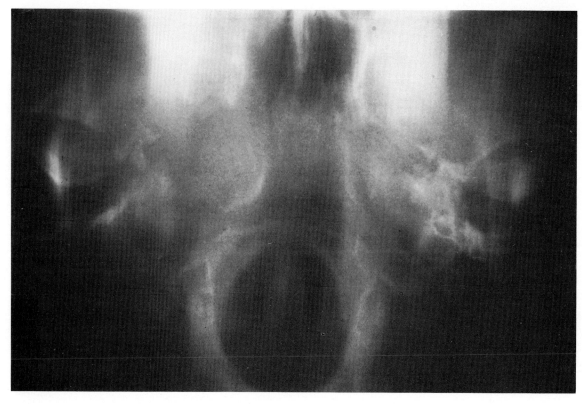

(b)

Figure 215. There is a large well circumscribed erosion of the floor of the middle fossa, undermining and also shortening the petrous apex but not arising primarily from the jugular foramen. It was a rhabdomyosarcoma. (a) Base view. (b) Tomogram of base (cont.)

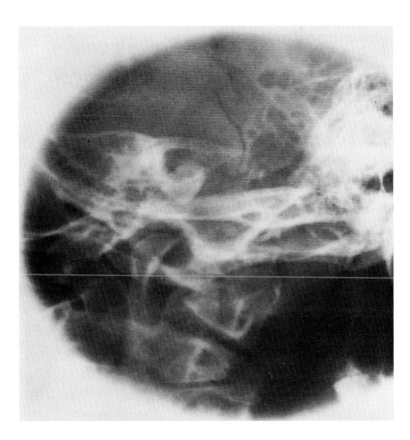

(c)

*Figure 215 (cont.). (c) Stenver's view.
(d) Tomogram of petrous bone*

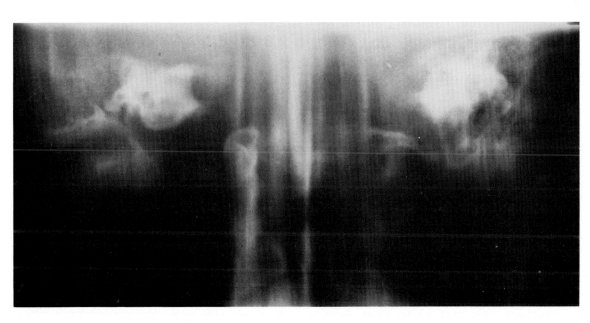

(d)

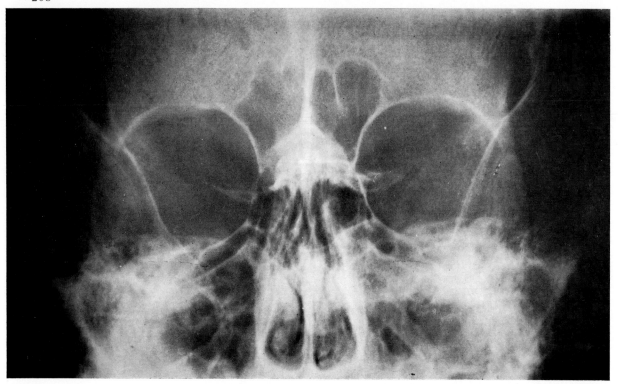

Figure 216. Flattening of the upper surface of the lesser wing of the sphenoid. The right lesser wing is flattened from above. There is an hyperostosis in the midline. The left lesser wing is either normal or slightly thickened. A meningioma arose in the midline and lay over the left. The right lesser wing was affected by long-standing intracranial pressure. Knowledge of the clinical findings (a Foster Kennedy syndrome with left optic atrophy) are essential before the picture can be fully interpreted

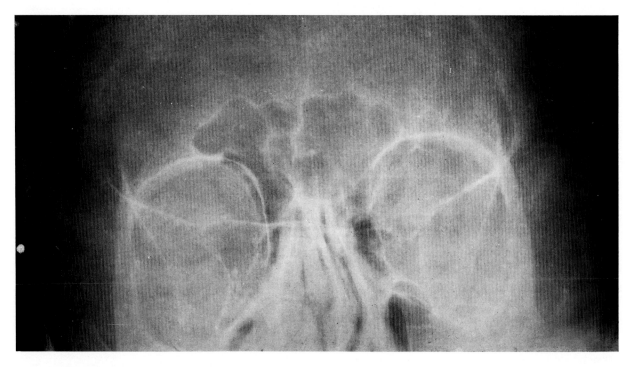

Figure 217. Postero-anterior view of a parasellar aneurysm. The right sphenoid fissure is expanded and the remains of the lesser wing of the sphenoid elevated

WIDENING OF THE SPHENOID FISSURE

Recognition

Asymmetry of size and shape of the sphenoid fissure of the two sides is extremely common. Small degrees of asymmetry, particularly if the lesser wings of the sphenoid are also asymmetrical in position and the bone texture is normal, are best ignored. Grosser degrees of expansion of the sphenoid fissure may present more difficulties of interpretation. If the visible parts of the lesser and greater wings of the sphenoid of the two sides are symmetrical in shape and position, asymmetry of size of the sphenoid fissure is rather more likely to be pathological.

The clinical signs are of the greatest importance in attempting to interpret the radiological features. Most of the lesions which produce expansion of the sphenoid fissure cause palsy of the muscles supplied by the third, fourth or sixth nerves, or sensory changes in the distribution of the ophthalmic division of the fifth. Many of the patients also have some degree of proptosis on the abnormal side. In the absence of clinical localization to the area, asymmetry of the sphenoid fissures should be interpreted with the greatest caution.

The lesions which expand the sphenoid fissure usually leave a smooth bone edge. Obvious ragged erosion of either the lesser or greater wings is most uncommon, but the edges of a large sphenoid fissure (either normal or abnormal) are sometimes so ill-defined in places that the true margin of the fissure is very difficult to see. A 'slits' coned view or views with a slightly different angulation may be of assistance in these cases.

Causes

ANEURYSM (*Figure 217*)

An aneurysm of the internal carotid lying in the cavernous sinus may become of such a size that it causes pressure erosion of the greater and lesser wings of the sphenoid and expansion of the sphenoid fissure. This is probably the commonest cause of pathological enlargement of the sphenoid fissure. Most of these aneurysms contain a certain amount of calcification but the calcium may not be easy to define in the postero-anterior projection.

MENINGIOMA

Meningiomas arising from the middle fossa usually cause hyperostosis of the sphenoid wings, often with narrowing of the sphenoid fissure; but sometimes there is also erosion, so that in rare cases an abnormally wide fissure may be bounded by unusually dense bone. Even more rarely, meningiomas fail to excite an osteoblastic reaction at all, and erosion is then the predominating sign. (For systematic reading on meningioma, turn to page 219.)

PITUITARY ADENOMA (*Figure 218*)

Rarely, pituitary adenomas expand sideways to such an extent that the bone around the sphenoid fissure is eroded. Calcification in these tumours is very uncommon but the appearance cannot be distinguished with certainty from that due to an aneurysm.

CRANIOPHARYNGIOMA

Craniopharyngioma — in which calcification is relatively common — also occasionally enlarge the sphenoid fissure by protruding sideways from the sella. The differential diagnosis from aneurysm and from pituitary adenoma may be impossible without the aid of angiography.

CHORDOMA (*Figure 219*)

A similar change may be found in occasional cases of chordoma. Calcification in these tumours may be massive and sometimes, in addition, the bones in the neighbourhood show increase in their density so that the differential diagnosis to be considered is chiefly that of a meningioma.

NEUROFIBROMA

Neurofibromas are very occasionally encountered on the nerves passing through the sphenoid fissure, and in such cases the fissure may be enlarged. Sometimes the texture of surrounding bone will be altered and may show coarse trabeculation or areas of density. Unless there are other manifestations of neurofibromatosis a diagnosis is not likely to be made from the radiograph.

CHRONIC SUBDURAL HAEMATOMA, TEMPORAL GLIOMA, LOCALIZED HYDROCEPHALUS OF THE TEMPORAL HORN, TEMPORAL LOBE AGENESIS WITH AN OVERLYING CEREBROSPINAL FLUID COLLECTION, AND NEUROFIBROMATOSIS

These conditions may all cause widening of the sphenoid fissure by expanding the whole of the middle fossa. They are described in the chapter dealing with alteration in shape of the vault (*see* page 126).

EROSIONS OF THE GREATER WING OF THE SPHENOID WITHOUT DEFINITE ENLARGMENT OF THE SPHENOID FISSURE

Recognition

Some difference is commonly seen between the translucency of the greater wings of the sphenoid. In the normal this is often due to differences in the thickness of the superimposed vault bones in the posterior part of the head. In doubtful cases a radiograph with slightly different angulation may resolve the problem.

Sometimes confusion is caused by the soft tissues of the orbit surrounding the translucent palpebral fissure, particularly after head injury causing an orbital haematoma. The characteristic shape of the palpebral fissure is visible on close examination.

The distinction between areas in which the greater wing of the sphenoid is merely thinned and areas in which complete erosion has taken place is sometimes

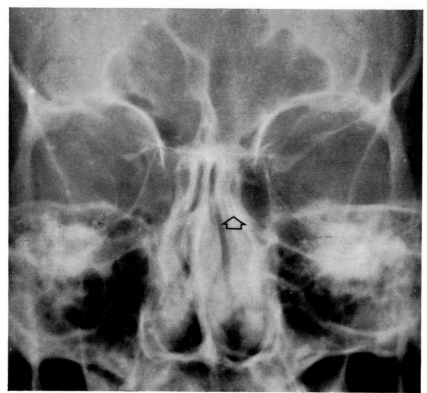

Figure 218. The postero-anterior view of a chromophobe adenoma confirms the parasellar position of part of the mass. Half of the floor of the pituitary fossa (open arrow) is absent (which is why only a 'ghost' is seen in lateral projection). The right lesser wing of sphenoid is much thinned and therefore very translucent. The right ethmoid air cells are opaque

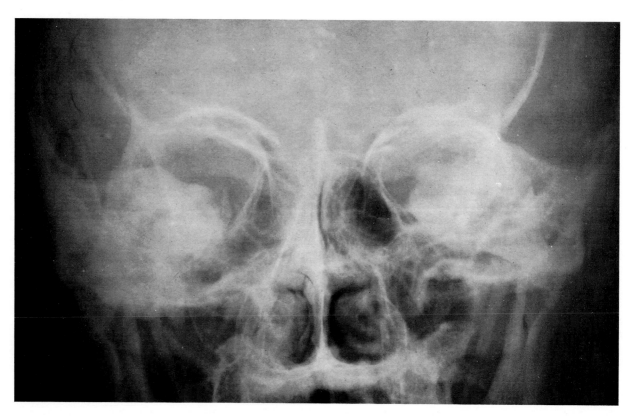

Figure 219. Chordoma. The right sphenoid fissure is enlarged

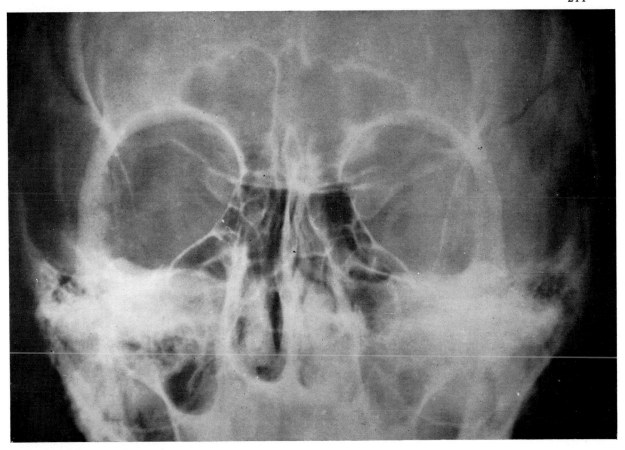

(a)

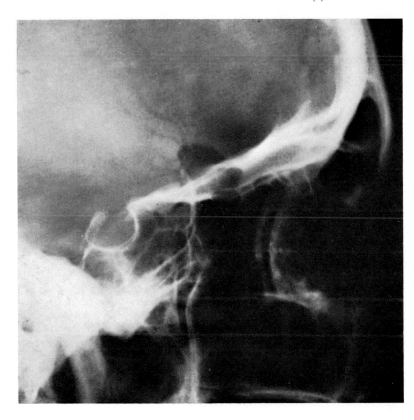

Figure 220. Metastatic deposit from carcinoma of the breast. There is destruction of parts of the greater and lesser wings of the sphenoid on the right. (a) Postero-anterior view. (b) Lateral view (cont.)

(b)

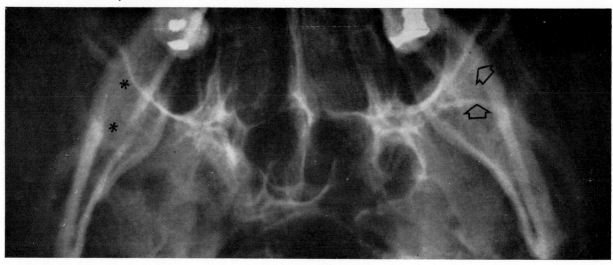

(c)

Figure 220 (cont.). (c) Full axial view showing loss of the anterior wall of the middle fossa and the postero-lateral wall of the orbit

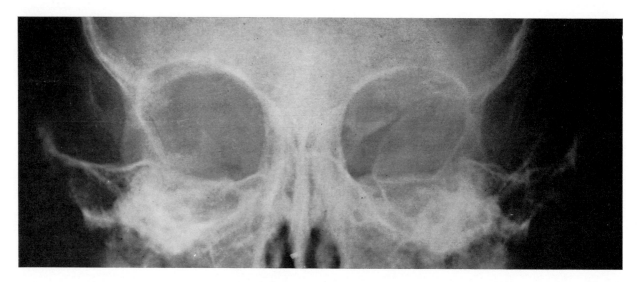

Figure 221. Eosinophil granuloma of the sphenoid wings in a patient aged 3 years who developed thirst and polyuria. Destruction of the lesser wing of the sphenoid is complete and there is also erosion of the greater wing. Note the complete absence of a sclerosed edge of the destruction; this is the rule. Similar lesions were seen in the vault and the clavicle. A biopsy was taken

impossible. The remaining bone may be thin and the edges of a defect therefore ill-defined and not sharply outlined on the radiograph.

Causes

Erosion of the greater wing may result from any of the causes described in the immediately preceding section, but these almost invariably also cause widening of the sphenoid fissure. The following are additional causes for consideration.

CONGENITAL DEFECT (*Figure 303*)

A congenital defect in the greater wing of the sphenoid is sometimes seen; it may be unilateral or bilateral, and may be an isolated phenomenon or accompany neurofibromatosis.

NEUROFIBROMATOSIS

There may be a plexiform neuroma of the orbit with or without orbital expansion. The middle fossa may also be enlarged.

LONG–STANDING RAISED INTRACRANIAL PRESSURE (*Figure 23*)

More or less sharply defined areas of thinning of one, or both, of the greater wings may be seen in patients who have other radiographic evidence of long-standing raised intracranial pressure.

MALIGNANT DEPOSITS (*Figure 220*)

Malignant bone deposits may produce erosions which appear sharply defined as well as those in which the surrounding bone seems infiltrated. If the edge of the erosion is ragged, the diagnosis of a metastatic growth is suggested, but if the erosion is sharp, it may not be possible to distinguish the cause from others in this section. (For systematic reading on malignant disease, turn to page 222.)

XANTHOMA (*Figure 221*)

Xanthomatous deposits and eosinophil granuloma may be found in the greater wing of the sphenoid. Characteristically, they produce clear-cut erosions with little or no surrounding bone sclerosis, and in this situation they look exactly like osteolytic metastatic deposits.

7 INCREASED DENSITY OF THE BASE

Because the bones of the base are more difficult to see than, for instance, those of the vault, and because their structure is more complicated, it is often impossible to make out exact limits to an area of increased density.

Problems of differential diagnosis are therefore liable to present themselves in certain particular situations where the bone is most clearly seen. These areas are the body of the sphenoid (as observed in the lateral radiograph), the sphenoid wings (as seen in the postero-anterior radiograph), and the region of the mastoid air cells and middle ear (in the full axial view).

When such an increase in opacity of the bone is observed in one of these regions, examination of the other radiographs should reveal whether the change is widespread or localized.

A practical approach to the discussion of the differential diagnosis may be made under two main headings: first, a widespread or generalized increase in density of the base of the skull; and secondly, increase in density as observed only in particular localized situations.

WIDESPREAD OR GENERALIZED INCREASE IN DENSITY

PAGET'S DISEASE

In lateral view it may be apparent that the vault of the skull is also affected and a skeletal survey may demonstrate other bones involved. The density of the base tends to obscure its texture, but the bones are always increased in their thickness, and the typical coarse trabeculation of Paget's disease can frequently be observed. The sphenoid and ethmoid sinuses and the air shadows of the mastoid cells disappear in the proliferating bone. Foramina become narrowed but they are, in any case, difficult to see. There may be basilar invagination because of bone softening (*see* page 229). (It is a mistake to think of this deformity only in terms of upward displacement of the odontoid process. The whole of the base of the skull is affected.)

Deafness associated with Paget's disease may be sensineural or conductive, or both. Petasnick (1969) recorded that 12/42 patients showed thickening of the footplate of the stapes but 2/3 with conductive deafness did not have detectable middle-ear changes.

Paget's disease of the base of the skull must be distinguished from fibrous dysplasia which it sometimes resembles: the coarse trabeculation of Paget's disease usually being sufficient to make the distinction. Typical lesions which are probably present elsewhere in the skeleton are also of help in making the diagnosis. (For systematic reading on Paget's disease, turn to page 287.)

FIBROUS DYSPLASIA (*Figure 122, 124*)

Fibrous dysplasia may affect the whole or only part of the base of the skull. The bones appear very much thickened and are either uniformly dense or may show a mixture of areas of increased density with other areas of hypertranslucency. In both instances, the abnormal bone is lacking in trabecular structure and has been described as exhibiting a ground-glass appearance due to semi-translucency — in spite of its great thickness.

If the base is widely affected it is likely that there will also be fibrous dysplasia of the facial bones and perhaps also of the vault. In the polyostotic form the changes will be found elsewhere in the skeleton.

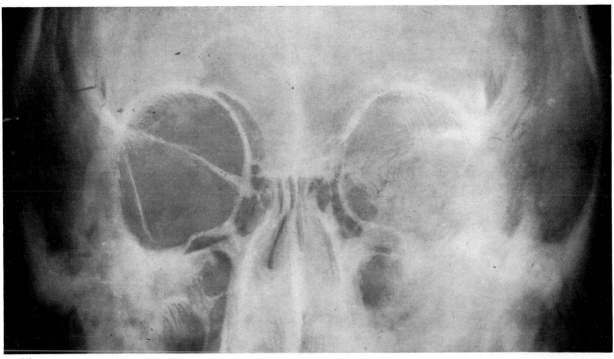

(a)

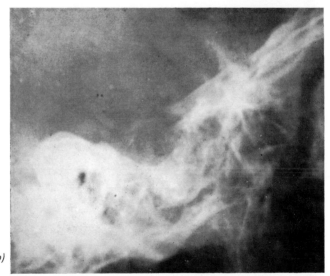

(b)

Figure 222. Meningioma of the middle fossa. This patient had been blind in the left eye for 12 years. The left eye was removed 5 years before these radiographs were taken because of proptosis. She had recently had headaches, suffered from mental deterioration and become drowsy. A large soft meningioma filled the left middle fossa. (a) Postero-anterior view. The greater and lesser wings of the sphenoid show a dense hyperostosis. It contains some trabeculae. The sphenoid fissure is narrowed. The expansion of bone affects half the planum sphenoidale and also the left anterior clinoid process. (b) Lateral view. The texture of the basisphenoid is abnormal. (c) Towne's view. The left petrous bone is denser than the right

(c)

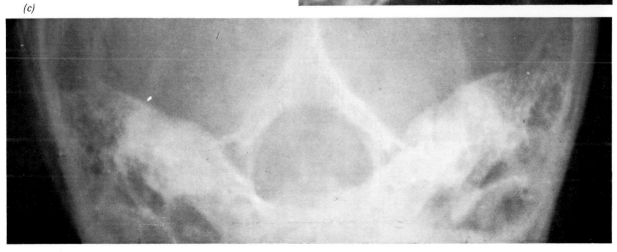

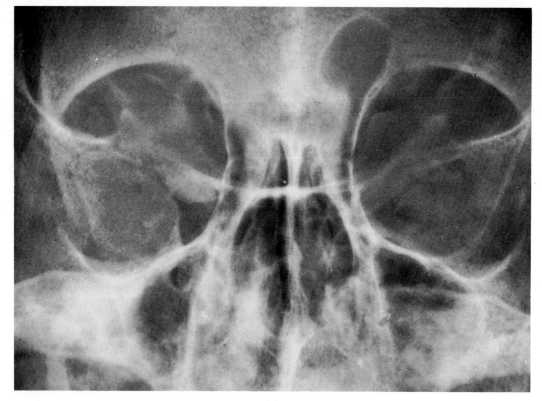

(a)

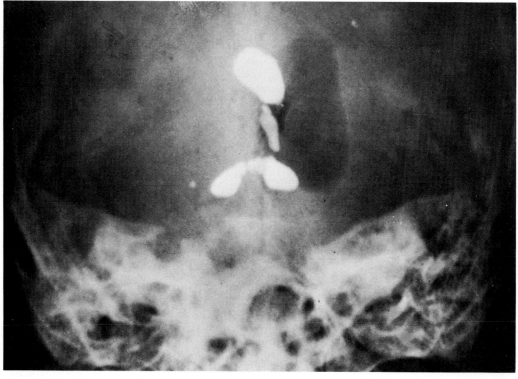

(b)

Figure 223. (a) Right-sided middle fossa meningioma. The combination of hyperostosis of the lesser wing of the sphenoid and expansion of the sphenoid fissure is very characteristic. (b) This tumour extends back as far as the petrous bone which it has eroded. Note the displaced third ventricle and aqueduct outlined with Myodil

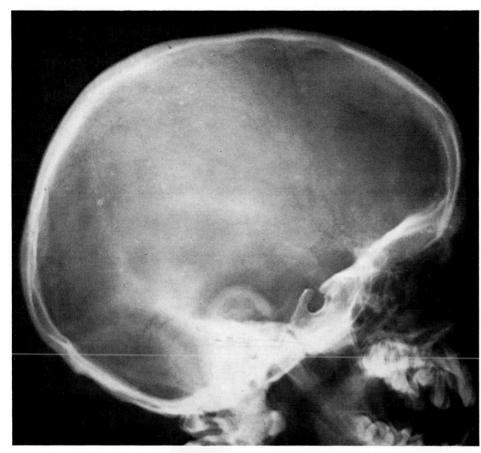

(a)

Figure 224. Osteopetrosis (marble-bone disease) in a child. Although the rest of the skeleton is affected, the vault is unaltered and the base would pass as normal. Severe changes usually take a long time to develop in the skull. (a) Lateral view of the skull. (b) Dorsal spine, ribs and sternum

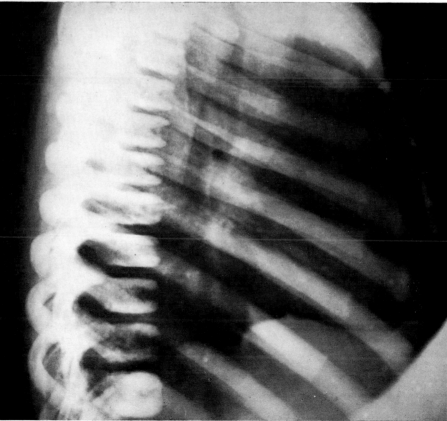

(b)

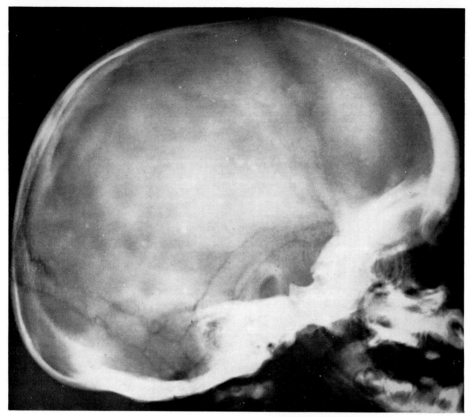

(a)

Figure 225. (a) and (b). Idiopathic hypercalcaemia in an infant, showing the typical skull features of increased bone density. It is most obvious in the base and the upper anterior orbital margins

(Reproduced by courtesy of the Hospital for Sick Children, Great Ormond Street, London)

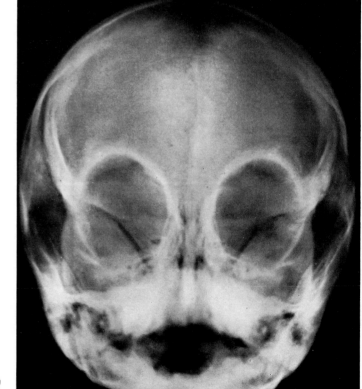

(b)

MENINGIOMA (*Figure 222*)

The hyperostosis due to a meningioma may also be very widespread and involve, for instance, one half of the floor of the middle fossa, including both sphenoid wings on that side, as well as the basi-sphenoid and basi-occiput, but it rarely affects as much of the opposite side.

The bone may be almost uniformly dense or there may also be areas of erosion bordered by hyperostosis, and this leads to confusion with the picture of fibrous dysplasia.

Although the clinical findings often distinguish the two conditions, even very widespread areas of hyperostosis may be associated with meningioma *en plaque* in which evidence of raised intracranial pressure may be absent.

An important differential point between the two is the bone texture. Hyperostosis due to meningioma is usually very dense but may retain a trabecular pattern, while the very greatly expanded bone of fibrous dysplasia is, thickness for thickness, less dense and has no obvious trabeculae. (For systematic reading on meningiomas, turn to page 253.)

NEUROFIBROMATOSIS

The many ways in which neurofibromatosis may affect the skull include thickening with alteration of the architecture of the bones of the base and face. The changes may be widespread but are rarely symmetrical. The bone is dense due to its thickness rather than an increase in the calcium content, and shows coarse trabeculation. There may be involvement of the overlying soft tissues, and there are often other manifestations of the disease.

MARBLE-BONE DISEASE (ALBERS-SCHÖNBERG DISEASE) (*Figures 109, 124*)

Very great generalized increase in density of the base of the skull associated with similar changes in the vault and spine without very much increase in thickness are due to marble-bone disease. The basal foramina are difficult to see through the superimposed dense shadows. They may be narrowed by slight overgrowth of bone. The appearance of the skull in advanced marble-bone disease is characteristic but in the early stages in childhood, when the sclerotic process may be more or less confined to the sphenoid bone, confusion may arise. It is resolved by a skeletal survey.

PROGRESSIVE DIAPHYSEAL DYSPLASIA (ENGLEMANN'S DISEASE)

A high proportion of the children who develop this rare condition exhibit generalized sclerosis of the base of the skull similar to that seen in marble-bone disease. The vault bones are less commonly and less severely affected.

HEREDITARY MULTIPLE DIAPHYSEAL SCLEROSIS (RIBBING'S DISEASE)

This may be the adult form of Englemann's disease which it closely resembles.

CRANIOMETAPHYSEAL DYSPLASIA

This is another very rare condition, discussed more fully in Chapter 11, in which patchy thickening of the bones of the base occurs as well as of the vault. The mastoid air cells and paranasal sinuses disappear.

MELORHEOSTOSIS

Changes in the skull, not invariably present, consist of a rather patchy sclerosis, predominantly of the base. The diagnosis is made by examination of the rest of the skeleton.

TOULOUSE-LAUTREC SYNDROME (PYKNODYSOSTOSIS)

This is more fully described elsewhere in the book (Chapter 11). The base of the skull is thickened. There is non-pneumatization of paranasal sinuses and straightening of the angle of the mandible.

CRETINISM

In cretinism, a moderate increase in the density of the bones of the base may be observed. The vault is thick and the sutures remain open for an abnormal length of time. There is hypoplasia of the paranasal sinuses and of the nasal bones.

TUBERCULOUS OSTEITIS

A few cases of increase in density of the bones of the base have been thought to be due to tuberculous osteitis. This is somewhat remarkable and very unlike the usual behaviour of tuberculosis of bone elsewhere in the skeleton.

VITAMIN D POISONING

Hypervitaminosis D, due either to overdosage or to abnormal vitamin D metabolism, may lead to a generalized increase in bone density of the whole skull. Some patients show premature synostosis of the sutures.

CHRONIC IDIOPATHIC HYPERCALCAEMIA (*Figure 225*)

The skull shows an exactly similar change to that in hypervitaminosis D. The premature fusion of sutures in the base may result in a deformity of the face (elfin facies).

VITAMIN D RESISTANT RICKETS (*Figure 111*)

Under treatment the porotic bones may become dense, and premature fusion of sutures occur.

HYPERPARATHYROIDISM (UNDER TREATMENT)

A patchy but widespread increase in bone density may occur.

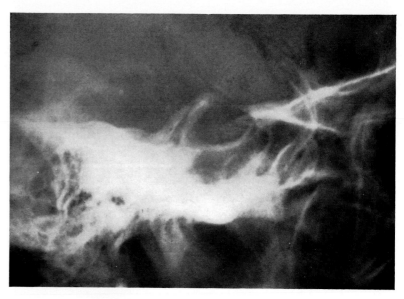

Figure 226. Meningioma in a woman aged 62 years with a history of 20 years of right-sided ptosis. She had had several attacks of giddiness and falling but without loss of consciousness. In the year before admission, investigations revealed an extensive meningioma of the right parasellar region and the floor of the middle fossa, and a partial removal was undertaken. The lateral radiograph shows an increase in density of the whole of the sella. One anterior clinoid is normal but the other is affected. There is also hyperostosis of the clivus and the petroclinoid ligaments are densely ossified. The appearance is typical of a meningioma

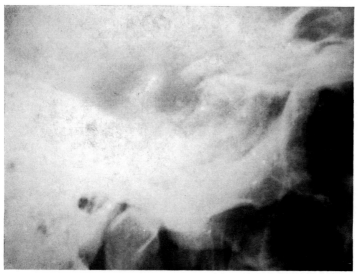

Figure 227. Secondary carcinoma. The primary growth was in the breast. Osteoblastic metastases are uncommon in the skull. Here there is a mixture of sclerosis and erosion which might well be due to a meningioma

RENAL RICKETS (UNDER TREATMENT) (*Figure 112*)

In some of these patients skull changes are seen which may occasionally include increase in density, particularly after treatment.

CHRONIC FLUORINE POISONING

The skull bones also show a rather patchy, slight increase in density in some cases, as do other bones of the skeleton.

INCREASE IN DENSITY OBSERVED ONLY IN PARTICULAR LOCALIZED SITUATIONS

THE REGION AROUND THE SELLA TURCICA

If in the lateral view the bone around the sella turcica is abnormally dense, examination of the other radiographs may show that the pathological change is more or less restricted to the basisphenoid, dorsum sellae and perhaps anterior clinoid processes; or an even more localized

hyperostosis may involve a small part of the planum sphenoidale or be attached to one of the anterior clinoid processes.

Increase in density affecting a large part of the bone around the sella is easy to see, but may be due to several different conditions.

MENINGIOMA (*Figure 226*)

A small, localized hyperostosis is easily overlooked, but when observed almost certainly indicates the presence of a meningioma. A blister-like expansion may sometimes be found extending into the hyperostosis from the subjacent sphenoid sinus. A similar appearance may apparently be seen after a fracture (Bonneville *et al.* 1978). The more widespread type of increase in density may also be due to a meningioma, either *en plaque* or perhaps a massive tumour extending into the middle fossa but other conditions must be considered. (For systematic reading on meningioma, turn to page 253.)

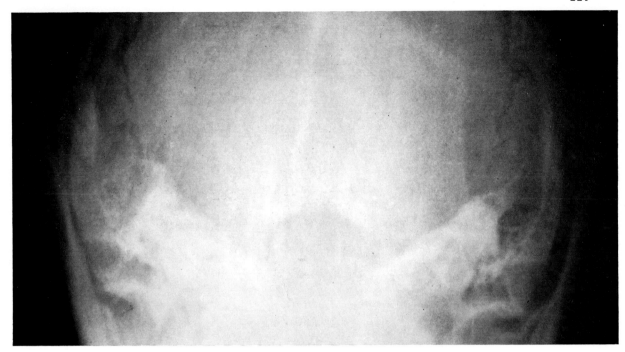

(a)

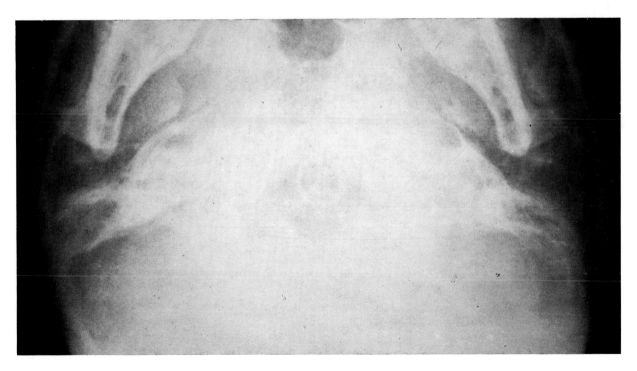

(b)

Figure 228. Acute otitis media. The normal left mastoid is largely diploëtic, although there are a few air cells. On the right side there is a general diminution in translucency of the whole area (including the middle ear). The drum appeared normal. At operation a little thin pus was found in the middle ear. There was no mastoid air cells, and the general opacity must be ascribed to the considerable overlying soft-tissue swelling

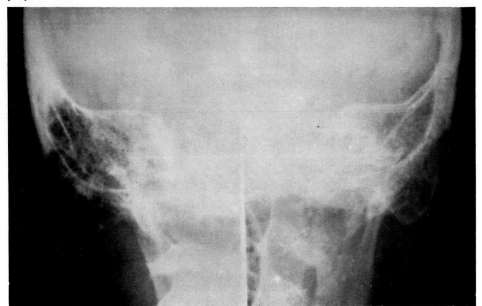

Figure 229. Acute mastoiditis. The air cells in the left mastoid bone have clouded opacity, but their walls are intact. Pus was found in them 3 days later

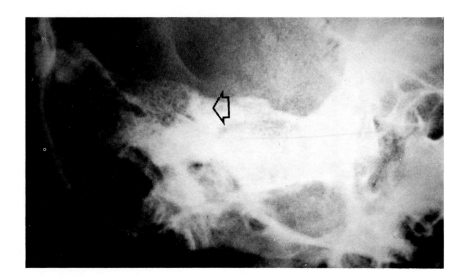

Figure 230. Otosclerosis. There was very severe otosclerosis on both sides. The left ear had been operated on. This view shows the condensed bone around the superior semicircular canal most clearly. Other radiographs showed its extent in the region of the cochlea. It is only in rare and very severe cases that a radiological abnormality may be detected

CHORDOMA (*Figure 200*)

Another possibility where the increase in density though of slight degree is fairly widespread, particularly if there is some associated erosion, is that of a chordoma. Differentiation between meningioma and chordoma on the grounds of the bone appearance may be impossible.

Two much less likely causes of increase in density should also be considered. These are metastatic carcinoma and low-grade chronic inflammatory change.

METASTATIC CARCINOMA (*Figure 227*)

Metastatic carcinoma in the skull generally produces lytic lesions, but from time to time patients are encountered in whom the secondary deposits are osteoblastic. In such cases, rather ill-defined increase in density of the sphenoid bone may be observed in the lateral view; but it is not always easy to see that there are probably similar disseminated metastases elsewhere in the base and in the vault.

LOW-GRADE INFLAMMATORY CHANGES

Very rarely, chronic sinusitis may lead to low-grade inflammatory changes in the bone around the sinuses and this may give the appearance of an increase in density of the sphenoid bone. The sphenoid sinus is almost certain to be opaque and other radiographs will show more widespread disease in the paranasal sinuses.

CHONDROMA

Chondromas occasionally grow from bones of the base, and may involve the region of the sella. They may be recognized by their typical type of calcification, but confusion with chordoma is possible.

THE TEMPORAL BONE

MENINGIOMA *(Figure 199)*

A meningioma, arising from the base of the skull near the tentorial attachment of the petrous bone, usually causes hyperostosis mixed with erosion. Overlying calcification in the tumour or in the tentorium may make it difficult to see details of the affected bone.

ACUTE AND CHRONIC MASTOIDITIS *(Figures 228, 229; see also page 196)*

Diploëtic mastoids throw a denser shadow than those which are cellular.

The degree of development of the air cells in a normal person is usually the same on the two sides of the head; but a history of long-standing infection in one ear is almost invariably accompanied by the presence of less well-developed cells and denser bone. Sclerosis and replacement of air in any remaining cells and in the middle ear by pus, oedema or fibrous tissue tends to mask areas of bone destruction.

Acute mastoid infection also causes an increase in opacity due to swelling of the mucosa, and if there is accumulation of mucus and pus in the larger mastoid air cells and in the middle ear they have a veiled look of semi-translucency, but oedema of the overlying soft tissue tends to exaggerate the increase in density.

In considering acute and chronic mastoid-cell infection the following points may be remembered.
(1) Acute mastoiditis is rather less likely to follow middle-ear disease in the diploëtic than in the cellular type.
(2) When, however, acute mastoiditis does occur in the diploëtic type, it is probably more likely to lead to intracranial infection by spreading through the bone.
(3) Chronic mastoiditis is very unlikely to be found in patients who have well-pneumatized temporal bones.

Valuable information may be given the surgeon by an examination of the radiographs. Points to note are as follows.
(1) The general shape of the bone and the distance between the sigmoid sinus plate and the anterior margin of the petrous in the lateral view.

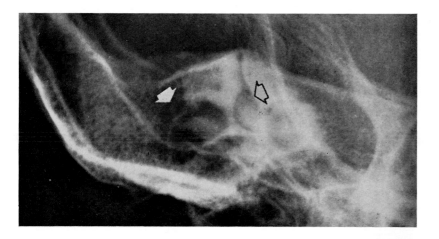

(a)

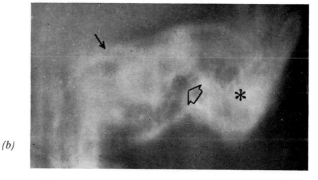

(b)

Figure 231. Congenital abnormality of the ears in a child aged 2 years whose mother had taken thalidomide. and who was born with atresia of the external auditory meatuses and deficiency of the pinnae. She was almost completely deaf and had facial weakness. (a) Right, Stenver's view shows an enormous lateral semi-circular canal (closed arrow). The vestibule is also large (open arrow). The superior semi-circular canal is more normal. There appeared to be a slit-like middle-ear cavity with abnormal ossicles. The internal auditory meatus was extremely narrow but the cochlear was present. (b) Antero-posterior tomogram on left side. There is a small very deeply placed middle-ear (open arrow) cavity. Other cuts showed an ossicular mass, possibly fused to the anterior wall of the cavity, while others showed clearly some features only dimly seen here—the very narrow internal auditory meatus (small arrow), the normal superior semi-circular canal, the short blunt lateral semi-circular canal, and the cochlear. There is a huge atretic plate (asterisk). The plain radiographs were also of the greatest importance in defining the position of the middle ear and the labyrinth

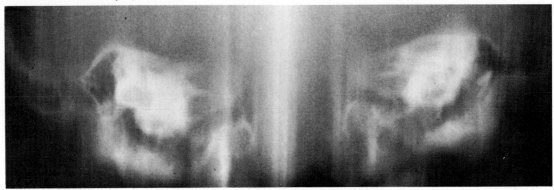

Figure 232. On the right side the vestibule and lateral semi-circular canal make one large cavity. There is probably a small round window. There was a double I.A.M. and malformation of the ossicular chain on the left side. The duplication of the I.A.M. is shown in the cut as well as a deformed incus

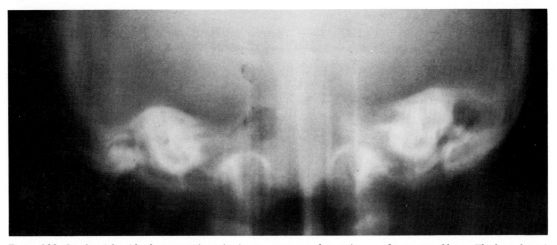

Figure 233. On the right side the tympanic cavity is very narrow and contains two fragments of bone. The lateral semi-circular canal is short. The I.A.M. is double. On the left side the thick atretic plate is shown as well as the abnormalities. There is no oval window. Note the facial canal

(2) The extent of cells — zygomatic, mastoid tip, peritympanic and perhaps petrous tip — and the distribution of those which are opaque.

(3) The extent of any erosion which may be present and, if possible, something about its nature.

(4) Whether there is definite destruction of the ossicles.

(5) The position of the facial canal. The vertical portion is usually visible in the full axial view, and it may be seen in part of its course in other views also.

(6) Opacity in the region of the external auditory meatus which may be due to a small osteoma or occasionally a more severe stenosis following infection or trauma.

OSTEOMA (*Figure 127*)

A well-defined, dense excrescence from the petrous bone may be an osteoma. It usually lies behind the pinna. The texture of the bone can only be appreciated when a tangential view is obtained because of the superimposition of other shadows in most of the routine radiographs. The diagnosis is made clinically, most patients complaining of the presence of a hard bony lump, and the radiographs serve only to confirm the diagnosis and establish the position of the osteoma. Such tumours are not common

but are also occasionally seen arising within the external auditory meatus and from other bones of the base (for example, in the pterygoid region).

CONGENITAL ABNORMALITIES

Opacity in the region of the external auditory meatus (as seen in the full axial, the lateral and the per-orbital views) may be due to congenital absence of the bony meatus. Congenital atresia of the bony meatus will be accompanied by abnormal position or development of surrounding structures such as the temporo-mandibular joint. The importance of radiology in congenital atresia, either bony or fibrous, is that it allows the surgeon a pre-operative examination of the structure of the middle and inner ear, which may, in fact, be normal. Advances in surgery now allow the correction of some congenital defects and a very detailed examination is demanded. The ossicles and labyrinth are best shown by a very high definition technique combined with tomography by special apparatus.

The most important elements of the technique are a short object-film distance, a very fine focus (usually 0.3 mm) and absolute immobility of the head (requiring

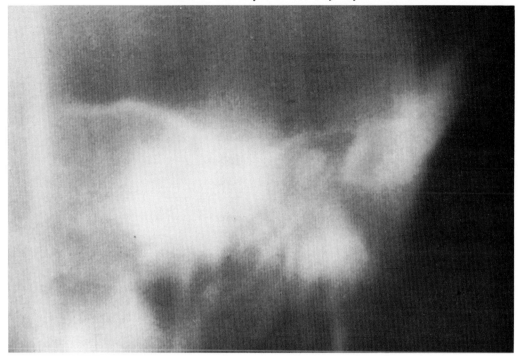

Figure 234. A deformed mass of ossicular tissue and a thin atretic plate

anaesthesia or heavy sedation in infants and young children).

There are several tomographic apparatuses available which are capable of producing adequate films. Some are better than others and a hypercycloidal movement, although not essential, may sometimes be very helpful. A great deal of information may, however, be obtained with linear movements only. A wide arc is essential (of the order of 50 degrees) and it is most important to have cuts spaced very close together in the region of the ossicles and labyrinth (2 or 3 mm apart at most). The 0.3 mm focus is used whenever possible.

Points of importance are as follows.

(1) Are the incus and malleus present, of normal shape, or are they represented by a shapeless mass of bone (the stapes cannot always be identified)?

(2) Is there a pharyngo-tympanic tube?

(3) What is the exact relationship of the facial canal to the middle ear?

(4) How well are the semi-circular canals developed? The lateral one, for instance, may form a large cavity which may be inadvertently perforated at operation, or deliberately fenestrated.

(5) Is the vestibule in a normal position of absent? Is the oval window identifiable?

(6) Is the cochlear of normal size, small or absent altogether?

(7) What is the state and size of the internal auditory meatus?

In order to answer these questions, multiple projections will be required. The most useful plain radiographs are the full axial, the Stenver's view, the lateral oblique

and the per-orbital. The most useful tomographic positions are the antero-posterior, the Stenver's position and the lateral.

SPHENOID WINGS

Asymmetry of shape and inequality of density of the sphenoid wings as seen in the postero-anterior projection in the normal subject is discussed in the chapter devoted to erosions of the base, and will not be repeated here in detail. Unless there is an alteration of texture of the bone, in addition to the increase of opacity, it is unwise to pay much attention to the asymmetry. If, however, the bone texture is not normal and the patient's symptoms suggest the possibility of a lesion on the side on which an increase in opacity has been observed, the following two conditions must be borne in mind.

MENINGIOMA (*Figures 235, 237, 238*)

Hyperostosis due to a meningioma may affect the lesser wing of the sphenoid alone. Sometimes the increase in opacity involves the greater wing of the sphenoid as well, but it is uncommon to see the greater wing affected while the lesser wing remains normal. Occasionally, a very small hyperostosis near the base of one anterior clinoid process may be seen through the ethmoid sinuses, but the presence of such an hyperostosis should be confirmed in the lateral view.

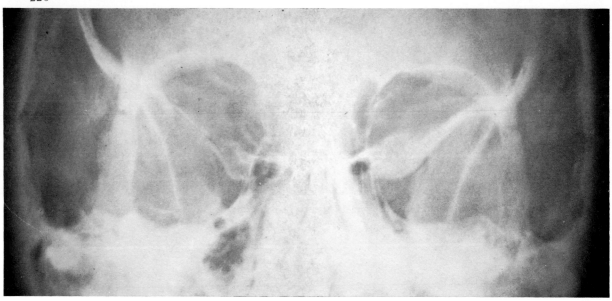

Figure 235. Meningioma in a woman aged 52 years. There was a history of 12 months' pain in the left eye and 4 months proptosis. An extensive flat tumour covered the whole sphenoid ridge and disappeared beyond the midline. The extent of the hyperostosis does not necessarily indicate the extent of the intracranial tumour, nor can the distinction be drawn between a massive meningioma and a meningioma en plaque

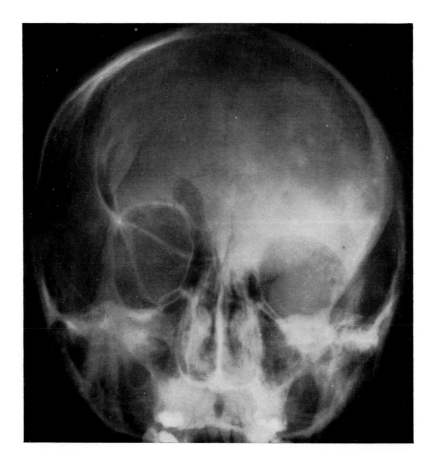

Figure 236. Fibrous dysplasia. The bone is expanded and dense but not with the opacity of ivory bone. There are a few translucent areas. The diseased regions appear structureless

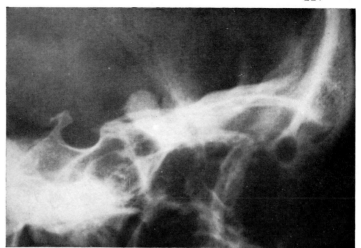

(a)

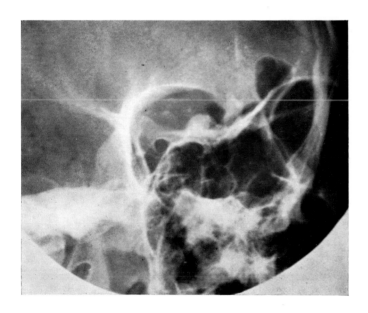

(b)

Figure 237. Meningioma in a woman aged 50 years who for 3 years had noticed visual deterioration and was found to have a defect in the temporal half and part of the upper nasal quadrant of the left visual field. There is a dense hyperostosis of the base of the left anterior clinoid and around the upper part of the optic canal. The tumour was about 1½ inches in diameter. (a) Lateral view. (b) and (c) Right and left ethmoid sinus views

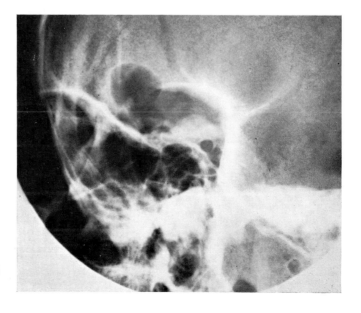

(c)

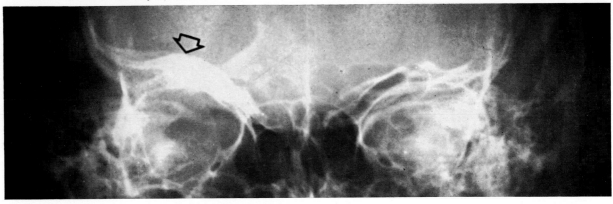

*Figure 238. Meningioma of the orbital plate of the frontal bone in a woman aged 61 years. Notice that the hyperostosis contains trabeculae.
A well-defined architecture may or may not be present in the bone affected by a meningioma, but is never seen in fibrous dysplasia*

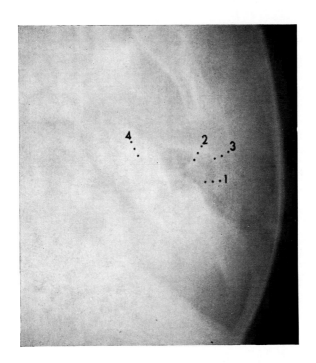

Figure 239. The normal middle ear. 1. The short process of the incus. 2. The head of the malleus. 3. The lateral wall of the epitympanic recess. 4. The cochlear

Hyperostosis of the lesser and greater wings of the sphenoid due to meningioma has the characteristics of hyperostosis elsewhere. The bone may be very dense. It sometimes contains a number of recognizable trabeculae and is usually increased in size, perhaps at the expense of the superior orbital fissure. The extent of the hyperostosis does not necessarily indicate the extent of the intracranial tumour, nor can the distinction be drawn between a massive meningioma and a meningioma *en plaque*.

FIBROUS DYSPLASIA (*Figure 121, 236*)

An increase in the density due to fibrous dysplasia of the sphenoid wings is usually less marked than the increase in density due to meningioma, although the bone may be more enlarged. The texture of the diseased bone is completely abnormal and there are no visible trabeculae. If the sphenoid bone is affected, there is often also a much more widespread change in the bones of the base. Fibrous dysplasia of the sphenoid wings is far less common than meningioma.

8 ABNORMALITIES OF THE SIZE AND SHAPE OF THE BASE

The plan adopted here is to discuss: (1) basilar impression and related conditions; (2) asymmetry due to any cause; (3) overgrowth of part or the whole base other than that which produces asymmetry; and (4) deficient growth.

BASILAR IMPRESSION AND RELATED CONDITIONS

Basilar impression (*Figures 99, 240–244*)

Basilar impression consists of an upward displacement of the bones of the base around the foramen magnum so that to a greater or lesser extent they invaginate the cavity of the skull. The deformity may be congenital (primary) in which cases it is likely to be complicated by the presence of other bony abnormalities, or acquired (secondary) due to bone softening.

In the normal skull, an almost completely smooth curved surface is presented by the clivus and the anterior part of the upper cervical canal. The foramen magnum and the spaces above and below it permit a certain amount of play for the brainstem during movements of the head upon the neck. The cerebellar tonsils do not protrude below the plane of the foramen magnum.

Basilar impression may disturb all these relationships and therefore result in a variety of symptoms due to restriction of movement or actual compression of the upper cervical cord or medulla. There may be interference with the function of the cerebellum and there may also be signs probably resulting from the distortion and elongation of cranial nerves.

Small degrees of basilar impression usually affect the antero-lateral parts of the foramen magnum. In more severe degrees there is also a marked upward and inward displacement of the posterior edge of the foramen. Deformity is likely to result in upward displacement of the medial ends of the petrous bones, and this may be recognized in the Towne's and postero-anterior radiographs.

It should be remembered that the normal has wide variations and, in the absence of symptoms, some discretion has to be exercised in the diagnosis of mild degrees of basilar impression. There are two salient features which help in its recognition, and a large number of measurements may be made which will demonstrate the degree of the impression. The two features by which basilar impression is usually recognized are: *in the lateral radiograph* – (1) an abnormally high position of the odontoid peg in relation to the base of the skull, and *in the postero-anterior projection* – (2) the displacement upwards, well above the horizontal plane, of the medial parts of the petrous bones.

As a measurement of the degree of basilar impression in more extreme cases, McGregor's modification of Chamberlain's line is often of value. Chamberlain's line joins the posterior margin of the hard palate to the posterior lip of the foramen magnum. McGregor's line is drawn (on a lateral radiograph centred over the atlanto-occipital articulation) starting from the posterior edge of the hard palate and passing at a tangent to the lowest point of the occipital bone. As a rough guide, the tip of the odontoid should not lie above Chamberlain's line. It should not protrude more than about 6 mm above McGregor's line, and frequently lies below it.

Numerous other measurements have been described, but the idea of basilar impression as an entity rather than one of the features of a complex developmental anomaly should not be so emphasized. Foramen magnum stenosis is probably the most important single feature of these congenital anomalies.

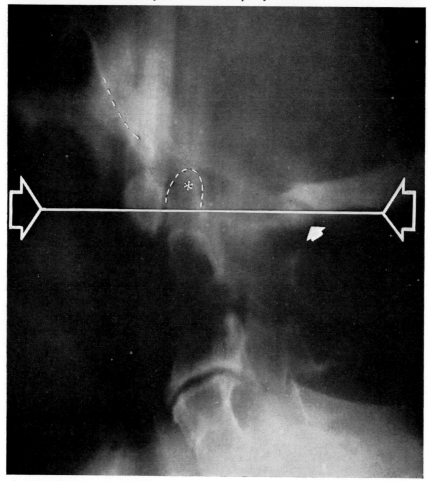

Figure 240. Basilar impression. A lateral tomogram shows that not only is the odontoid process (asterisk) high in relation to the modified Chamberlain line (→————←) but it encroaches slightly on what should be a smooth curve running from the clivus into the cervical canal. The foramen magnum is somewhat smaller than normal. Associated congenital abnormalities in this case are fusion of C 4 and 5 and C 6 and 7 with a lower cervical spina bifida. The two halves of the posterior arch of the atlas (closed arrow) have not fused with each other, and lie close to the occipital bone. There is disc degeneration and arthritis

CONGENITAL

Congenital (primary) basilar impression is found only occasionally as an isolated abnormality. Usually it is seen in association with one or more of the following additional defects. (*a*) Failure of fusion of the posterior arch of the atlas; (*b*) assimilation of part or the whole of the atlas to be occiput; (*c*) Klippel–Feil deformity; (*d*) atlanto-axial dislocation with or without congenital separation of the odontoid; and (*e*) stenosis of the foramen magnum.

Many other defects are seen from time to time.

ARNOLD–CHIARI MALFORMATION

All the abnormalities may be found in association with Chiari and Arnold–Chiari malformations. The latter (also known as Chiari Type 2) is found in the presence of a meningocoele and bone defects at the occipito-cervical region may be very gross. There may be signs of hydrocephalus. Chiari Type 1 malformation is largely confined to the cerebellar tonsils which are elongated into the cervical canal. Bone abnormalities may be completely absent or very slight. Enlargement of the foramen magnum is the commonest. Kruyff and Jeffs (1966) also described scalloping of the postero-medial aspects of the petrous bones. Hydrocephalus is uncommon.

ACQUIRED

Acquired or secondary basilar impression may result from: (*a*) Paget's disease; (*b*) renal rickets and hyperparathyroidism; (*c*) osteogenesis imperfecta; (*d*) the delayed or defective ossification accompanying chondro-osteodystrophy and cleidocranial dysostosis; and (*e*) severe and usually fatal trauma.

Other causes of basilar impression have also been mentioned in the literature, but there is doubt about the criteria upon which the diagnosis has been made in cases of rickets, senile osteoporosis, and in cretinism as well as in chronic hydrocephalus.

In order to arrive at a diagnosis, a routine skull radiograph may be supplemented by a lateral view centred at the atlanto-occipital junction, but in both primary and secondary basilar impression a full demonstration of the anatomy of the region may only be possible after tomography in both the sagittal and coronal planes.

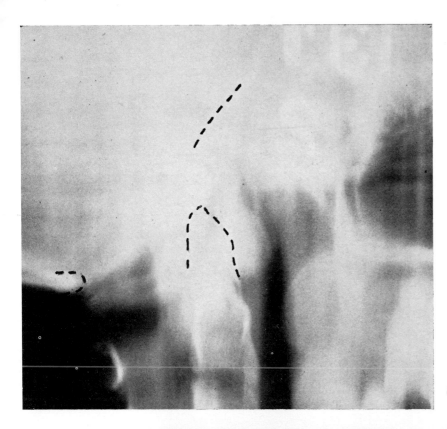

Figure 241. Basilar impression. (a) Although the odontoid process lies well above the Chamberlain line, the smooth curve of the clivus and upper cervical canal is not encroached upon. (b) In the half axial projection the petrous bones (particularly the right one) point in an abnormally horizontal direction. The patient suffered from tinnitus, headache, cerebellar ataxia and mild long-tract signs. At operation there was very little abnormal posteriorly. Anteriorly there was more invagination. No C 1 posterior root was present and the posterior root of C 2 coursed downwards at a much more oblique angle than normal

(a)

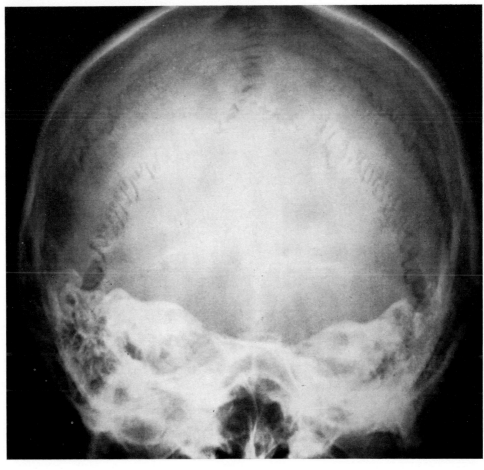

(b)

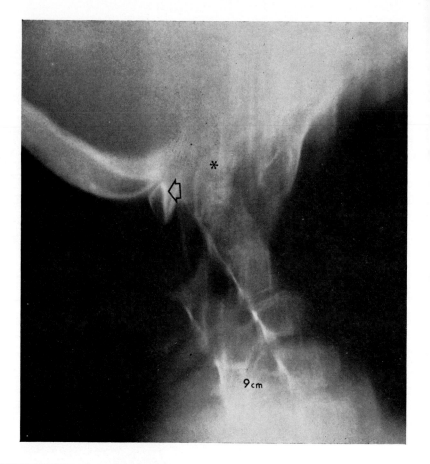

(a)

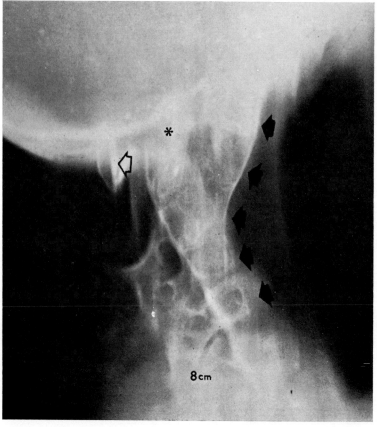

(b)

Figure 242. Occipitalization of the atlas in a boy aged 13 years with life-long torticollis. He had been paraplegic since an injury, but did very well after a decompressive and corrective operation. (a) The lateral tomogram shows the deformed posterior arch of the atlas (arrow) close to the occiput to which it was partly fused by fibrous tissue and by bone. The anterior arch of the atlas, the body of C 2 vertebra and the basi-occiput form a single segmented bar which is also fused to C 3 and C 4 (closed arrows in (b)). The odontoid appears to lie in the centre of the foramen magnum in this view; but (b) in reality is far over to the left

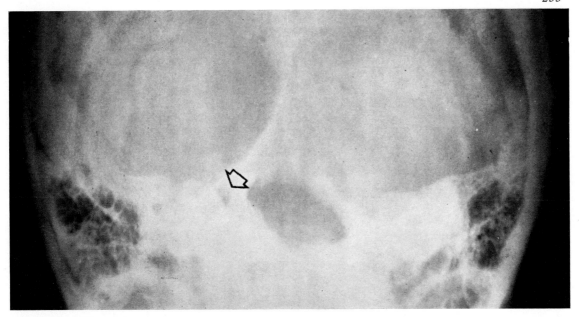

(a)

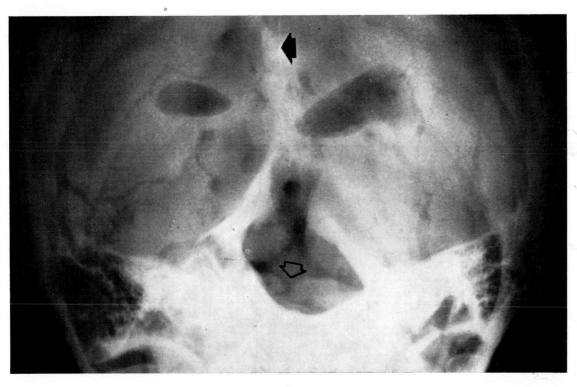

(b)

Figure 243. Developmental asymmetry of the foramen magnum and the posterior fossa. The patient, aged 40 years, had a history of left occipital pain and paraesthesia in the distribution of the left fifth nerve, mild deafness in the left ear and frequent vertigo. On examination, in addition to impaired sensation in the left fifth nerve and C 2 distribution there was mild ataxia. Contrast examinations were all negative. (a) There is elevation and flattening of the right side of the foramen magnum. (A well-formed posterior condylar foramen (open arrow) is present on this side.) (b) One film taken during encephalography. An unfused posterior arch of the atlas is shown (open arrow). The falx is seen edge on proving that the view is straight (closed arrow)

234

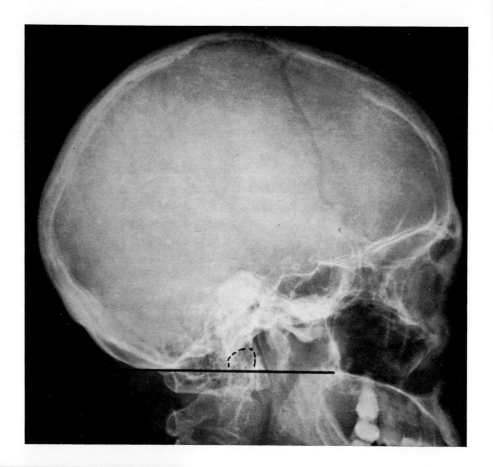

(a)

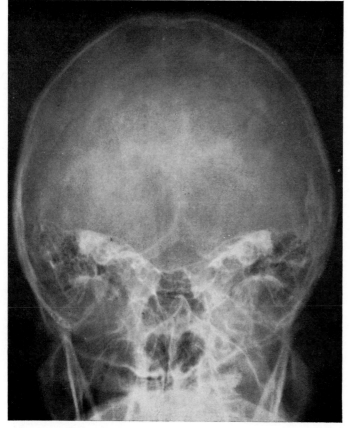

(b)

Figure 244. Osteogenesis imperfecta, adult. A mild case, unrecognized until the age of 64 years when the skull was examined for some other purpose. She has basilar invagination (McGregor's modification of Chamberlain's line has been drawn). The bones are thin, lacking in trabeculae and therefore translucent. (a) Lateral view, (b) Towne's view. Note the elevation of the medial ends of the petrous bones

The term basilar 'invagination' is also used to describe this condition and may be considered an exact synonym. Some confusion is also caused by the use of the word 'platybasia'. It seems better, as McGregor suggested, to reserve the term 'platybasia' for the deformity described in the next section.

Platybasia

The term 'platybasia' has often been used as an alternative to basilar impression, but it probably better described the condition in which the floor of the anterior fossa and the clivus make an angle which approaches 180 degrees. Platybasia in this sense may accompany basilar impression but it is not always present, even in severe degrees of the condition, and it may be present as an isolated deformity. It is frequently a normal variant and of itself is of no clinical significance.

Boogaard, who in 1865 described most of the features of basilar impression, also proposed an angle by which the degree of flattening of the base of the skull might be measured. Boogaard's angle remains the most satisfactory criterion of platybasia. It is measured on the lateral radiograph and is the angle formed at the centre of the pituitary fossa between lines running to the nasion and to the anterior lip of the foramen magnum. Subsequent workers have drawn these lines with slight variations and the point of the angle has been placed on the tuberculum sellae and on the top of the dorsum sellae. Whichever variant is used, there is a wide range of normal values, but an angle greater than 143 degrees is generally considered abnormal.

Other congenital abnormalities around the foramen magnum

As elsewhere, severe congenital abnormalities tend to occur together. Logically the abnormalities of the skull base may be grouped like those at other transitional regions of the spine into those which are assimilations of atlas to occiput and those due to incomplete development of extraspinal elements. On the one hand are found all degrees of atlanto-occipital fusion, and on the other partial or complete segmentation of the basi-occiput, and the group of abnormalities which are described under the general heading of 'Manifestations of the occipital vertebra', that is to say, the third condyle, the paracondyloid process, the basilar processes and other accessory detached or fused bone elements between atlas and occiput. Anatomical variants also include the inconstant posterior condylar foramen, which may be mistaken for an erosion when seen in the Towne's view. Irregularities of the posterior margin of the foramen magnum are sometimes seen and may be explained as minor developmental abnormalities.

PERSISTENT CRANIOPHARYNGEAL CANAL

The oblique line representing this passing through the sphenoid to the sella is seen in 1 per cent of neonates (Lowman, Robinson and McAllister, 1966).

ASYMMETRY

Postural asymmetry (*Figure 131*)

This is described more fully in the chapter devoted to abnormalities of shape of the vault.

The base of the skull is involved in the general asymmetry, but the volumes of the two halves of the head remain equal. Postural asymmetry resulting from scoliosis beginning early in life is a cause of severe distortion of the base.

Cerebral hemiatrophy (*Figures 132–134*)

In severe degrees of hemiatrophy the deficient growth stimulus from the atrophic hemisphere is responsible for asymmetry of the base as well as for the small size of the affected half of the vault. The petrous bone on the abnormal side is higher than on the other. The middle fossa may be shallower and there may also be an unusually large frontal sinus on the same side. All of these asymmetrical features contribute to the smallness of the affected half of the head.

Plagiocephaly

The primary cause and greatest manifestation is in the vault. The base may show compensatory changes in shape (*see* page 133).

OVERGROWTH

Hydrocephalus

In severe hydrocephalus beginning in infancy or childhood, there may be overgrowth of the skull base to carry the increase in size of the vault with alteration in the shape of the sella, depression of the mid-part of the floor of the anterior fossa and perhaps platybasia. The squamous occipital bone may occasionally bulge downwards to mimic basilar impression.

Ocular hypertelorism (*Figures 11, 24, 245, 328*)

It is an elementary axiom in portraiture that 'the distance between the eyes has the width of an eye'. The term 'ocular hypertelorism' literally means that the eyes are too far apart, and has been used to describe a wide variety of cases in which the eyes may be laterally displaced. It has also been used as a descriptive term for those normal variations from the average in which the eyes lie further apart than an eye's width, but in whom there is no evidence of a pathological cause.

However, the term 'ocular hypertelorism' was originally coined to describe 2 cases of gross deformity of the skull in mental defectives in whom one of the most striking features was the great width between the orbits. Other features included increased depth of the anterior fossa, brachicephaly associated with overgrowth of the lesser wings of the sphenoid and a persistent craniopharyngeal canal. In the absence of a description of the

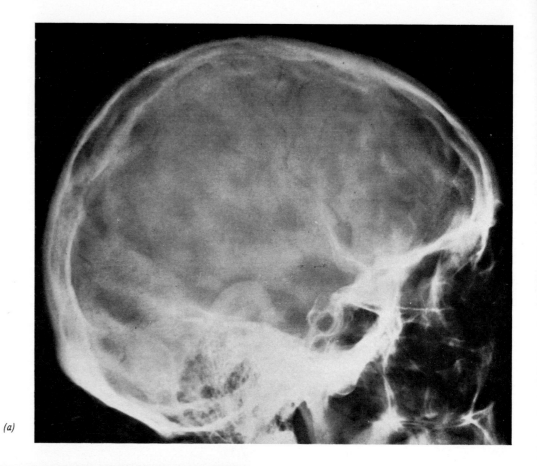

(a)

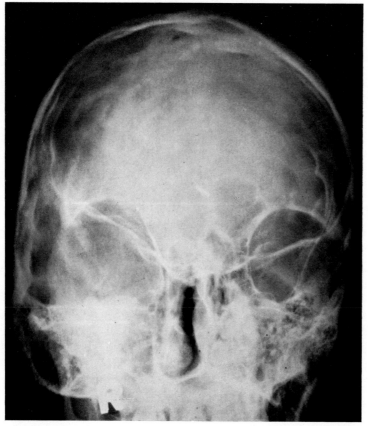

Figure 245 (a) and (b). Hypertelorism (a clinical diagnosis). Cause unknown, but note that the cranium is small and the sagittal and coronal sutures are fused

(b)

cranial contents in these cases, the nature of any associated cerebral deformity remains in doubt.

Hypertelorism has been precisely defined as a distance between the lamina papyracea of the orbit on a postero-anterior film taken at 100 cm F.F.D. of more than 2–3 cm. It has to be distinguished from telecanthus, in which only the medial canthus, rather than the orbit or the eye, is laterally displaced.

Hypertelorism accompanies other facial abnormalities in the syndromes of median cleft nose, prolabium and premaxilla. In these cases there is cranium bifidum occultum frontalis and there may be a superficial midline lipoma. Mental defect in this syndrome is uncommon.

Frontal dermoids, lipomas and teratomas, and occasionally other tumours, may be more deeply placed between the orbits and involve the anterior fossa. The skull radiographs should be examined carefully in cases in which the eyes appear too far apart for signs of such midline tumours. Chronic hydrocephalus and craniostenosis of the coronal suture may produce a superficially similar deformity, so may an anterior meningocoele. Fibrous dysplasia of midline structures has been known to push the eyes apart.

Hypertelorism is also a feature of several named syndromes, for instance, familiar metaphyseal dysplasia (Pyle's disease) and 'bird headed' dwarfism. Lateral displacement of the epicanthal folds, as in mongolism, may give a false impression of hypertelorism, even in hypoteloric cases.

Craniostenosis

Primary craniostenosis of the vault, oxycephaly and scaphocephaly cause secondary changes of shape of the skull base that may be classified as overgrowth, determined in childhood by the brain's advancing size. Somewhere the skull has to expand. Overgrowth may not, of course, be possible when craniostenosis is part of a more generalized condition involving premature fusion of basal sutures too.

DEFICIENT GROWTH

The bones of the base of the skull and face are likely to be hypoplastic in all forms of dwarfism, and in the following conditions, most of which are dealt with more fully in Chapter 11.

Gargoylism (Hurler's syndrome, dysostosis multiplex) (*Figures 246, 247*)

The skull is sometimes normal in other mucopolysaccharidoses. There is often considerable disproportion between the base and the vault because of the enlargement of the calvaria, particularly when hydrocephalus is present. Depression of the sulcus chiasmaticus gives the appearance of a long, flat sella in the lateral view. There may be true enlargement of the sella turcica in those patients who have hydrocephalus.

Chondro-osteodystrophy (*Figure 249*) Morquio-Ulbrich's disease (keratosulphate is found in the urine), Morquio-Brailsford disease (this may represent a mixed group)

The skull is generally normal, but occasionally there may be platybasia and basilar impression. Hydrocephalus has been described as a complication of the picture.

Achondroplasia (*Figure 248*)

All the bones of the base are underdeveloped and premature synostosis of the occipito-sphenoid suture occurs. The vault is of normal size and of brachicephalic shape. The appearance, therefore, somewhat resembles that seen in hydrocephalus. True hydrocephalus also occurs, and is believed to be associated with stenosis of the foramen magnum due to premature fusion of the ex-occipital and supra-occipital portions of the occipital bone.

Thanatophoric dwarfism

This is a severe and invariably fatal form of dwarfism in which the skull base is shortened. The root of the nose is depressed and the frontal bone appears to bulge.

Achondrogenesis

The skull is similar to that of a thanatophoric dwarf, but the skeletal ossification is extremely retarded.

Crouzon's disease (craniofacial dysostosis)

This name is probably best reserved for those cases of craniostenosis of the vault in which there is also extreme facial bone hypoplasia, but in which there are no limb abnormalities. The combination of craniostenosis and facial bone hypoplasia may cause such difficulties for the growing brain that the orbits are forced to grow apart (hypertelorism), the optic nerve may be stretched and possibly compressed.

Acrocephalosyndactyly (Apert)

This condition adds syndactyly to the syndrome of craniofacial dysostosis.

Acrocephalopolysyndactyly

This also adds polydactyly. The skull abnormality may be mild.

Orbital hypotelorism with arrhinencephaly and trigonocephaly

There is a whole spectrum of deformities which, at their least, consist of no more than narrowing of the interorbital distance because of early fusion of the metopic suture, and scarcely merit inclusion in this chapter. This mild abnormality is hypotelorism alone.

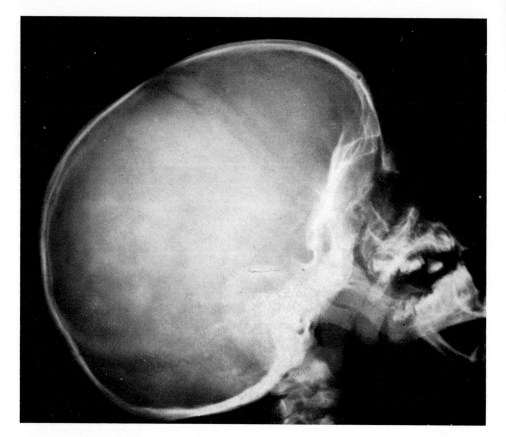

Figure 246. Gargoyle. In about 25 per cent of cases of gargoylism the head is not enlarged. This was a child aged 13 months without evidence of hydrocephalus but with Hurler's syndrome. Note the convolutional impressions restricted to the posterior part of the head, suggesting that the child usually lies on its back

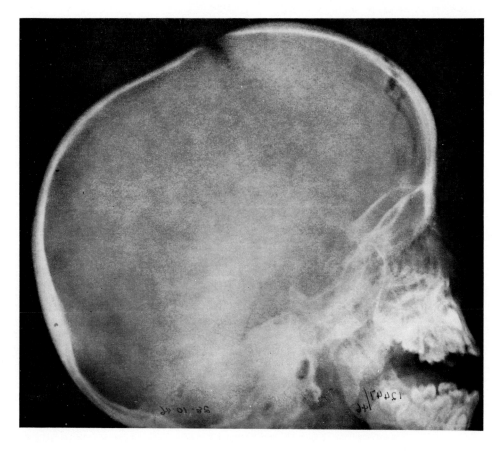

Figure 247. Gargoyle. A typical abnormal skull. The head is large, but in spite of some evidence of hydrocephalus the vault is thick. In the frontal bone there are some prominent venous channels—a common accompaniment of gargoylism

(Reproduced by courtesy of The Governors of the Hospital for Sick Children, Great Ormond Street, London)

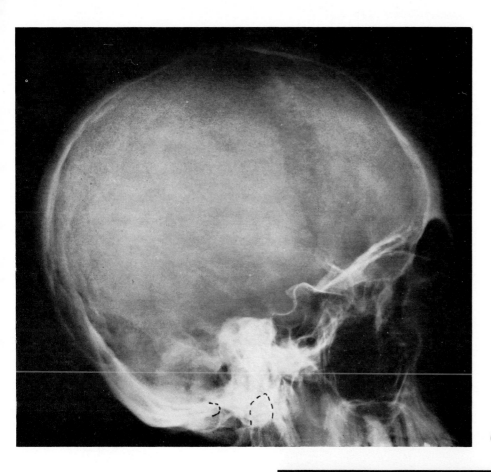

(a)

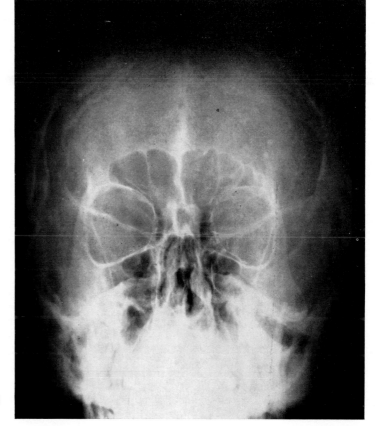

Figure 248. Achondroplasia. The vault is large, the base mildly hypoplastic. This is the typical appearance of achondroplasia. Some cases are complicated by hydrocephalus, which is said to be associated with stenosis of the foramen magnum. In this patient hydrocephalus was probably present. There is basilar invagination and the foramen magnum is small. (a) Lateral view. The odontoid and the posterior lip of the foramen magnum have been outlined. The clivus is short. Extreme pneumatization masks the fact that parts of the maxilla and the basi-occiput are small. (b) Postero-anterior view. Note the upward tilt of the petrous bones resulting from hypoplasia of the occipital bone and indicating the degree of basilar invagination

(b)

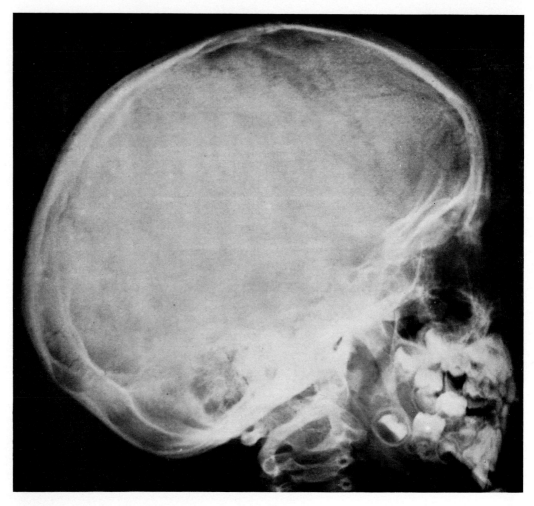

Figure 249. Chondro-osteodystrophy (Morquio type). Occasionally, as in this case, there is some basilar invagination. Usually the skull is normal

Reproduced by courtesy of The Governors of The Hospital for Sick Children, Great Ormond Street, London)

The next severer form, which includes neurological abnormality, is arrhinencephaly with trigonocephaly. To early closure of the metopic suture are added microphthalmia, absence of the olfactory nerve and a rudimentary fore-brain. Trigonocephaly should alert the observer to the possibility of associated fore-brain abnormality, so that the manifestations of trigonocephaly may usefully be mentioned here. They are, in addition to hypotelorism, a small anterior fossa with a dense, beaked anterior ridge at the site of the metopic suture.

More severe still are arrhinencephaly with lateral cleft lip and palate; arrhinencephaly with medial cleft lip; cebocephaly (a rudimentary nose and possibly anophthalmia); ethmocephaly (absence of the nose); cyclopia in which the orbits are actually fused.

Dyscephalia mandibulo-oculo-facialis (Hallerman–Streiff syndrome)

There may be many associated abnormalities (Francois, 1958; Hoefnagel and Benirschke, 1965). The patients have large skulls, delayed closure of the anterior fontanelle and sutures, flattened skull bases and increased convolutional markings. The face, on the other hand, is small and malformed, small nose, small mouth, sometimes absent temporo-mandibular joints, maleruption and sometimes premature eruption of teeth.

Dwarfism is usual and the children may show localized baldness, microphthalmic congenital cataract, nystagmus, squint, motor and mental retardation, underdevelopment of the external genitalia.

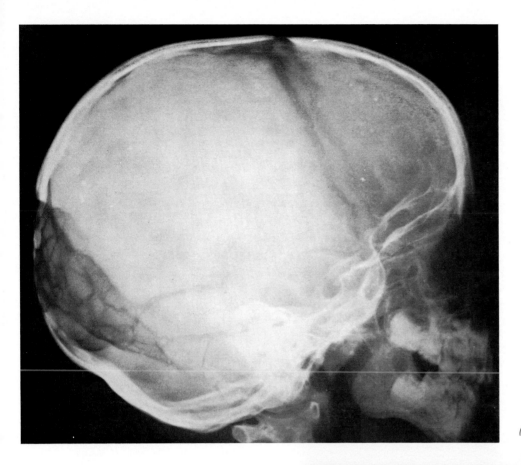

(a)

Figure 250 (a) and (b). Cleidocranial dysostosis in a child aged 3½ years who presented with difficulty in biting due to underdevelopment of the mandible. The clavicles were represented by disorganized bone islands, and there are also metaphyseal deformities in long bones. The skull shows wide sutures, partly filled by discrete islands of bone, but although the facial bones are small, the cranium is not, and the main parts of the calvaria are of normal thickness

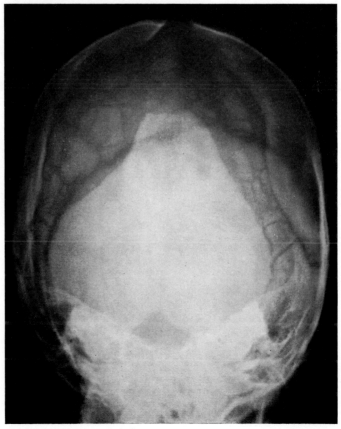

(b)

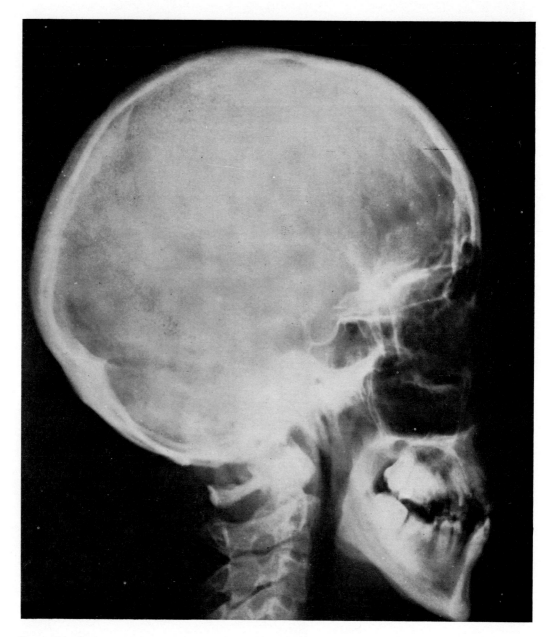

Figure 251. Cleidocranial dysostosis an adult case. The cranium is small. The sutural gaps have filled up. The very small size of the maxilla is shown by the crowded teeth

Cranial dysostosis and cleidocranial dysostosis (*Figures 250, 251*)

In this condition there is underdevelopment of the bones of the base in association with slow and imperfect ossification in the membrane bones of the vault. The basal sutures remain open for an unusual length of time, and the vault usually fails to attain a normal size.

Conradis disease, chondrodystrophia calcificans congenita, congenital stippled epiphyses

Fifty per cent of these children show a saddle nose. Many more severe abnormalities have been described, including a high arched palate, craniostenosis, both microcephaly and macrocephaly, hypertelorism and micrognathism.

Cretinism

In cretinism the bones of the base develop slowly and incompletely and the sutures tend to remain open; but, unlike the appearance in other hypoplastic conditions, the bones are usually rather dense and the pituitary fossa is of a more normal shape.

Autosomal trisomy syndromes

Trisomy 13-15 (D) — The brain is nearly always abnormal, arrhinencephaly being the commonest malformation. The skull is poorly ossified. Death occurs in the first few months.

Trisomy 18 — Microcephaly or hydrocephalus and lumbar meningocoele, with abnormal gyri and various cerebellar malformations are found.

Trisomy 21 — Down's syndrome; mongolism. The basi-occiput and basisphenoid may be short and the head slightly microcephalic. It is brachycephalic.

Chromosome anomalies (Klinefelter's syndrome)

Klinefelter's syndrome (with one additional X chromosome) shows no obvious skull abnormality, but with further additional X chromosomes there is progressively more mental retardation, genital hypoplasia and skull deformity such as vault thickening, sclerotic sutures, hypertelorism and prognathism.

Other conditions are described in Chapter 11.

9 INTRACRANIAL CALCIFICATION

INTRODUCTION

Calcification may be a normal feature in the pineal, the choroid plexus, the falx, tentorium and other ligaments, and in the dura over the vault. There is also a very large number of abnormal conditions in which calcification may be observed.

This chapter deals first with recognition of normal calcified structures and their displacement by disease processes. In the second half of the chapter the calcification of abnormal structures is described.

Although the interpretation of opacities within the head presents so many difficulties, the recognition of the *presence* of calcification is often of the greatest importance in indicating the necessity for further investigation and sometimes pointing to the investigation which would be most profitable. It cannot be emphasized too strongly that first-class radiographs are essential for this purpose. Radiography of the skull is dealt with more fully in the appropriate chapter, but a few of the main points as they affect the demonstration of intracranial calcification are repeated here.

(1) Reasonably fine grain intensifying screens should be used.
(2) The intensifying screens should be meticulously clean. Whether this cleaning is carried out as a regular routine or only when a mark is noticed on the radiograph must depend upon the circumstances of the x-ray department, but confidence must be felt that a small shadow is not an artefact.
(3) The focal spot of the tube should be small – of the order of 1 mm² or less.
(4) For demonstration of small areas of calcification within the head at some distance from the film, a longer focus-film distance is more effective than a shorter one.

(5) An efficient grid must be properly used.

The introduction of C.T. scanning has radically altered the statistics of incidence of calcification, both normal and abnormal, but, although much smaller concentrations of calcium can be seen on a C.T. scan, their shapes are not clearly revealed. Plain radiographs are invaluable in interpretating the significance of the C.T. finding. In any case, it is not practicable to carry out C.T. scanning on all patients for whom some sort of cranial radiological examination is required.

NORMAL INTRACRANIAL CALCIFICATION

Calcification in the pineal (*Figure 252*)

Calcification is seen on the plain radiographs in some part of the pineal in 50–70 per cent of all adults, and may also be found from time to time in children even before the age of 10 years. Its physiological significance is unknown but it is of great radiological importance, providing a landmark for the position of the midline structures and giving an indication of the presence of tentorial pressure cones. Other authors have suggested lower frequencies, for instance, 49 per cent in men and 39 per cent in women (Bruch, Bushe and Gregl, 1965). C.T. scanning shows calcification in almost all pineal glands of adults and in a high proportion of children.

It may consist of a single faint speck, a collection of specks or, more rarely. a ring of calcification up to 1.0 cm in diameter. Calcified structures in this region larger than 1.0 cm diameter are probably pathological (either pinealoma or aneurysm of the great vein of Galen).

A faint spot of calcification in the pineal is more easily observed in the lateral view than in any other. It

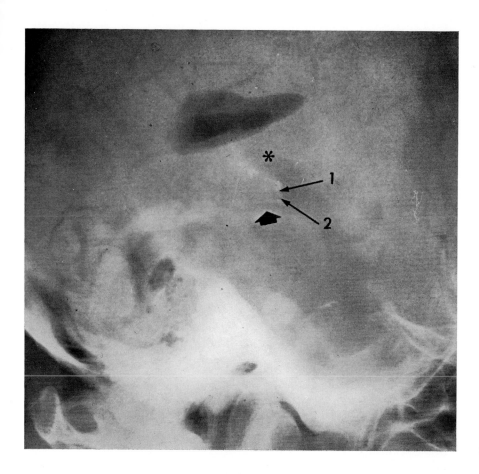

(a)

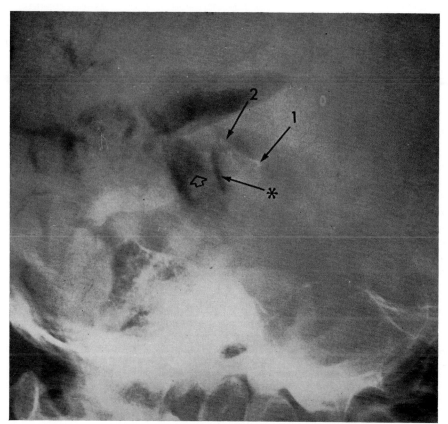

Figure 252. Normal calcification in the habenular commissure. (a) Note the relationships of the suprapineal recess (asterisk), pineal recess (arrow-one), posterior commissure (arrow-two) and aqueduct (closed arrow). (There is a large intrasellar and parasellar tumour.) (b) After the introduction of more air, there is partial outlining of the quadrigeminal plate (open arrow) and air around the posterior surface of the pulvinar on one side (arrow-asterisk). Air also lies over the cerebellum. Habenular commissure (arrow-one). Pineal (arrow-two)

(b)

usually lies about 2 inches vertically above the external auditory meatus. The exact area in which it may be expected varies greatly from patient to patient, depending to a considerable extent on the shape of the skull. Measurements, particularly those of Vastine and Kinney (1927), provide a basis for ascertaining whether the pineal seen in the lateral view is displaced upwards or downwards, but an experienced eye is probably more reliable.

In the lateral view in this general area three normal structures commonly contain calcium. They may be met with singly or together and they are: posteriorly, the glomus of the choroid plexus of the lateral ventricle; in the middle, the pineal; and anterior to it the habenular commissure.

The habenular commissure has a characteristic shape in the lateral view consisting of a 'C', reversed or otherwise, or some part of such a figure, and in an axial projection the form of an incomplete circle. The choroid plexus may be distinguished in these axial projections because it lies so far to one side of the midline. Approximately midline calcification will be either pineal or habenula, and although the distinction between these two can usually be made by the shape of the calcification it is of little importance since displacements usually affect both equally.

If pineal calcification is visible in the lateral view it is important to try to visualize it in one of the axial views as well, but if there is no pineal calcification shown on the lateral projection attempts to demonstrate it in other positions will be unsuccessful.

In the Towne's projection, if the calcified pineal lies in the midline, its shadow may well be lost in that of the dense bone in the middle of the occiput, while in postero-anterior projections a small fleck of calcium in the pineal tends to be confused with shadows of the frontal sinuses and the crista galli. The best single radiographic view for the demonstration of the calcified pineal in axial projection is the straight antero-posterior film. In this, the bony walls of the frontal sinuses are somewhat blurred by their distance from the film, while the translucent air spaces provide a window through which the opaque pineal may be viewed against a relatively thin part of the occiput. The definition of the view may be further increased by using a smaller cone or diaphragm, but it is important that this diaphragm should include the vault at the sides of the head in order to allow measurement. A slit-shaped diaphragm is commonly employed and the radiographic projection is therefore known as 'slit A.P.'. Other authors have stated that as few as 30 per cent of calcified pineals may be demonstrated in axial projection, but there is no doubt that careful technique with modern apparatus employing, where necessary, this extra 'slit A.P.' projection is more successful. The pineal is demonstrable in this plane in some 80 per cent of those who show any calcification in the lateral.

The habenular commissure

The habenular commissure lies in the posterior margin of the third ventricle, just above the pineal recess. Calcification in the edge of the commissure is not uncommon and the appearance produced by this calcification has already been described. It is usually a faint shadow but it may be found in the absence of pineal calcification and, since it lies so close to the pineal and is displaced in the same manner by expanding and contracting processes in the cerebral hemispheres, its localization has the same radiological importance.

On rare occasions the calcification at the back of the third ventricle may also include a thin line around part of the suprapineal recess and in the margin of the posterior commissure as well.

DISPLACEMENT OF THE PINEAL (AND HABENULA) IN AXIAL VIEW (*Figures 253, 254*)

In axial projection the pineal lies very close to the midline of the head and minor normal degrees of asymmetry of the skull do not disturb this relationship. The distance of the centre of the calcified pineal from the vault should be measured on both sides. It is of little importance in most cases whether the inner or the outer tables of the vault are used as the point from which the measurement is taken. The outer table will be easier to identify, but on theoretical grounds measurement from the inner table is probably desirable. The author's practice is to measure the line from the outer table to the centre of the pineal from each side in all cases in which the thickness of the vault is symmetrical, but to use the inner table where there is a large discrepancy between the thickness of the vault on the two sides.

The pineal should lie within 2.5–3.0 mm of the midline. Displacements from the midline in excess of this are nearly always evidence either of a space-occupying lesion or of unilateral shrinkage and loss of brain substance.

To be properly certain of displacement of the pineal it is essential that the radiograph should be really straight. However, in many cases the axis of rotation of the head passes close to the pineal gland. The maximum biparietal diameter at right-angles to this rotational axis is also usually close to the pineal, while the curvature of the vault, anterior and posterior to the maximum biparietal diameter, is more or less uniform. For these reasons small degrees of rotation from the true antero-posterior position may not throw the pineal very far from the apparent midline by measurement.

Since the pineal gland may occasionally be as much as a centimetre in diameter and calcification can take place in any part of it, the centre of the pineal may seem a difficult point to mark on the radiograph. However, in practice, when only one dot of calcification is visible, this is almost invariably in the middle of the pineal, but if the periphery of the pineal is calcified it tends to be calcified all around the circumference. The centre of the pineal can, therefore, be ascertained with some accuracy in the great majority of cases.

The interpretation of displacement of the pineal to one side of the midline must depend largely on other factors, particularly the clinical picture. Not all cerebral tumours cause lateral herniation of the brain. The tendency to displace the pineal will be greater when the tumour lies in the parietal or posterior temporal regions than when it is anteriorly situated.

Displacement of the pineal after a head injury may be an important pointer to the presence of a haematoma, and to the side on which it lies. When, therefore, there are clinical grounds suspecting that a haematoma is

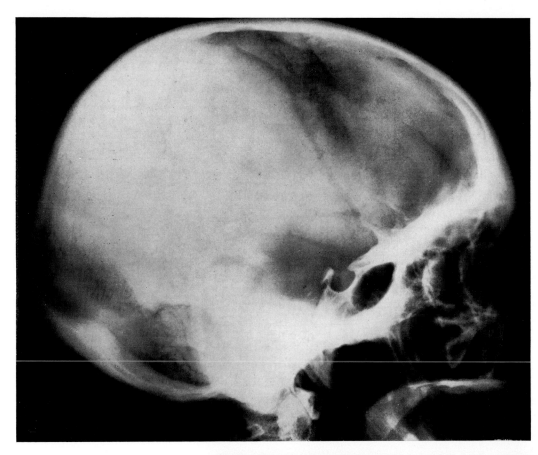

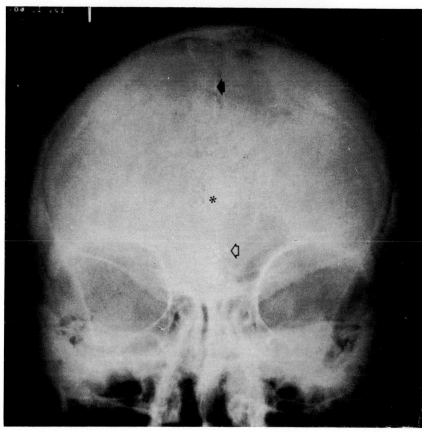

Figure 253. Displaced pineal. (a) Lateral view. The pineal is calcified. (Note also calcifications in the pectro-clinoid ligaments.) In the antero-posterior view it is seen clearly through the frontal sinus (open arrow). By measurements the centre of the area of calcification is found to lie 3 mm to the left of the midline. Such a displacement is very probably significant as it was in this case. The radiograph is correctly positioned. Not only is the lambda (asterisk) in line with the midpoint between the orbits (b), but the falx can be seen edge on (closed arrow)

(a)

(b)

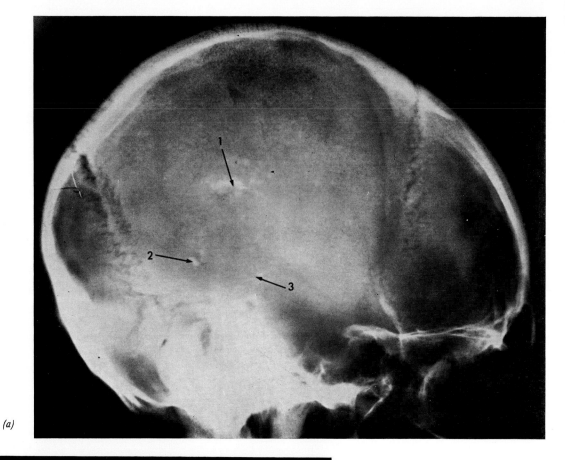

(a)

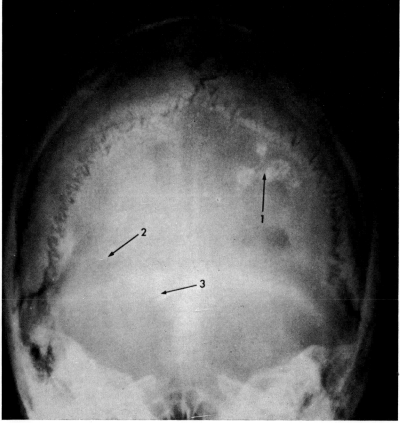

Figure 254. Calcification in a glioma. Lateral radiograph of the skull of a young man. (a) There are three areas of calcification, as follows. (Arrow-one) A dense collection of amorphous material. This lay in the very benign part of a tumour which elsewhere showed the characteristics of a Grade III astrocytoma. (Arrow-two) The calcified choroid plexus in the opposite lateral ventricle. (Arrow-three) The pineal gland displaced markedly forwards. (b) The half axial radiograph shows lateral displacement of the pineal. The tumour lay below the trigone of the left lateral ventricle, and the choroid plexus was adherent to its upper border. It may be that some of the left-sided calcification is in this choroid. Much of it, however, was shown histologically to be amongst the astrocytic tumour cells

(b)

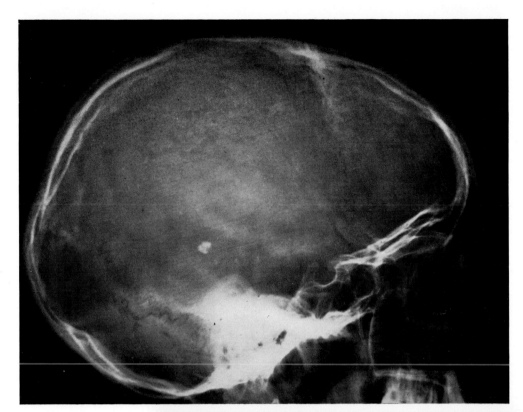

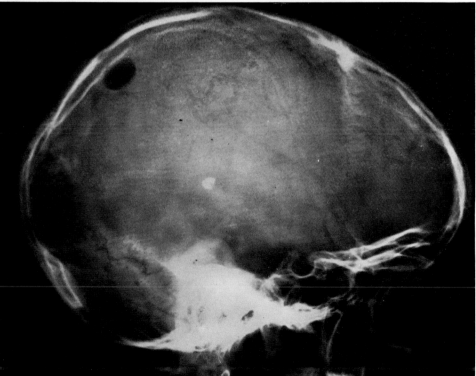

Figure 255. Pineal displacement in a boy aged 13 years with a 7 months' history of drowsiness and visual disturbance. (a) The lateral skull radiograph showed the pineal displaced downwards. It also lay well to the right of the midline. The patient was found to have a tumour in the region of the quadrigeminal plate causing obstruction at the posterior end of the third ventricle, hydrocephalus and consequently tentorial herniation. (b) One month later, after a ventriculo-cisternostomy to overcome the obstruction, the tentorial herniation has been reduced and the pineal has risen. It remains displaced to the right by the tumour mass in its immediate vicinity

present, demonstration of the position of a calcified pineal can be of great value. Ward radiographs are almost always inadequate for this purpose, and since the patient is likely to be less disturbed by a journey to the x-ray department than by the manipulations necessary when trying to obtain a radiograph in bed, there should be no hesitation in moving him to adequate apparatus. In such cases for pineal localization, a brow-up horizontal-ray lateral view and an antero-posterior projection are sufficient, although other pictures may be necessary to demonstrate depressed fractures.

Very occasionally, in patients with hydrocephalus due to obstruction of the midline ventricular pathways, the lateral ventricles may be so unequal in their dilatation that the pineal is pushed to one or other side.

Acquired cerebral atrophy of sufficient degree and asymmetry to produce pineal displacement is only rarely seen. In cases of hemiatrophy, however, where the skull growth has been affected, the diminished volume of one-half will be reflected in the short measurement from vault to pineal on the affected side. This is due as much to flattening of the vault as to displacement of midline structures towards one side.

DISPLACEMENT OF THE PINEAL (AND HABENULA) IN THE LATERAL VIEW (*Figures 254, 255*)

In the lateral view the pineal may be displaced upwards, downwards, forwards or backwards (with or without lateral displacement as seen in one of the other projections). The recognition of this displacement may be learned quickly by experience. The use of Vastine and Kinney's measurements to predict the normal position for the pineal in any skull leads to too many false-positive diagnoses.

If there is doubt about the position of the pineal in the lateral view, help may sometimes be given by a free-hand sketch in grease pencil of the expected situation of the third ventricle, aqueduct and fourth ventricle, made directly on the lateral skull radiographs. Prediction of the normal position of the aqueduct and fourth ventricle by measurement of the skull is more accurate than a prediction of the position of the pineal. An attempt to draw the ventricular system in normal relationship both with the skull and with the calcified pineal often helps to decide whether the pineal is, in fact, displaced.

The pineal may be displaced upwards or downwards along with tentorial herniation of the brain. Downward displacement is more common than upward and may be due to hydrocephalus, or to a cerebral tumour. The presence of a lateral displacement in addition is evidence strongly in favour of a tumour.

The association of an enlarged sella with a short or eroded dorsum, and downward displacement of the pineal is common in chronic obstruction of the posterior ventricular pathways by lesions other than posterior fossa tumours – aqueduct stenosis, for example.

Upward displacement of the pineal is occasionally due to a local tumour, but much more commonly the result of reversed tentorial herniation and an upward displacement of the whole brainstem. The commonest cause is probably a tumour extending into the midline anterior to the pons in the tentorial opening. For instance, a medially extending acoustic neuroma will often produce this radiographic sign, but any posterior fossa tumour may be responsible.

Backward or forward displacement severe enough to be recognized on the lateral radiograph is nearly always the result of a tumour in the immediate vicinity, but it may be remembered that slight backward or forward displacement may accompany severe upward and downward displacement, depending upon the exact cause of the tentorial herniation. Such small degrees of displacement are difficult to assess.

Calcification in the choroid plexus

Calcification in the choroid plexus is seen in a large proportion of adult skull radiographs. It is uncommon in children but may occur in the normal, even before the age of 10 years. By far the commonest site for calcification in the choroid plexus is the glomus which lies in the trigone of the lateral ventricle. Occasionally, calcification is seen further forward in the body of the lateral ventricle or in the temporal horn. The calcification is frequently symmetrical in position, shape and density on the two sides, but this is not invariable as sometimes the glomus of the choroid plexus lies in a slightly different situation in each ventricle and may be mobile; at other times the part of the choroid plexus which is calcified is not the same on the two sides of the head. Sometimes only one choroid plexus shows calcification. CT scanning shows calcification in nearly all skulls.

The calcification may take various forms. The commonest appearance is that of a sphere or ovoid between 0.5 and 1.0 cm in diameter, consisting of a large number of small, dense dots. Sometimes only the periphery of the sphere is calcified and throws a ring shadow. In other cases there may be a few small nodules or even a single nodule of calcification on one or both sides.

When typical spherical or ovoid calcification lies symmetrically on the two sides in the proper situation for the choroid plexus, its recognition presents no difficulties. Even a single nodule of calcification on both sides in this situation is very unlikely to be due to anything else. However, when the calcification occurs in the body of the lateral ventricle or the temporal horn and is thus asymmetrical, or when it is unilateral and consists of no more than a small nodule or flake, the possibility of some other and pathological cause must be borne in mind.

DISPLACEMENT OF THE CHOROID PLEXUS (*Figure 254*)

The calcified part of the choroid plexus will be displaced when a tumour, haematoma, abscess or cyst displaces the posterior part of the lateral ventricle. Such displacement may be recognized on lateral and axial radiographs, but since some asymmetry may be a normal feature, displacement should be beyond the normal range of position of the lateral ventricle before the diagnosis of a space-occupying lesion is made. Owing to the relationships of the trigone, downward displacement is often due to brain herniation beneath the falx and therefore not necessarily due to tumour lying about the ventricle.

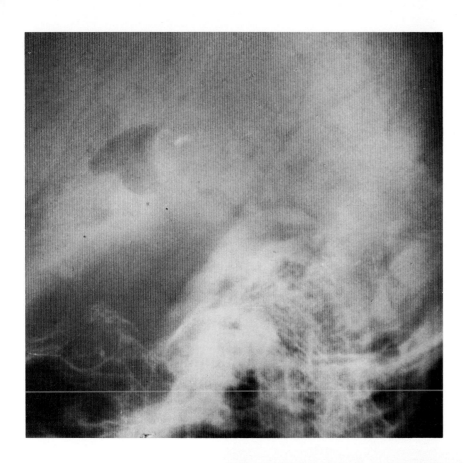

Figure 256. A single picture from a pneumo-encephalogram showing an elevated pineal and evidence of a small mass indenting the back of the third ventricle. It was a secondary deposit. Diagnosis of the presence of the tumour was made from the plain radiograph

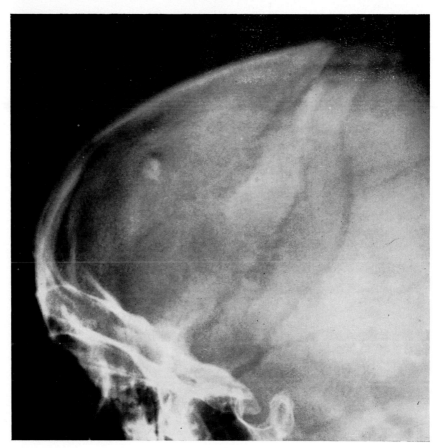

Figure 257. Pacchionian granulations with associated calcification. Calcification is seen in Pacchionian granulations on rare occasions

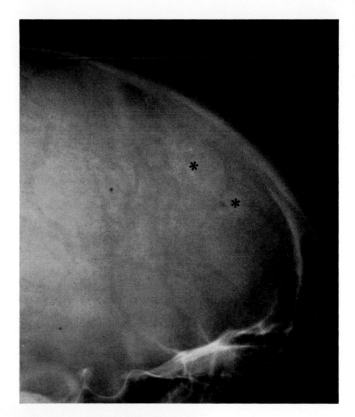

(a)

Figure 258. Calcification in the falx. (a) Lateral view. (b) Full axial view

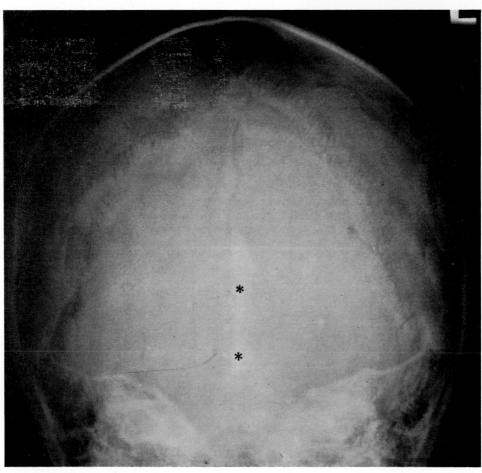

(b)

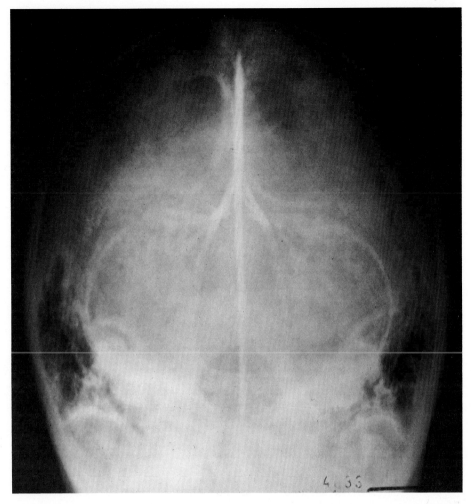

Figure 259. Extensive calcification of the tentorium and falx due to secondary hyperparathyroidism

(Reproduced by courtesy of Dr. Besigye)

Calcification in the dura

Large and small flakes of calcification or bone form in the dura in many places, particularly with advancing age. They are recognized by their situation which conforms to the distribution of the dura, and they very rarely give rise to serious confusion with pathological processes (*see* Calcification in meningioma on pages 263 and 283, Calcification in the carotid siphon on page 258, and Calcification in subdural haematoma on page 258). However, a meningioma in the neighbourhood occasionally provokes a marked degree of ossification. This is particularly obvious in the petroclinoid ligaments with petrous ridge tumours.

THE DURA LINING THE VAULT (*Figure 257*)

A dense area seen through the vault may represent a flake of calcium or bone in the dura which lines it. Careful scrutiny of other radiographs, particularly a tangential view, may show a line of opacity deep to the contour of the inner table and there may be more than one such area in the skull under examination. This is the only other situation in which dural calcification gives rise to serious confusion with calcification in the base of a meningioma, the diagnosis of which may rest on the presence of hyperostosis and vascularity of the vault, or on other evidence of the presence of an intracranial tumour. Multiple areas of dural calcification are unlikely to be due to multiple meningiomas. The history and clinical signs will probably dispel any confusion.

THE SUPERIOR SAGITTAL SINUS (*Figure 366*)

Along the walls of the superior sagittal sinus, single or multiple areas of calcification may be seen close to the midline in the Towne's and postero-anterior projections, and as ill-defined areas of opacity near the top of the skull in the lateral view. In the Towne's and postero-anterior projections the shape of the calcium suggests one or both lateral walls of the superior sagittal sinus with its triangular cross-section.

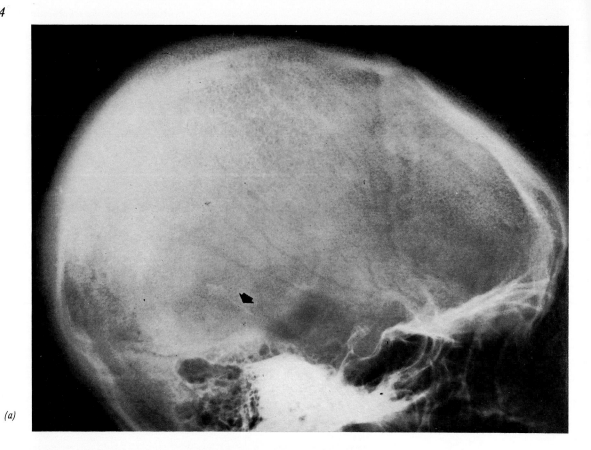

(a)

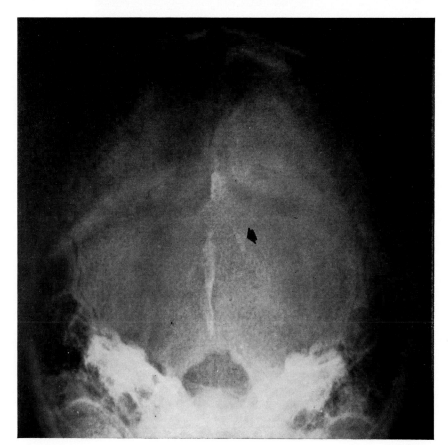

Figure 260. Calcification at the free edge of the tentorium (arrow). There is also calcification in the falx. (a) Lateral view. (b) Half axial view

(b)

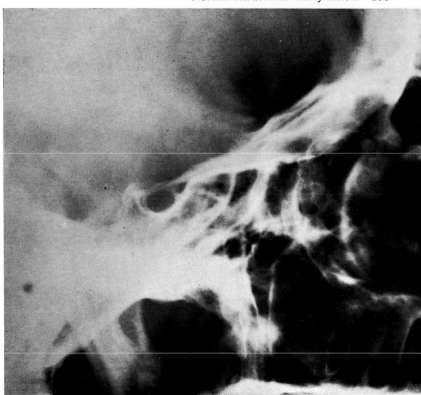

Figure 261. Ossification in all the interclinoid ligaments (see also Figure 177)

Calcification may be seen in any part of the falx as well as in the layers from which it springs around the lateral walls of the superior sagittal sinus. Calcification is commonest in the anterior part of the falx, but dense flakes and bony islands may also appear as rather ill-defined opacities well away from the anterior and upper surface of the vault in the lateral view. In axial views these areas are seen in or very close to the midline but are not always linear. Many of the calcified or bony islands are surprisingly thick, projecting to one or other side of the falx with a rounded or spiked prominence. The falx itself, even when uncalcified, is commonly visible in well-centred postero-anterior radiographs as a thin, vertical white line. Very occasionally it may be seen to be displaced 2–3 mm to one side by an expanding lesion, and with it any calcification that it carries.

Calcification has also been observed on a few occasions in the free edge of the falx in the lateral view, where it produces a long, curved streak whose shape suggests its situation.

Exaggerated calcification in the falx is seen in Gorlin's syndrome, a rare inherited condition in which the patients have multiple basal cell epitheliomata, jaw cysts, bifid ribs, scoliosis and mesenteric cysts (Mills and Foulkes, 1967).

Calcification in the tentorium (*Figure 260*)

Many mammals have bony tentoria as a normal feature. The development of a few areas of bone in the human falx and tentorium is not particularly surprising.

Except around the anterior attachments to the sphenoid bone, calcification in the tentorium is much less common than in the falx. Occasionally a flake may be seen projecting posteriorly from the upper surface of the petrous bone or lying in the free edge of the tentorium. Such a small flake can be confused with a displaced pineal or with pathological calcification, and the difficulty may only be resolved by further investigation of the patient.

Calcification in ligaments around the pituitary fossa

Calcification and ossification occur commonly in the petroclinoid ligaments and the interclinoid ligaments.

THE INTERCLINOID LIGAMENTS (*Figures 177, 261*)

These are shown in the lateral projection as complete or incomplete bony bridges between the anterior and posterior clinoid processes. In a true lateral the interclinoid ligaments of the two sides should be superimposed, but if the radiograph is oblique the ligaments will be seen one above the other and the lower one will partly obscure the pituitary fossa. Complete ossification of the interclinoid ligaments leads to the appearance described as a 'bridged' sella but the 'bridge' lies lateral to the diaphragma sellae. There may also be calcification in the ligament which joins the middle and the anterior clinoid processes.

Calcification in the interclinoid ligaments has to be distinguished from abnormal calcification around the sella. This is usually easy because of the shape and attachments of the ligament. It bears only a superficial resemblance to the calcification seen in atheromatous arteries and in aneurysms (which is nearly always curved, frequently lower in position and does not have the characteristic line of direction of the interclinoid ligament).

THE PETROCLINOID LIGAMENTS

The petroclinoid ligaments project downwards and backwards from the posterior clinoid processes towards the apices of the petrous bones. When calcified they are usually seen as one or two incomplete lines of opacity lying at an angle of about 45 degrees to the coronal plane. Any part of the ligament may be calcified, and its shadow may or may not fuse with the shadow of the posterior clinoid processes.

Sometimes there is a second line of calcification running towards the posterior clinoid processes at a slightly higher level, making an angle with the petroclinoid ligament. This lies nearer to the free edge of the tentorium at its anterior attachment.

Distinction from calcification in a pathological process is made by the shape and position of the shadow, except in one instance. The presence of a meningioma in the region sometimes leads to an asymmetrical increase in petroclinoid calcification. The diagnosis should not be suggested without other supporting evidence.

ABNORMAL CALCIFICATION IN THE HEAD

Consideration of the *position* of abnormal calcification within the skull is of some value in arriving at a diagnosis. The *shape* of the calcification provides additional help, but even after full consideration of all the radiological findings it is frequently impossible to tell with certainty the cause of the shadow. In the following pages, brief consideration will first be paid to the position in which the calcification lies, in so far as that provides some help towards the diagnosis. The various forms of calcification will then be described in more detail under six main morphological headings. It will be seen that a number of conditions appear under more than one heading. In order to avoid excessive repetition, cross-references are often used in these cases.

DIAGNOSTIC VALUE OF POSITION OF ABNORMAL INTRACRANIAL CALCIFICATION

CALCIFICATION IN AND AROUND THE SELLA

This subject has been dealt with in detail in the chapter dealing with radiology of the sella turcica. A list of the causes of calcification in and around the sella turcica includes some which are never, or only very rarely, found elsewhere in the head. These are atheroma, craniopharyngioma, arterial aneurysm and pituitary adenoma.

CALCIFICATION EXTENDING DOWN TO OR VERY CLOSE TO THE SURFACE OF THE BASE OR VAULT (*Figure 262*)

Some diseases of the meninges give rise to calcification and these are rarely found at any distance from the bone surface. They are meningioma, chronic subdural haematoma and, rarely, extradural haematoma. Other conditions which arise primarily in the bone and by expansion mimic the appearance of intracranial calcification are described in the chapters dealing with disease of the vault. The distinction between primarily intracranial calcification and an intra-osseous expanding lesion will probably depend upon a good tangential radiograph aided perhaps by tomography.

MIDLINE OR SYMMETRICAL CALCIFICATION IN THE REGION OF THE PINEAL (*Figure 265*)

Large cyst-like structures lying more or less symmetrically across the midline in the region of the pineal are usually aneurysmal dilatations of the great vein of Galen, which sometimes occur in association with an arteriovenous malformation. A pinealoma may also calcify and present with solid or cystic shape in this region, but is rarely greater than an inch in diameter, while aneurysm of the great vein of Galen may be considerably larger than this.

SYMMETRICAL CALCIFICATION OF THE CORPUS CALLOSUM (*Figure 292*)

In lipoma of the corpus callosum two curved bands of calcification, one on either side of the midline with their concave surfaces towards each other, are characteristic and are best shown in the Towne's projection.

INTRAVENTRICULAR CALCIFICATION

On rare occasions calcification is seen which is clearly forming a cast of some part of the ventricular system (which may be dilated). If the calcification does not transgress the ventricular boundaries, the cause will probably be a choroid plexus papilloma. The calcification resembles that seen in the normal choroid, but the diagnosis may be suggested when the size of the calcified shadow is too large to have been produced by a normal choroid. Other partly intraventricular tumours, for example, an ependymoma, do not show the same sharply circumscribed edges. Extensive choroid plexus calcification is occasionally found in neurofibromatosis.

TYPES OF CALCIFICATION AND THEIR CAUSES

Five distinct types of calcification are described here and, in addition, there is a further group in which mixed types are discussed. This scheme is used, not because of any special pathological basis for different formations

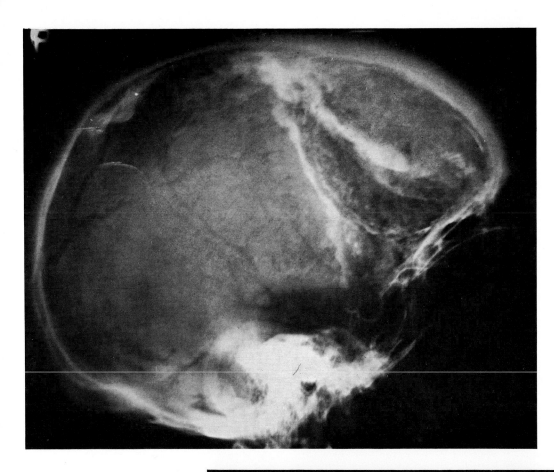

(a)

Figure 262 (a) and (b). Subdural haematoma. The patient was a man aged 69 years who had had occasional epilepsy since a head injury 13 years before. The radiographs show extensive calcification over both frontal and parietal lobes, clearly outlining deep extra-cerebral spaces. Calcification is uncommon even in very chronic subdural haematomas. At operation thick membranes were found with fluid below

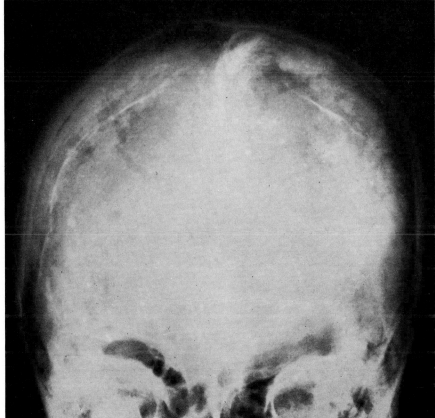

(b)

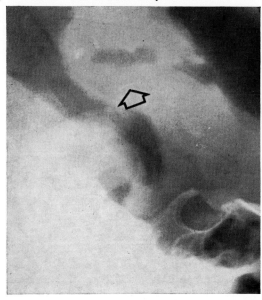

(a)

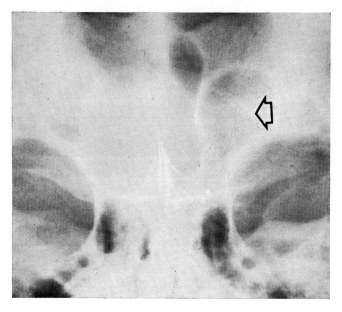

(b)

Figure 263 (a) and (b). An aneurysm, with calcificiation in its wall, in a man aged 52 years who presented with 9 months' progressive right hemiparesis, left ptosis and miosis. 'Cystic' calcification of this type in this situation might well be due to a craniopharyngioma (but it is unusual in that tumour to find 'cystic' calcification without some amorphous material). Other possibilities include chromophobe adenoma (very improbably if the sella is normal), angioma (which nearly always also shows amorphous calcification), toxoplasmosis, a hydatid cyst (both very uncommon), or even a glioma

of calcification but because it offers some assistance in the diagnosis. The types are as follows:

(1) Complete and incomplete cyst-like shadows.
(2) A single nodule, a group of nodules or an amorphous mass of calcium.
(3) Two or more disseminated areas of calcification.
(4) Band-like calcification.
(5) Faint homogeneous calcification.
(6) Mixed types of the above.

Complete and incomplete cyst-like shadows

Except for atherosclerosis in the carotid, cystic calcification confined to one area and without other forms of calcification in the vicinity, is extremely uncommon, for some conditions characteristically produce this appearance but are themselves rare, whilst a number of more commonplace diseases produce calcification which is only very rarely of this particular type. An attempt is made to group the conditions more or less according to their incidence.

Atherosclerosis Calcification commonly occurs in the carotid siphon beginning in the elastic lamina (Fisher *et al.*, 1965) in patients suffering from atheroma, but is very rarely seen in any other artery in the head. The calcification conforms to the shape of the internal carotid but may not be extensive enough to be recognized as a tube. Commonly, there are one or two curved lines of calcification in the lateral view superimposed upon the shadow of the sella turcica, and in the postero-anterior

view a complete or incomplete circle may be seen showing through the ethmoid air sinuses. The differntial diagnosis is chiefly from aneurysm or craniopharyngioma and is dealt with in the section entitled Calcification Around the Sella (*Figures 184, 185*).

Aneurysm Complete rings or segments of circles as well as more oval cyst-like shadows are sometimes the result of calcification in the walls of aneurysms or in the haematomas which surround them (*Figure 263*). The cystic shadows may be of almost any size but will be found related to the position in which the circle of Willis and its branches lie. The most commonly calcified aneurysm is that which arises from the intracavernous portion of the carotid where the calcification may be half obscured by overlying bone, and there may be erosion of the side of the pituitary fossa and of the sphenoid wings. The differential diagnosis is discussed in more detail in the section on Calcification Around the Sella.

Haematoma Long-standing intracerebral and extracerebral haematomas resulting from head injury as well as from ruptured aneurysms may calcify. Such an intracerebral haematoma will have a complete or incomplete cyst-like outline. Some are very large. If there is no history to suggest the diagnosis, no certain differentiation from other causes in this group can be made.

Very uncommonly the outer layers of a chronic subdural haematoma may contain shells of calcium, and the size of the haematoma will then be evident on the plain radiograph (*Figure 262*)

Even less commonly a small haematoma, never operated upon, heals with the growth of a shell of bone

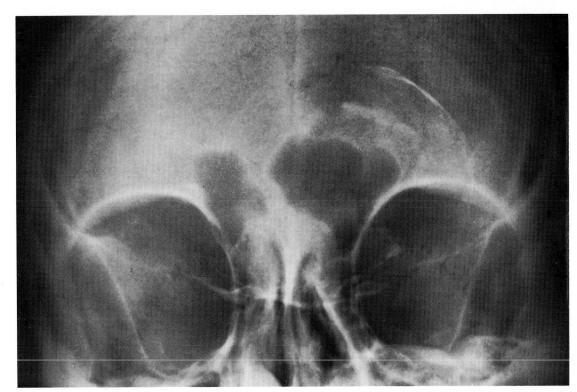

(a)

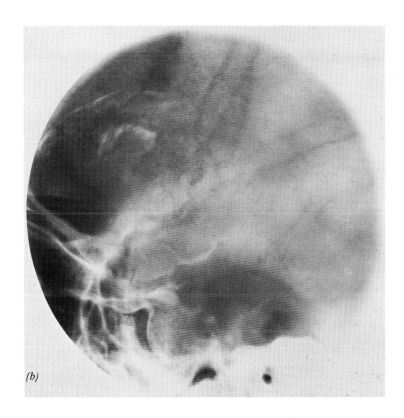

Figure 264. A calcified aneurysm of the
supraclinoid portion of the carotid. (a)
antero-posterior view. (b) Lateral view

(b)

over its inner surface, continuous with the inner table of the skull. It is known as an internal cephalhaematoma. There may be other evidence of an old fracture.

Craniopharyngioma Cystic calcification (usually an incompletely outlined cyst) is frequently seen in a craniopharyngioma, but there is nearly always some nodular calcification as well. The position of the calcification in the midline or close to it and more or less above the sella in most cases is an important diagnostic point. The calcification sometimes extends into the cavity of the pituitary fossa. The sella turcica itself may be normal in shape, show flattening without enlargement, or very occasionally it may be expanded. The differential diagnosis is dealt with under Calcification Around the Sella (*Figure 179*). The most important differentiation is that from an aneurysm. Other authors have stated that cystic calcification in craniopharyngiomas may be of surgical importance because such a cyst may be easily collapsed by tapping during operation. This is not necessarily true since cystic calcification may occasionally be seen around what is later proved to be a solid portion of tumour.

Angioma (arteriovenous malformation) Sixteen to thirty per cent of all intracranial arteriovenous malformations show some calcification on radiography, generally of a mixed type. It is only on rare occasions that incomplete 'cystic' forms are demonstrated without associated fine nodules. The 'cysts' consist of the partially calcified walls of dilated arterialized veins. They may be found anywhere in the head and be of almost any size. Not uncommonly there may be segments of more than one circle due to calcification in different parts of the dilated venous drainage. A particular case of this condition is the aneurysm of the great vein of Galen which may be more than 5 cm in diameter and is typical in its position (*Figures 265, 266*). Calcification in angiomas shows up more easily on C.T. scanning, but the resolution of C.T. scans is not good enough to reveal fine details of its morphology.

Epidermoid, dermoid and teratoma These are all rare intracranial tumours; teratoma is very rare, but is considered to be the pathological basis of most pinealomas. Epidermoids and dermoids may arise within the bones of the skull or, more rarely, they may lie entirely within the cranial cavity. Calcification in them is uncommon. Those which expand into the cranial cavity from an extra-osseous origin may be surrounded by curved flakes of the displaced inner table of the skull or dural calcification, and a number of the published examples of intracranial calcification due to epidermoid tumours appear to be of this nature. In such cases tangential radiographs demonstrate not only the position of the mass but also give a great deal of assistance in making the diagnosis as there are very few conditions which have a similar appearance. For details of the differential diagnosis refer to the sections on Translucencies in the Vault and Erosions of the Base (pages 82 and 186).

Pituitary adenoma Between 1 and 6 per cent of chromophobe adenomas are said to show calcification, and in the majority of these cases the form of the calcification suggests the wall of a cyst. There may be a single curved flake which usually stands up, projecting the line of the dorsum sellae, but may lie distinct from the dorsum over the surface of the tumour. More rarely, a complete cystic form may be encountered extending far into the cranial cavity. The pituitary fossa is nearly always expanded. Nodular calcification in a chromophobe adenoma is even less common. For details of the differential diagnosis refer to the section on Calcification Around the Sella (*Figure 268*).

Toxoplasmosis When calcification is present in cases of toxoplasmosis it usually consists of multiple disseminated areas, some of which are nodular while others consist of curved flakes of as much as 2 cm in length. Some are suggestive of the shape of a cyst. In others the thickness of the calcification is greater than with most of the causes of cystic calcification so far described. The areas of calcification may be found in any part of the brain; but are most common in the basal ganglia and near the walls of the (frequently dilated) ventricles. The most important differential diagnosis of a single area of calcification is that of a glioma. The patient may have chorioretinitis and there may be a positive complement fixation test and a family history of the same condition (*Figure 269*). The differential diagnosis includes torulosis and cytomegalic inclusion disease.

Cytomegalic inclusion disease (*Figure 270*) Fine nodular calcification in and near the walls of the dilated lateral ventricles in infants and young children who present with fits or cerebral haemorrhage may be due to this disease. The distribution of the calcification suggests the wall of a cyst — in reality the hydrocephalic ventricles. The appearance of toxoplasmosis may be almost identical.

Congenital rubella Rubella, too, in the neonate may be found to have caused calcification looking like toxoplasmosis or cytomegalic inclusion disease.

Hydatid cyst Very few cases of intracranial hydatid cyst are encountered in England. In those that are seen, calcification is not a usual feature, but it has been described. The cyst may be several centimetres in diameter, may appear folded or collapsed, or may closely resemble the calcification of large aneurysms or haematomas in the vicinity of aneurysms. If angiography excludes the presence of an aneurysm or angioma and there is a history suggesting the possibility of Echinococcus infestation, the diagnosis may be tentatively suggested.

Tuberose sclerosis The calcification which is seen in the brain in tuberose sclerosis is pleomorphic and may be disseminated, but from time to time single isolated areas are encountered and a cyst-like form has been described. The diagnosis is made on clinical grounds.

Glioma Very rarely a glioma may present in this way (*Figure 271*).

A single nodule, a group of nodules or an amorphous mass of calcification

There are a number of causes of amorphous calcification of this kind. The position of the calcification may sometimes be of help in suggesting the likely diagnosis, but apart from the situation of the calcium the various causes produce an indistinguishable picture. They are described here in two main groups. The first group are all relatively common and are arranged in an approximate order of frequency. The second group are all rare causes of calcification.

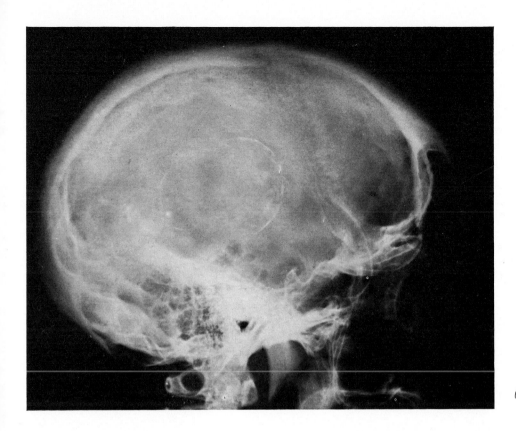

(a)

Figure 265. Aneurysm of the great vein of Galen. The patient was a woman who 17 years before began to grow above average height. Eleven years ago she first noticed weakness of the left arm and leg which had since increased, and she had suffered from headaches since that time. Eight years ago she was found also to have incomplete left hemi-anaesthesia and a calcified cyst was discovered in her skull by radiography. For the last year she had had more severe headaches, and deteriorating vision. She also had a right ptosis. Her heart was considerably enlarged and her blood pressure 110/65. (a) The lateral radiograph shows the calcified wall of the aneurysm. (It completely opacifies during the late phase of carotid angiography). Note the enormous size of the vertebral artery canal across the posterior arch of the atlas. Full axial view also showed huge carotid canals and the arterial hypertrophy was confirmed by angiography. An angiomatous malformation extends through most of the head. The large head and thick skull are part of a generalized giantism the reason for which is not understood. (b) The aneurysm protrudes more to the left than the right

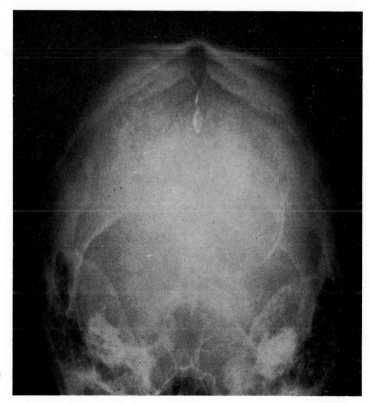

(b)

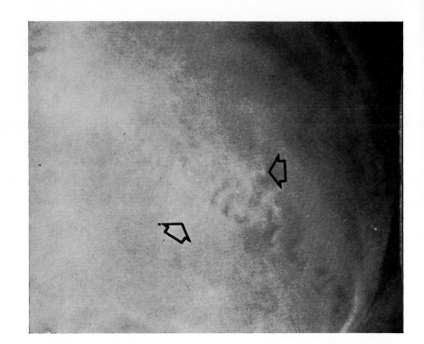

Figure 266. Angioma. The calcification usually consists of a mixture of dots and curved lines

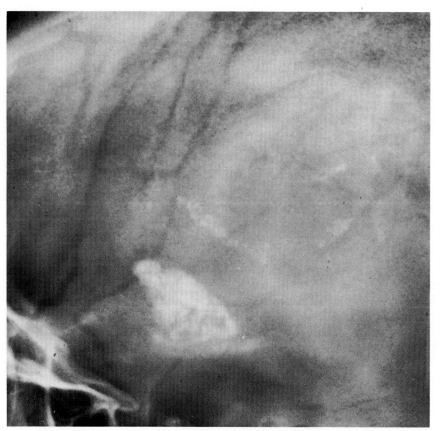

Figure 267. Not all angiomas have such typical calcification. Sometimes it is very hard indeed to distinguish it from the calcification in a glioma

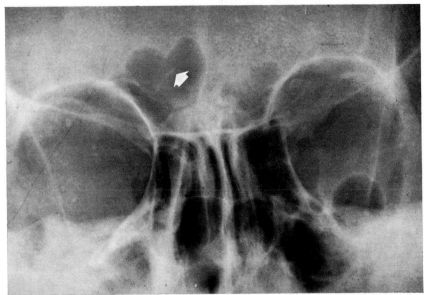

Figure 268. Calcification in the capsule around a chromophobe adenoma

(Reproduced by courtesy of the Editor of *Br. J. Radiol.*)

GROUP 1

Glioma With the exception of atheroma in the carotid siphon, gliomas are the commonest cause of pathological intracranial calcification. Calcification may be found in all forms of gliomas above and below the tentorium, It is more easily demonstrated and more frequently recognized in the supratentorial part of the brain, but this may be due partly to the difficulties of recognizing calcification in routine radiographic projections in the posterior fossa through the dense overlying bone.

Calcification is found more often in patients who give long histories than in those in whom the course of the disease is a rapid one, but the presence, nature and extent of calcification bear no relationship to the type of glioma as demonstrated at biopsy or necropsy except for the rarity of calcification in medulloblastoma (*Figures 272–275*).

Craniopharyngioma This is fully dealt with in the section describing Calcification Around the Sella (*Figure 276*).

Scarring From time to time small and large areas of calcification, often of considerable density, are discovered by change on the skull radiographs taken for reasons which cannot be connected with the incidental finding of calcification. In other cases, similar shadows have been demonstrated in patients suffering from epilepsy, and in a few of these exploration has demonstrated a discrete area of dense calcification surrounded by some gliosis.

Some have been considered the end-result of birth trauma or injuries later in life which have produced intracerebral haematomas. Others have been ascribed to the late results of scarring after cerebral abscess and after tuberculoma. Clear evidence of the nature of these discrete dense areas of calcification is usually lacking. They are sometimes multiple.

Meningioma Isolated nodules or dense conglomerations of calcification are sometimes seen in meningiomas. The great majority of these tumours lie close to the vault or base of the skull, and in many cases there will be associated bone changes, either hyperostosis or erosion, as well as some evidence of hypervascularity of the bone, but the nature of this type of calcification itself is of no help in making the diagnosis (*Figures 277, 278*). Extremely rare cases of neurofibromatosis have been described (Zats, 1968) in which choroid plexus calcification is more extensive than usual. In one of these there were multiple intraventricular meningiomata. (For systematic reading on meningiomas turn now to page 253.)

GROUP 2

Angiomata The calcification in angiomas is usually typical (*see* above) but some cases are encountered in which only a few small nodules are recognizable (Figure 37).

Chordoma A dense mass of calcification close to the base of the skull may be a chordoma. This is more fully described under Calcification Around the Sella, and Basal Erosions (*see* pages 169 and 222).

Chondroma Chondromas do occur, though they are very rare. They may arise from the precursor of bone at the skull base and can be mistaken for chordomas. Calcification is generally scanty. Chondromas also occur, but even more rarely, in association with the choroid plexus of the lateral ventricle (Forsythe *et al.*, 1947).

Hamartoma An amorphous mass of calcification has been seen in hamartomas. There is nothing to distinguish it from the calcification in a glioma. Hamartomas are extremely rare.

Pinealoma A tumour of the pineal gland is very uncommon but has been described as showing a well-defined, dense, rounded area of calcification larger than the shadow thrown by a normal pineal gland.

Choroid plexus papilloma These rare tumours when benign remain confined to the ventricle, although it may be dilated. Some calcify and by their shape and position

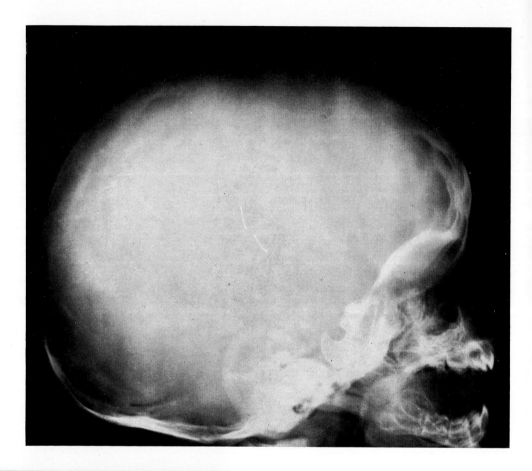

(a)

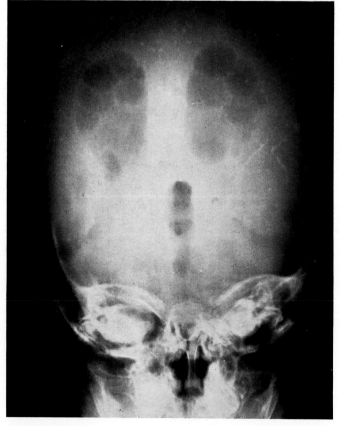

(b)

Figure 269. Toxoplasmosis. A boy aged 11 months who was normal at birth after a normal pregnancy. There was a history of vomiting for 2 weeks. The anterior fontanelle was bulging and the head large—circumference 16½ inches (normal at this age is about 14½ inches). There was evidence of chorioretinitis. Tests for toxoplasmosis in the mother and the infant were strongly positive. The boy subsequently deteriorated and died. (a) Lateral view shows widespread granular and curvilinear calcification. The vault bones are thin and the coronal suture and anterior fontanelle wide open. (b) Reversed half axial view at ventriculography shows the distribution of calcium (as well as the hydrocephalus) (cont.)

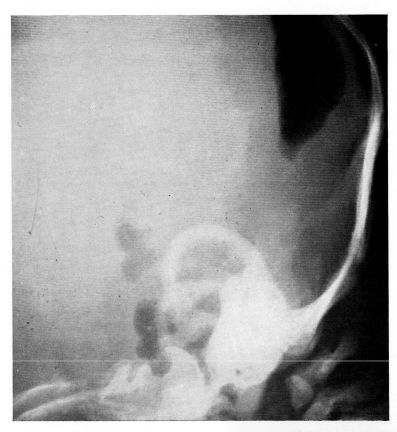

Figure 269 (cont.) (c) A brow-down lateral view at ventriculography also shows obstruction of the aqueduct. The front of the dilated third ventricle is lying on the diaphragma sellae. Autopsy findings were: (1) aqueduct atresia (1 cm gap); (2) widespread loss of nerve cells and gliosis with calcium deposits

(c)

Figure 270. Cytomegalic inclusion disease. The form of calcification may be indistinguishable from that in toxoplasmosis. The typical appearance is of a shell of sub-ependymal calcium outlining the dilated ventricles

(Reproduced by courtesy of the Hospital for Sick Children, Great Ormond Street, London)

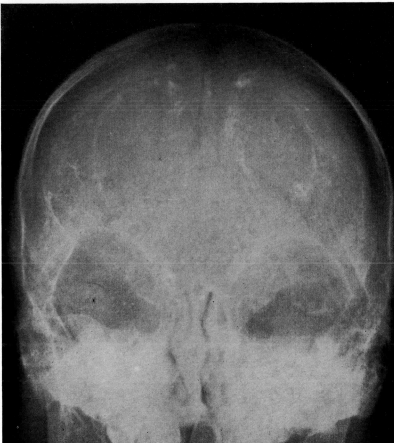

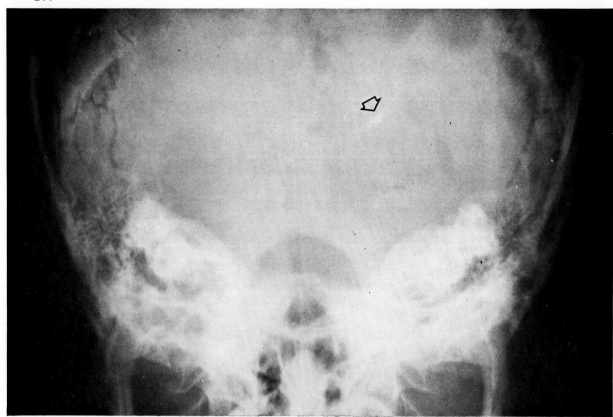

Figure 271, 'Cystic' calcification in a glioma. This child, aged 12 years had a large cerebellar astrocytoma. There is a thin shell of calcification in or near its edge. Calcification in posterior fossa gliomas is more common than is generally realized

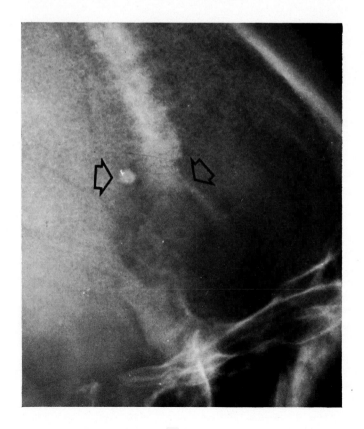

Figure 272. Astrocytoma in a man aged 41 years with a 6-year history of epilepsy. The calcification is of two types. There is a well-defined dense round nodule and a long fairly wide gently curving line. Partial removal of the tumour allowed a careful histological examination—astrocytoma, Grade 2

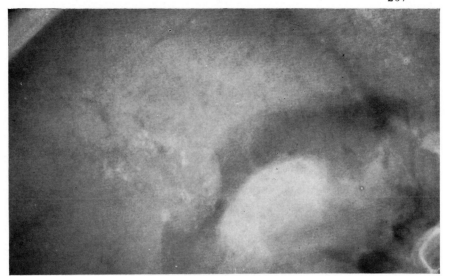

Figure 273. Ependymoma in a man aged 28 years who had recurrent attacks of weakness of his left leg. The partly intraventricular nature of the tumour is shown by this encephalogram. A macroscopically complete excision was achieved with good recovery. The calcification in this case consists of a collection of nodules

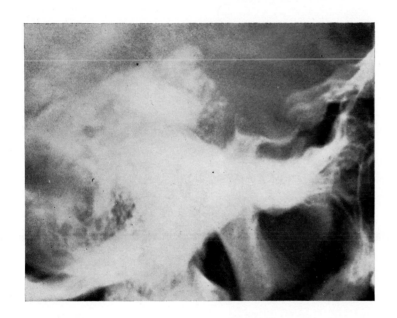

Figure 274. Astrocytoma in a girl aged 13 years with a temporal lobe astrocytoma. There is a great deal of dense, amorphous and nodular calcification in the tumour (the dorsum sellae is eroded and there may be early suture diastasis). (a) Lateral view. (b) Half axial view

(a)

(b)

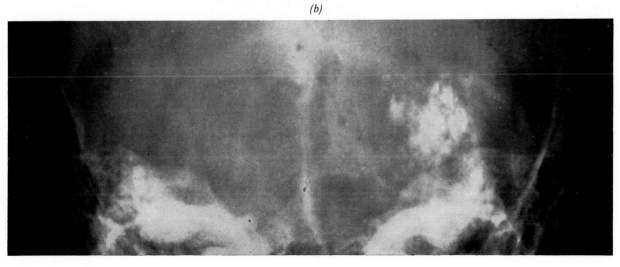

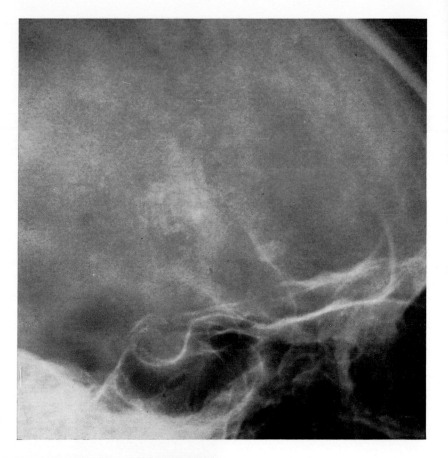

(a)

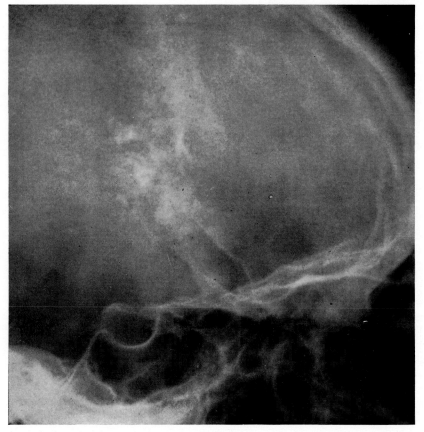

(b)

Figure 275. The patient, a man aged 42 years, was investigated for headaches and sensory epilepsy. (a) Nodular and confluent calcification was shown in the posterior frontal region. After further investigation the presumptive diagnosis of a glioma was made, but no operation attempted. (b) Three years later the patient was again examined radiologically during a review. The calcification had increased and now included a curved linear shadow (cont.)

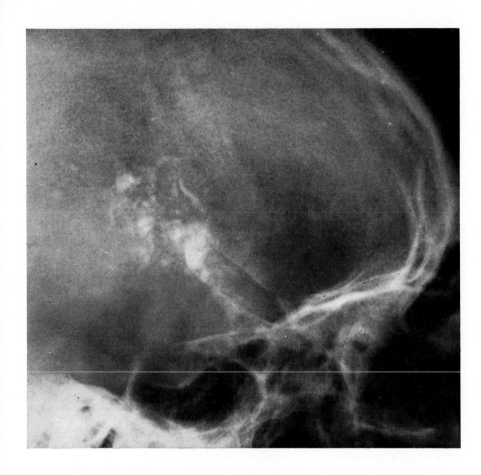

Figure 275 (cont.). (c) After a further 3 years he suddenly deteriorated. The lateral radiograph shows some increase in both the nodular and 'cystic' elements of the calcification. Exploration revealed a solid mass, part of which was a glioblastoma multiforme, but part showed typical features of oligodendrioglioma. The sella also shows progressive destruction

(c)

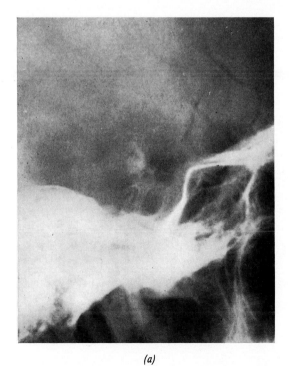

(a)

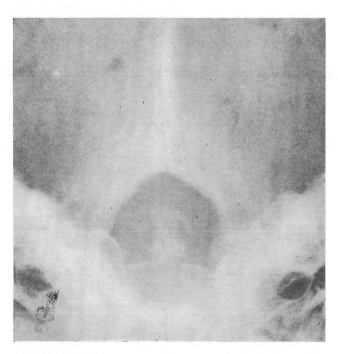

(b)

Figure 276. Craniopharyngioma. The patient was a fat girl, aged 17 years, who had primary amenorrhoea and bilateral optic atrophy. (a) The lateral view shows nodular (and linear?) calcification above and behind the sella. The radiograph was imperfectly centred and details of the sella are therefore obscured; but it is not grossly abnormal. (b) Half axial view proving that the calcification lies in the midline. It is superimposed upon the upper part of the shadow of the dorsum seallae

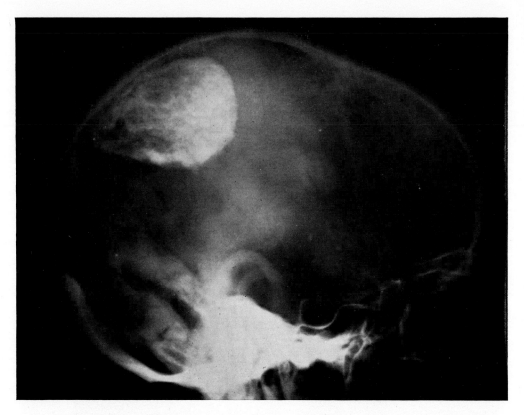

Figure 277. Meningioma. This heavily calcified tumour has a well-defined margin and a close relationship to the meninges, but these features, although suggestive, are not completely pathognomonic of a meningioma. The calcification is not homogeneous and might, for instance, have been in a glioma

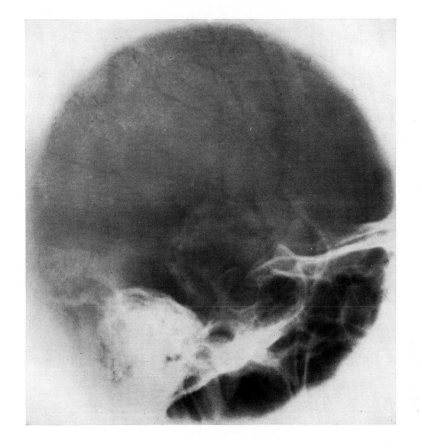

Figure 278. Calcification in a meningioma. The patient, aged 34 years, gave a history of fits for the past 20 years, and had been deteriorating mentally for the past 9 months. This tumour was partially removed. Its attachment to the dura was undoubtedly very limited and never identified with certainty; but probably lay in the region of the anterior clinoid process. The middle cerebral artery ran through the substance of the meningioma. The calcification is not sufficiently homogeneous to make a correct diagnosis possible from the skull radiography

are recognizable as intraventricular structures. If the margin is sufficiently clear-cut, the diagnosis may be suggested.

Rovit, Schechter and Chodroff (1970) found calcification in only 4.1 per cent of 234 accumulated cases, but C.T. scanning must radically change this statistic.

It is not uncommon to find a localized bulge of the parietal bone overlying the trigone of the lateral ventricle that contains a papilloma.

Tuberose sclerosis Isolated as well as multiple areas of calcification, both faint and dense, usually small in extent, may be found anywhere in the brain in tuberose sclerosis, but it occurs fairly late in the disease.

The commonest position for the calcium is in the paraventricular regions. Dense islands of bone in the skulls of some of these patients cause a certain amount of difficulty in the recognition and localization of intracranial opacities (*Figures 280, 281*).

Tuberculous granulation tissue Single and multiple areas of amorphous calcification, both faint and dense, are commonly found after tuberculous meningitis has been successfully treated. Most of the calcification lies in the basal exudate in the cisterns and Sylvian fissures. The patient's history provides the diagnosis (*Figures 187, 279*).

Toxoplasmosis Although the typical calcification is more suggestive of a cyst, some patients are seen in whom a nodule of calcification is the only radiographic manifestation (*Figure 283*).

Cysticercosis Calcification is only rarely discovered on the skull radiographs. When it is seen it nearly always lies in the scalp. However, a few cases have been described in which calcification has been shown in cerebral lesions; it is then usually a single, more or less rounded area (*Figures 284, 285*).

Other infestations Infestation by *Paragonimus westermanni* may sometimes produce granulomas in the brain with surrounding calcification. Oh (1968) noted calcification in about 50 per cent of cases and commented that it was not always characteristic. The cases described have occurred in Korea. In typical cases they present an appearance of large, lobulated, smooth-walled agglomerations of calcium.

Encephalitis, meningitis and cerebral abscess From time to time calcification has been described following infections by many different organisms. The cases are rare and proof is often lacking. In the neonate congenital herpes virus infection and possibly also rubella (Harwood-Nash, Reilly and Turnbull, 1970) may cause widespread intracerebral calcification which gives the impression of a cast of the brain, separated from the vault by an abnormally wide subarachnoid space.

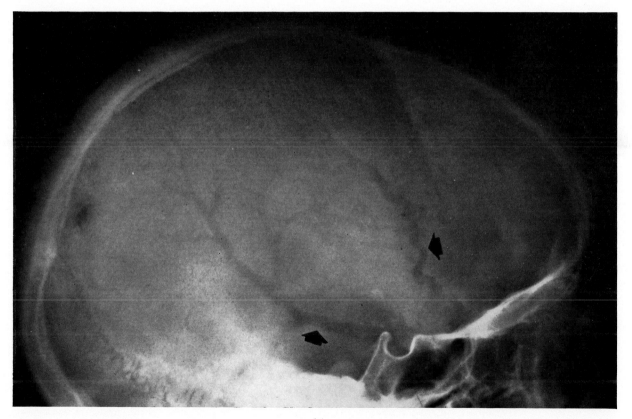

(a)

Figure 279. (a) Calcified tuberculous exudate. A boy aged 12 years who was treated for tuberculous meningitis at the age of 6 years. The calcification is dense and well defined now. For 3 years after his recovery from meningitis he suffered from behaviour disorder, consisting of outbursts of temper and moodiness. He had nocturnal enuresis and an electroencephalogram showed a diffuse abnormality. After precocious puberty at 9 years he is now a relatively stable and intelligent boy (cont.)

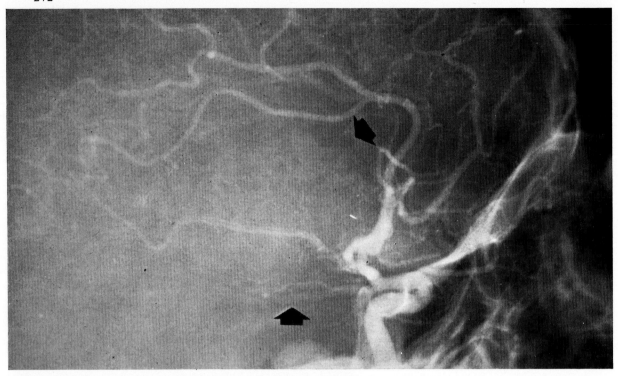

(b)

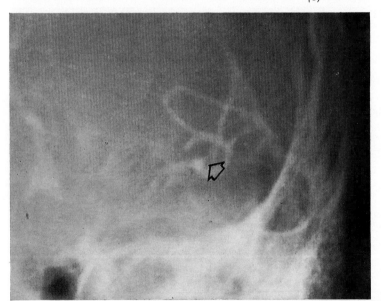

(c)

Figure 279 (cont.). The skull radiographs also show greatly enlarged channels for branches of the middle meningeal artery (closed arrows) and this is confirmed by arteriography (b) and (c) which also shows occlusion (open arrow) of branches of the middle cerebral and streaming of blood and contrast medium in one remaining one. It seems probable that the middle meningeal has taken over the missing cerebral blood supply which was cut off slowly by arteritis. A very unusual picture. (d) The hypertrophied foramen spinosum

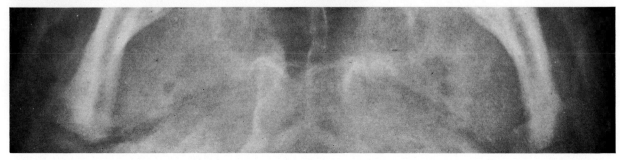

(d)

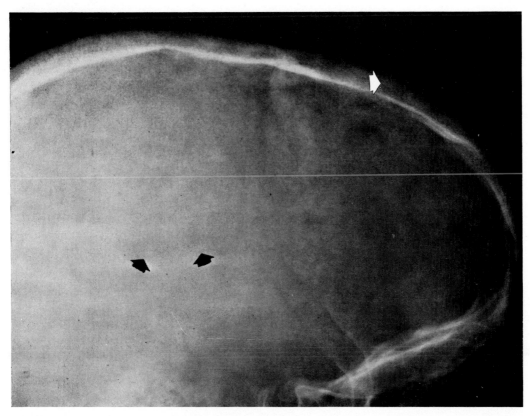

Figure 280. Tuberose sclerosis in a girl aged 11 years who had fits since the age of 5 years and adenoma sebaceum. She was otherwise normal. The lateral radiograph shows patches of increased density in the vault (open arrow) and some fine nodular calcification (closed arrows) which was proved by stereoscopic views to lie in the paraventricular region

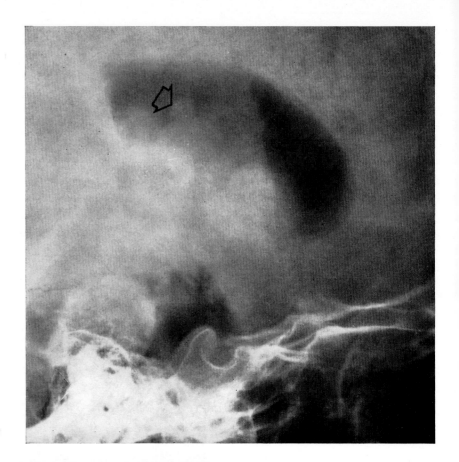

(a)

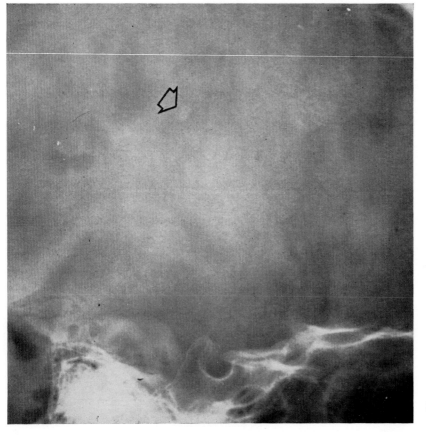

(b)

Figure 281. Tuberose sclerosis in a girl aged 4½ years, severely retarded and epileptic, with an atypical rash on the face and a very unusual condition of the skin and subcutaneous tissues on the chest. There was no family history of epiloia. Her sister was normal. At the age of 13 months this child's skull radiograph showed one faint spot of calcification. (a) An early picture during pneumoencephalography at the age of 4½. A number of faint calcified nodules are shown. (b) One at least of three nodules is shown to be lying within an area of gliosis protruding into the ventricle. CT scanning has shown that calcification is generally present at a very early age in patients with tuberose sclerosis

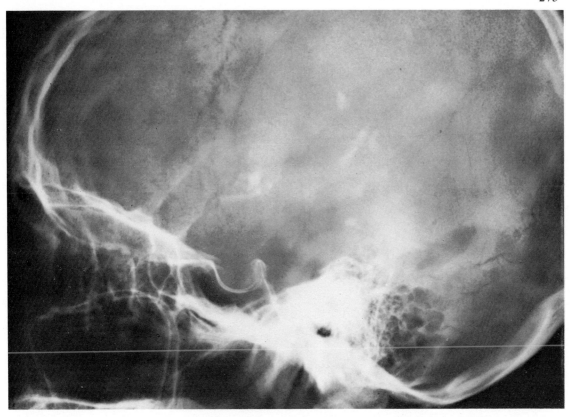

Figure 282. Much denser calcification may also be found

Figure 283. Toxoplasmosis in a young adult with a history of epilepsy for 13 years. He had had poor vision in his left eye since childhood and there was chorioretinitis of the left macular region. Toxoplasma antibody tests were positive. His mother was symptom-free but had a positive toxoplasma complement-fixation test. His sister suffered from major and Jacksonian epilepsy and had intracranial calcification, but her complement-fixation test was negative

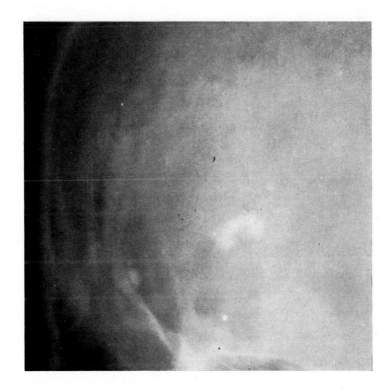

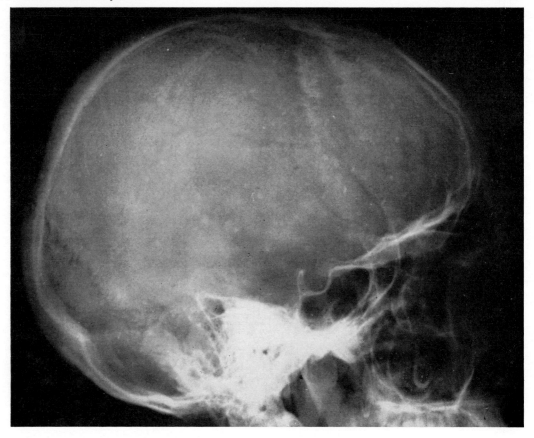

Figure 284. Cysticercosis in a man aged 39 years who lived for some time in India and has developed epilepsy. Some of these calcified cysticerci are in the brain

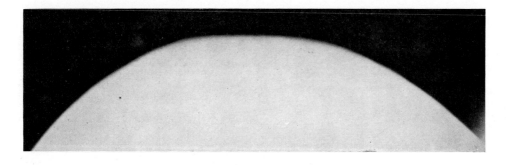

Figure 285. Cysticercosis. A solitary cystercus in the scalp. The patient was subsequently found to have many in the muscles of the limbs

Radiation damage

Calcification, usually finely scattered, may be found a long time after irradiation of the brain. It is likely to be recognized more frequently with the introduction of C.T. scanning.

Multiple areas of calcification

In many patients the cause of multiple areas of intra-cranial calcification is never established. Some presumably represent the late effects of previous infection. However,

multiple areas of calcification occur fairly typically in a number of conditions, and some of these may be recognized by their characteristics. Most are rare. The possible causes are as follows.

Tuberose sclerosis See above. Multiple areas of calcification are found in at least 75 per cent on plain radiographs.

Toxoplasmosis See above. In addition to the plaques and nodules in the cortex and subependymal brain, calcification may be seen in the choroid plexus and in the meninges.

Cysticercosis See above.
Scarring See page 263.

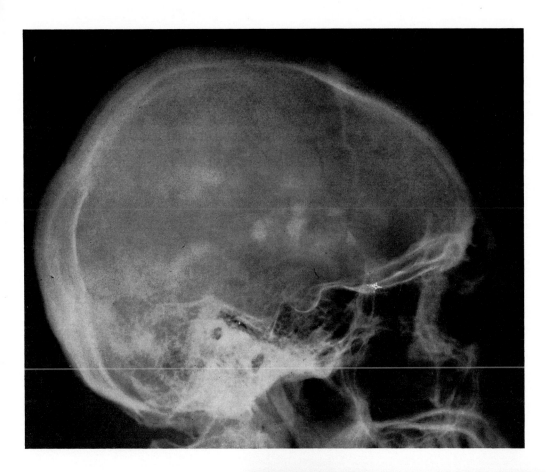

(a)

Figure 286 (a) and (b). Pseudohypoparathyroidism. The patient was aged 27 years at the time of examination. He has congenital cataracts, is mentally retarded and has in the last few years shown lethargy, ataxia and slurring of speech. He is said to have had frequent headaches with neck stiffness lasting for a very short time, and to exhibit jerky movements of his whole body when sitting. His arm ataxia is of cerebellar type, but he also has increased muscular tone. There is a history of one attack of hypoglycaemic coma. His sister has a similar condition. Both radiographs show calcification of a moderately dense and homogeneous nature in large confluent agglomerations in the caudate and dentate nuclei. Calcification in the brain in pseudohypoparathyroidism may also be very slight or obscure

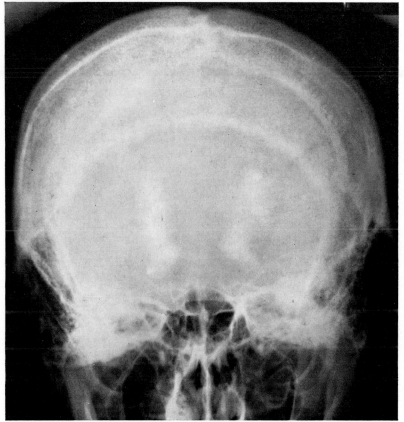

(b)

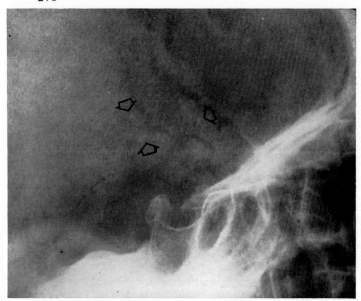

Figure 287. Primary hypoparathyroidism. A woman in her early thirties with hypoparathyroidism, probably primary, of unknown cause. There are fine specks of calcification in the basal ganglia (stereoscopic views were necessary for localization). She also had widespread skeletal changes

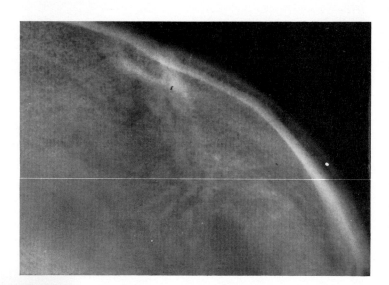

(a)

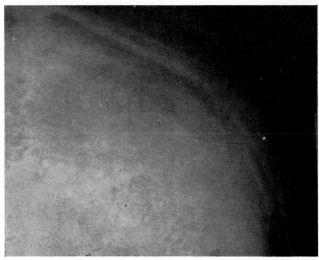

Figure 288 (a) and (b). Oligodendroglioma in a man aged 42 years with a history of 4–5 months' personality change and, more recently, fits. Radiographs show a collection of wavy lines of calcification high up in the left frontal region. This was proved after craniotomy to be an oligodendroglioma. Calcification of this type is found in about 50 per cent of oligodendrogliomas, but is also seen in about 25 per cent of astrocytomas which are much more common tumours. As an aid to the diagnosis of the pathological type of a tumour such an appearance is therefore of limited value

(b)

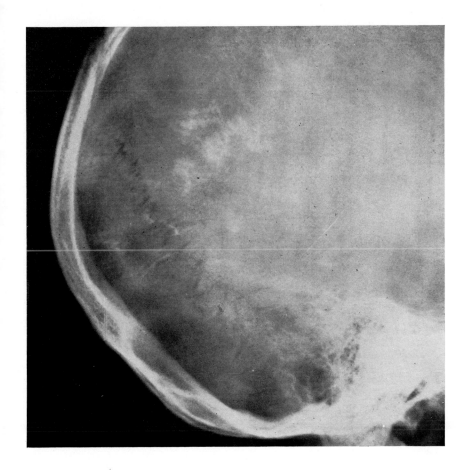

Figure 289. Sturge—Weber syndrome in a child aged 6 years. When calcification is not very extensive or fails to outline many cortical convolutions, the appearance may closely resemble that sometimes seen in a glioma

Tuberculoma and tuberculous granulation tissue Occasionally, after recovery from tuberculous meningitis, small areas of calcification are found over the cerebral cortex as well as in the basal cisterns, or even without basal calcification. The patient's history provides the diagnosis.

Sebaceous cysts of the scalp Calcification occurs in sebaceous cysts and these may be multiple in the scalp. Examination of suitable radiographs with a strong light will demonstrate that the areas of calcification lie in the soft tissues.

Foreign bodies Opaque foreign bodies in the scalp may easily be mistaken for intracranial calcification.

Calcification in the basal ganglia (Figures 286, 287) More or less symmetrical calcification may rarely be found in the corpus striatum and in the dentate nucleus. Most of the cases fall into three main groups: (1) those with hypoparathyroidism and pseudo-hypoparathyroidism; (2) those with a familial incidence but without hypoparathyroidism (Fahr's syndrome); and (3) those which

are isolated and unexplained phenomena, who may exhibit the same clinical picture as the familial type. A similar appearance may be seen after encephalitis lethargica, carbon monoxide poisoning and anoxia. The pathology and differential diagnosis have been revised by Muenter and Whismant (1968). The primary deposit is of acid mucopolysaccharides containing iron. Extrapyramidal motor deficit is present in about 25 per cent of patients with basal ganglia calcification but progressive neurological disease rarely develops after calcification is visible in those not aleady showing symptoms.

Calcification in the basal ganglia is also found in some cases of Cockayne's syndrome, a rare form of truncal dwarfism in which mental retardation begins in the second year of life. Retinal atrophy and deafness occur (Cockayne, 1936; Land and Nogrady, 1969).

C.T. scanning has revealed that symptomless calcification of small often symmetrical areas of the basal ganglia is much more common than had been believed.

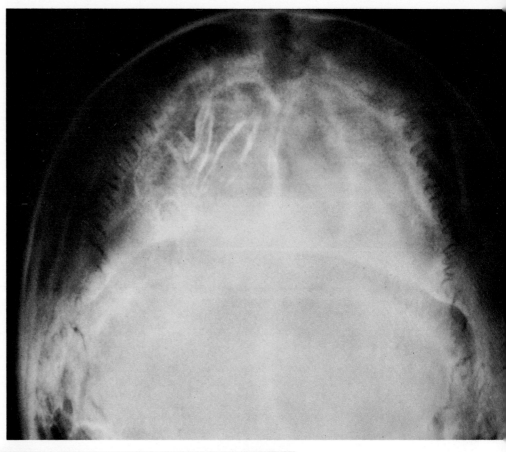

Figure 290. The calcification of Sturge—Weber syndrome is in atrophic brain. The corollary of atrophy is smallness of the affected part of the cranial cavity. If the cranial cavity is, on the other hand, expanded, as in this case, the diagnosis is more likely to be a slow-growing glioma, as this was. The calcification is not, in fact, really like Sturge—Weber on close examination. The gyri are swollen, not atrophic

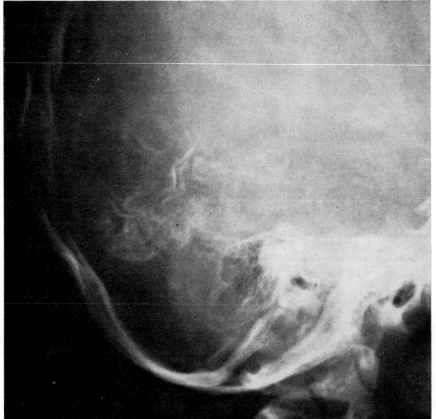

Figure 291. Sturge—Weber syndrome in a girl aged 2½ years. The distribution of calcification in the cortex of the occipital lobe is clearly seen. More deeply placed calcification may be found as well in some cases

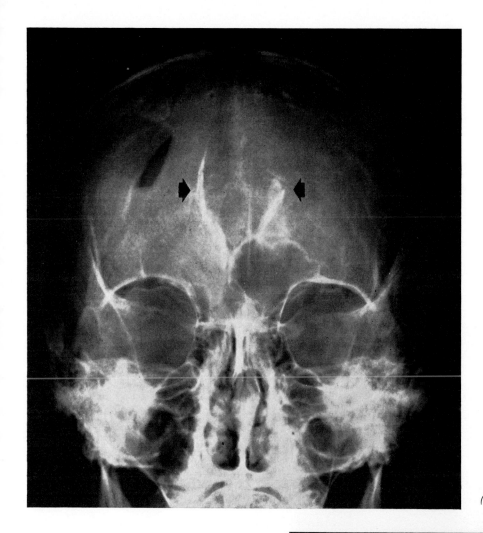

(a)

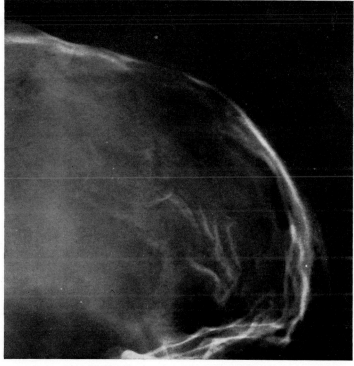

(b)

Figure 292. Lipoma of the corpus callosum. The patient, a man aged 25 years, had no symptoms referable to his head. On examination there was a 'cystic' swelling over the frontal region and another over the vertex. In addition to the lipoma of the corpus callosum—a presumptive diagnosis based on the presence of typical calcification—he has bone defects near the bregma and in the frontal region. The overlying soft-tissue lumps may be lipomatous. The presence of a meningocoele cannot be excluded. (a) Postero-anterior view. Note the typical form of calcification. Small islands of bone around the defects cast shadows resembling superficial calcification. (b) Lateral view. The shape of the vault around the defect shows pressure deformity due to the mass trapped below the galea

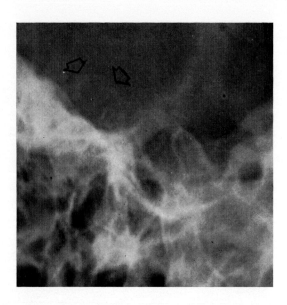

Figure 293. Meningioma. There is a small uniformly calcified tumour with a well-defined edge, characteristic of a meningioma. It arises near the base of the right anterior clinoid process where there is a hyperostosis. The patient had a left third nerve palsy which recovered after removal of this small tumour. A carotid angiogram was normal Pneumo-encephalography showed normal ventricles, but the tumour mass was outlined by air

(a)

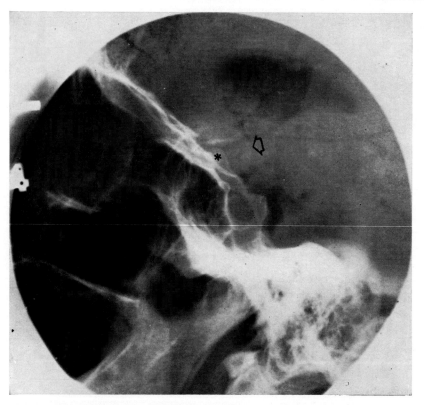

(a) Oblique view to show calcified tumour (arrows). (b) Lateral view at encephalography with the calcified tumour partly outlined by air (arrow), and the underlying hyperostosis (asterisk)

(b)

Band-like calcification

Glioma Bands of calcification of several millimetres in width are sometimes found in intracranial gliomas. They may be several centimetres in length and usually pursue an irregular course. This kind of calcification has frequently and correctly been considered typical of oligo-dendroglioma, but careful analysis of biopsy and necropsy material indicates clearly that exactly the same appearance may occur in other more common kinds of glioma (*Figure 288*).

Sturge-Weber's syndrome In cases with a capillary naevus of the meninges (usually associated with a naevus of the skin of the scalp and face), bands of calcification are frequently seen. These are usually about 2 millimetres in width and extend for long distances, often parallel with other similar bands and surrounded by a pattern suggesting the shape of cerebral gyri. These are areas of calcification in the superficial part of the cerebral cortex below the naevus. Calcification also probably occurs deep in the brain. The calcification, however, does not appear in the first few years of life, and should not be relied upon to make the diagnosis in infancy (*Figures 289, 291*).

Lipoma of the corpus callosum Two arcs of calcification, usually several millimetres in width, may be seen symmetrically placed about the midline in the anterior part of the head, their concave surfaces facing one another. The appearance is due to a lipoma of the corpus callosum and is unlike that produced by any other condition. There may be an associated meningocoele (*Figure 292*).

Faint homogeneous calcification

Meningioma A faint, truly homogeneous area of calcification with clear-cut margins is occasionally found adjacent to the bones of the base, particularly around the sella. There may be an associated hyperostosis. The appearance is due to a meningioma. The position of the mass and its smooth appearance with clear-cut margin makes the diagnosis certain (*Figure 293*).

Mixed types of calcification

The conditions in which two or more types of calcification may be present together have already been referred to under the appropriate headings. They will not be described again but are listed here for reference.

Glioma (nodules, masses, bands, cystic shadows)
Angioma (nodules, cystic shadows)
Craniopharyngioma (nodules, masses, cystic shadows)
Meningioma (nodules, masses, homogeneous calcification)
Tuberose sclerosis (nodules, cystic shadows; disseminated or single)
Toxoplasmosis (nodules, cystic shadows; disseminated or single)
Cysticercosis (nodules, cystic shadows; disseminated or single)

10 THE FACIAL BONES AND THE NASOPHARYNX

THE ORBIT

BONES

Three of the routine skull radiographic projections provide good views of the bony margins of the orbits.

In the *lateral view* the roofs of the orbits are seen clearly but are superimposed upon each other, and to view them separately a very slight degree of obliquity is sometimes required in the projection. This is best achieved by tilting the sagittal plane of the head a few degrees out of parallel to the film. The floor of the orbit is not so well shown because of its steep slope from medial to lateral side.

In the *postero-anterior projection* the whole of the anterior margin of the orbit is seen, but on the medial side, because of the delicate structure and shape of the bone, it may not always be easy to identify. Two fine white lines running more or less parallel to one another are often visible because the medial wall of the orbit is not flat but presents a depression for the lacrimal sac. In this radiological projection the apex of the orbit and the postero-lateral surface formed by the greater and lesser wings of the sphenoid, with the superior orbital fissure between them, are very well shown. All the other walls of the orbit are also demonstrated, but lying as they do, oblique to the path of the rays, they seem somewhat featureless. In addition, the medial wall of the orbit is confused by the complicated shadows of the superimposed ethmoid and sphenoid air cells.

A *full axial projection* gives a satisfactory picture of the whole length of the lateral wall of the orbit. Parts of the medial wall of the orbit are also visible but tend to be obscured by the superimposed nasal cavity and ethmoids.

Two other radiographic projections are of value — the occipito-mental and the optic canal view.

In the *occipito-mental view* a good picture of the anterior end of the floor of the orbit is seen, and in the *optic canal view* structures are shown at the extreme apex of the orbit which in other projections are obscured by their obliquity.

SOFT TISSUES (*Figure 294*)

An increase in the depth of soft tissues due to proptosis, oedema or contusion will cause a generalized decrease in translucency of the bony structures of the orbit, while on the other hand enophthalmos or enucleation of an eye results in an apparent increase in translucency of the affected side. In many postero-anterior radiographs, both normal and abnormal, and particularly when the eyelids are swollen, the general configuration of the soft tissues may be seen. In the centre of the orbit an oval or linear translucency represents the palpebral fissure, while above and below there may be translucencies showing pits above and below the eyelids. The swelling which accompanies severe contusion around the eye produces a fine, straight black line of translucency due to the closed palpebral fissure. This is easily mistaken at first glance for a fracture of the sphenoid wings upon which it is superimposed.

Abnormalities of size of the orbits (*Figures 295–300, 320*)

Normal growth of the orbit depends largely upon the presence of a normal eye. Congenital absence of the eye

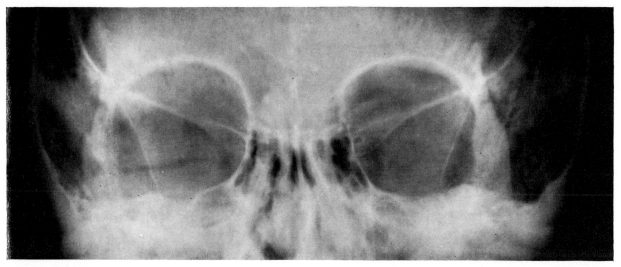

Figure 294. 'A black eye.' Swelling of the lids leaves a translucency to mark the position of the palpebral fissure. A linear translucency of this kind may be mistaken for a fracture

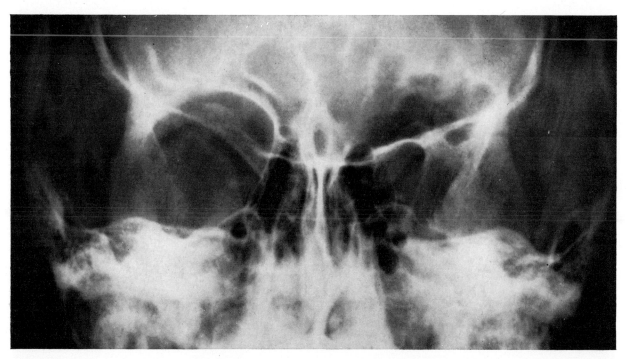

Figure 295. A woman, aged 21 years, who was found to have a bilateral retinoblastoma at the age of 15 months. Both eyes were removed before the age of 21 montsh. On the left a partial extenteration was performed, lids being kept to the cavity. She also had radium implanted in the left socket. The radiograph shows a small but otherwise normal right orbit. On the left the shape of the orbit has been altered by the operation, and in addition there is overgrowth of the ethmoid and frontal sinuses into the cavity

(anophthalmos), an abnormally small eye (microphthalmos), or enucleation of the eye before the bones of the skull are fully developed all result in the bony orbit remaining much smaller than its fellow.

In severe cases of craniostenosis, the general deformity of the skull may include forward bulging of the anterior walls of the middle fossa to such a degree that the posterior and lateral walls of the bony orbit are encroached upon, giving rise to exophthalmos.

The orbits may be diminished in size as a result of encroachment from neighbouring structures. For example, a mucocoele of the frontal sinus or an intradiploic dermoid in the frontal bone may displace the superior orbital wall downwards. Encroachment may also occur as a result of tumours or cysts in the nasal cavity or in the antrum.

The orbits may also increase in size (the more striking increases occur in infancy and childhood). The orbit

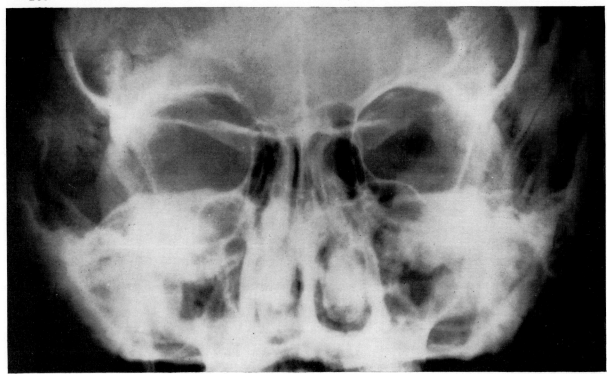

(a)

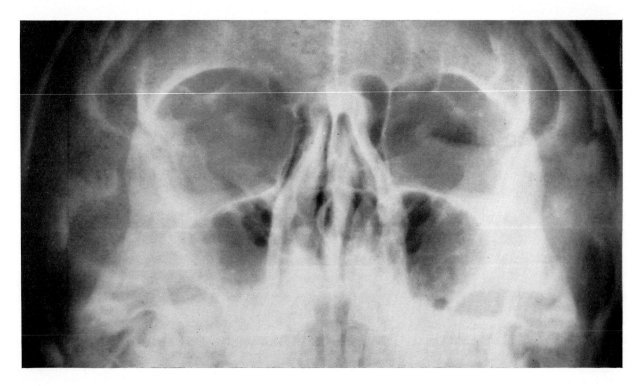

(b)

Figure 295 (a) and (b). The patient, aged 24 years, had her left eye removed at the age of 1 year because of a retinoblastoma. The right eye was treated with radon seeds. The radiographs show that the left orbit has failed to grow to a normal size. The neighbouring antrum and ethmoids on the other hand have developed at the expense of the orbital cavity. Air is shown in the orbit

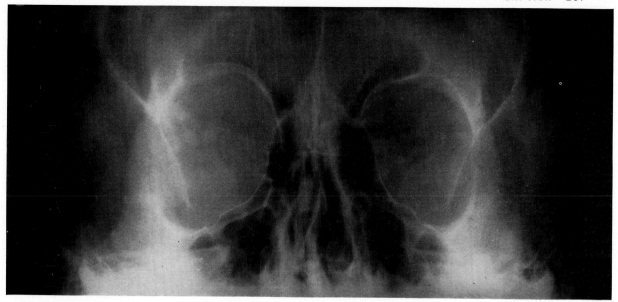

Figure 297. Orbital haemangioma in a young woman with a long history of increasing right proptosis. The expansion of the orbit visible here has occurred in the last few years. Earlier radiographs showed little abnormality. A cavernous haemangioma was subsequently removed

may be enlarged from birth in infants suffering from buphthalmos, or may become enlarged by the presence in the orbit of a tumour such as a haemangioma, a dermoid cyst, or a plexiform neurofibroma. Malignant tumours in childhood are rarely present for long enough to cause a demonstrable change in the size of the bony orbit.

In adults, a tumour has to be present for a year or more before change in size of the orbit can be seen on the radiograph. Even then it may be necessary to measure several orbital diameters for comparison with diameters of the other orbit before an enlargement may be detected. Exophthalmos of thyrotoxic origin can also expand the orbit, and mild enlargement is sometimes seen with large optic nerve gliomas.

Tumours of the lacrimal gland tend to cause a more localized type of orbital enlargement, and dermoid cysts may sometimes be encountered in a similar situation producing an identical appearance of ballooning of the outer part of the roof.

Hypertelorism

This has been discussed already (*see* Chapter 8, page 235).

Hypotelorism and arrhinencephaly

See page 324.

Fractures

See Chapter 12, Head Injuries.

Increase in bone opacity around the orbit (*Figures 121–124*)

Any of the conditions described in the chapters on opacity of the bones of the base and of the vault may be encountered, and these will not be described again here.

One of the commoner sites for fibrous dysplasia is the frontal bone over the orbit. When the changes are bilateral and affect other facial bones as well, the deformity has been called leontiasis ossea.

LEONTIASIS OSSEA

The term leontiasis ossea is, however, a clinical description and is not restricted to fibrous dysplasia of bone. Some cases are the result of Paget's disease.

MENINGIOMA

Meningioma may present as hyperostosis of the lesser or greater wings of the sphenoid or around the optic canal or of the orbital plate of the frontal bone (*see* page 219). Occasionally, meningiomas which began on the sphenoid wing or the cavernous sinus extend eventually as large growths invading the orbital cavity. Such cases usually seem to follow repeated attempts at removal.

CHRONIC PERIOSTITIS (*Figure 321*)

Rarely a low-grade inflammation of bone, having its original focus in one of the sinuses, may cause a widespread thickening and sclerosis of the bones comprising the orbital walls.

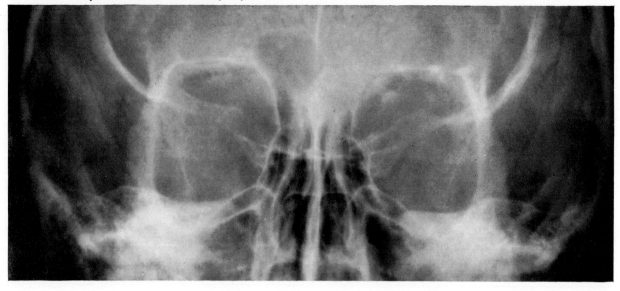

(a)

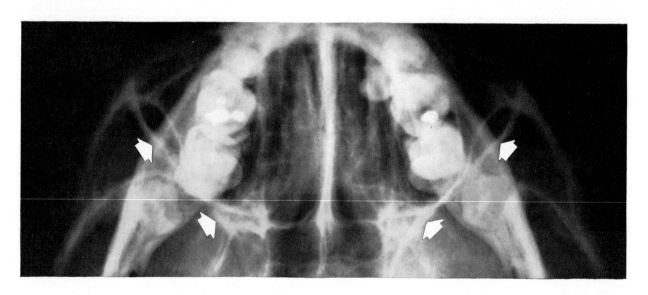

(b)

Figure 298 (a) and (b). Buphthalmos in a girl aged 15 years with bilateral glaucoma which had been present since the first year of life. There is a moderate enlargement of the right orbit and probably also of the left. The lateral orbital walls are indicated with arrows

MALIGNANT BONE TUMOURS

Malignant tumours, both primary and secondary, sometimes cause a mixture of sclerosis and erosion.

NEUROFIBROMATOSIS (*Figure 314*)

Areas of bone sclerosis may be found in association with plexiform neurofibroma of the tissues of the orbit, or sometimes with neurofibromas of the nerve running in the infra-orbital canal.

Erosions and translucencies of the orbital walls

DEFECTS IN THE GREATER WING OF THE SPHENOID
(*Figure 303*)

Radiologically, the appearance of a defect in the greater wing of the sphenoid is of a more or less featureless posterior orbital wall, and particularly when the orbit is enlarged this is aptly described by the term 'blank orbit'.

Such complete erosions may be difficult to distinguish from extreme degrees of thinning in which there is some bone preserved.

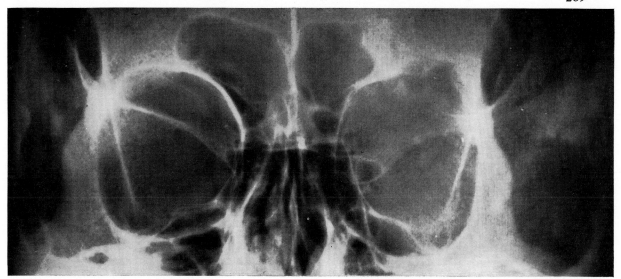

(a)

Figure 299. Intra-orbital dermoid in a patient aged 50 years with a left proptosis of many years' duration. (a) The postero-anterior radiograph shows a general increase in opacity of the left orbit due to soft-tissue swelling, and an increase in the vertical diameter of the orbit with a localized expansion of the upper and outer part. The transverse diameters of the two orbits are equal. (b) The oblique radiograph shows how well defined is the localized expansion of the orbit. It has a thin cortex of dense bone

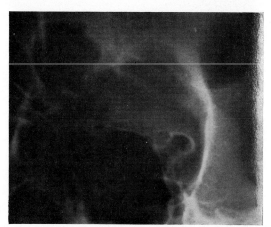

(b)

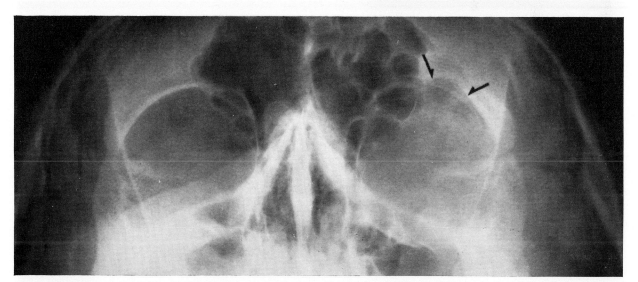

Figure 300. Lacrimal gland tumour. The patient, a middle aged man, had already had a local excision of a left orbital tumour. This recurred within a year. After this radiograph was taken a local mass was excised from the upper part of the orbit. The first tumour was reported to be a carcinoma, the second a benign mixed salivary tumour. The occipito-mental view shown here, and also other postero-anterior views reveal expansion of the upper lateral part of the orbit indicating the probable site. Soft-tissue opacity on the left is due to the proptosis

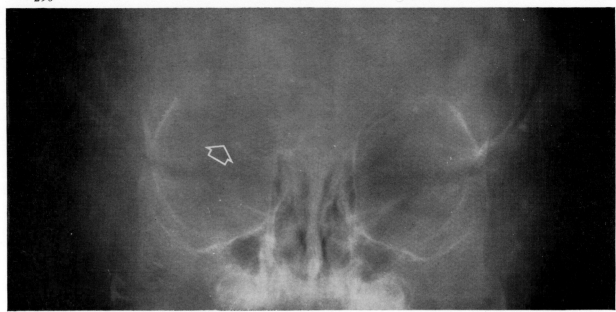

Figure 301. Neuroblastoma deposit. A young child with right proptosis and raised intracranial pressure (there is moderate suture diastasis). The right orbit is veiled by an increase in the soft-tissue opacity due to the proptosis. An erosion of the roof of the right orbit is present and this erosion shows a sharply defined posterior margin (arrow). Erosions of very thin bones nearly always have clear-cut edges whatever the cause. A neuroblastoma deposit does not necessarily cause new bone formation

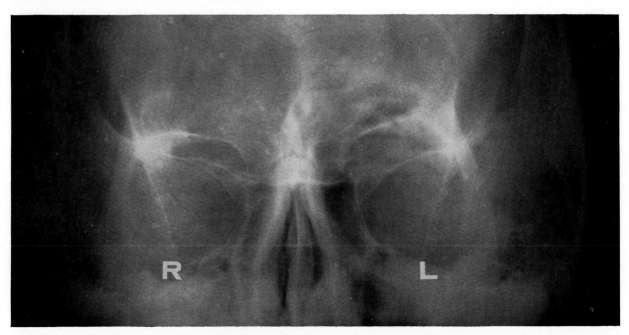

Figure 302. Reticulosarcoma. There is an erosion of the roof of the right orbit, but as the anterior margin of the orbit is preserved and the frontal sinus is opaque, this bone destruction is very difficult to recognize. The tumour is invading both the orbit and the frontal sinus

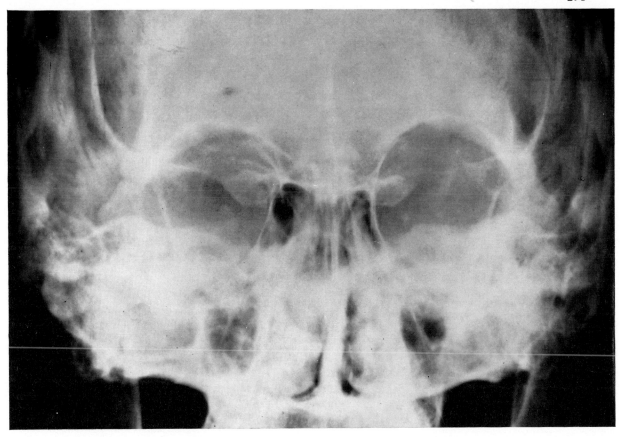

Figure 303. Orbital haemangioma in a man aged 34 years who complained of left proptosis brought on by stooping. There were many large venous channels in the orbit. In addition there are defects in the greater wing of the sphenoid through which the arachnoid was seen to protrude. Phleboliths are only rarely seen in the varicosities associated with some orbital haemangiomas

Figure 304. Optic nerve glioma in a woman aged 22 years who had her left eye removed 9 years before for a retrobulbar tumour. Seven months ago there was evidence of a recurrence in the orbit, and at operation after this radiograph was taken the tumour was found extending through the canal. There was an intracranial nodule about 0.5 cm behind the internal opening of the canal. 'Sections of the extreme posterior end of the intracranial portion of the optic nerve show that there are some fine strands of tumour cells in it.' The maximum diameter of this optic canal is between 8 and 9 mm. Any canal with a diameter greater than 6–7 mm on orthodox radiographs should be regarded with great suspicion. The optic canal reaches its adult size at the age of 4 years. Notice that the orbit appears to be well formed in spite of enucleation at the age of 13 years; and that the optic canal has a well-defined, corticated edge although it contains tumour. The tumour was a very slow-growing one

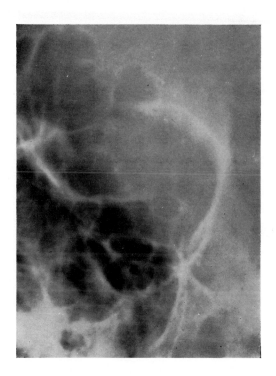

Thinning may occur as a result of very long-standing raised intracranial pressure, or due to a chronic subdural hygroma or some other long-standing space-occupying lesion, in which there will be other evidence of expansion of the middle fossa (*Figure 23*).

A defect in the greater wing of the sphenoid may occur as an isolated phenomenon and sometimes give rise to pulsating exophthalmos. Usually the meninges behind the defect are thickening but an orbital meningocoele or encephalocoele may occur. Such defects are also found in association with plexiform neurofibroma of the orbital tissues, and in many of these patients the orbit will also be enlarged.

Intra-orbital tumours — Other intra-orbital tumours are also occasionally associated with a defect in the greater wing. For instance, an orbital haemangioma has been found in which the greater wing of the sphenoid was perforated by a large number of small defects.

BENIGN AND MALIGNANT TUMOURS OF THE ORBITAL WALLS (*Figures 220, 301, 302*)

Any of the bony walls of the orbit may be the site of a primary or secondary bone tumour. In distinguishing between bone destruction due to benign and malignant growth it is unwise to consider a clear-cut edge to the erosion to be evidence of a benign tumour. The most malignant growth may present with erosions showing edges of clear-cut sharpness. The thinness of the orbital plates, for instance, ensures the most erosions involving them destroy at once the whole thickness of the bone, and appear rapidly.

Benign expanding lesions, on the other hand, may grow slowly enough to allow the bone to mould itself around them. On rare occasions, as already mentioned, a meningioma arising in the floor of the anterior fossa may grow downwards through the frontal or ethmoid sinuses towards or into the orbit. Like any tumour in this situation, it may block the drainage of the sinus so that the erosions are more or less masked by mucus or pus filling the air space.

NON-LIPOID HISTIOCYTOSIS (*Figure 221*)

Bone deposits are found in xanthomatosis and in eosinophil granuloma; they are indistinguishable radiologically from erosion by tumours. Sclerosis may follow treatment.

ENLARGEMENT OF THE SPHENOID FISSURE

This is discussed elsewhere (*see* page 203).

Intra-orbital opacities

C.A.T. scanning has revolutionized the diagnosis of intra-orbital soft-tissue masses, making them clearly visible for the first time.

FOREIGN BODIES

The recognition and localization of intra-orbital foreign bodies will not be discussed in this book.

INTRA-ORBITAL CALCIFICATION (*Figure 303*)

Calcification may be seen in the choroid and vitreous humour with atrophy of the eye after injury and infection. It may sometimes be seen in the lens in cases of cataract, and conjunctival and corneal calcification is described in hypercalcaemia.

Phleboliths occur in rare cases of haemangioma and are then found lying in the draining veins which may be of very large size.

Few intra-orbital tumours show recognizable calcification on the radiographs, but an irregular, mottled and granular appearance may indicate the presence of a retinoblastoma. An intra-orbital osteoma has an appearance similar to osteomas elsewhere in the body.

The optic canal (*Figure 304*)

This is often referred to as the optic foramen, but it has a length of several millimetres. The inner end is usually slightly oval with the long axis of the oval in a vertical plane. The orbital end of the canal tends to be more or less circular. Slight alterations of radiographic projection will therefore cause considerable changes in its shape on the radiographs. It usually appears more or less oval and the two canals may be very different.

Normal adult dimensions are achieved by the age of 4 years, and any diameter (as measured on the radiographs) in excess of 7 mm should be regarded as highly suggestive of enlargement. If the canal has two diameters of 7 mm enlargement is almost certain. Three anatomical variants occur. In one the optic strut forms above the ophthalmic artery, thus dividing the canal into two parts and separating the nerve from the vessel. In the second the posterior strut fails to develop and the foramen looks like a keyhole. The third arises from complete absence of the whole strut so that the optic canal and orbital fissure form a single opening.

Enlargement of the canal may take place within a few months in childhood, but occurs more slowly in the adult. It is usually due to a tumour of the optic nerve itself. There is evidence of the intracranial extension of an optic nerve glioma if the inner end of the canal can be shown to be enlarged. Other rare causes of enlargement are neurofibroma, meningioma and retinoblastoma. Enlargement of the canal in neurofibromatosis is not proof positive of the presence of an optic nerve glioma. The nerve may be enlarged by an increase in its fibrous stroma.

The canal may be narrowed by the hyperostosis of a meningioma, and sometimes by bone tumours. It may be seriously narrowed in severe cases of craniostenosis as part of the general deformity of the skull base. Any diameter less than 2 mm is usually associated with visual deterioration.

Blindness may follow fractures across the canal. When it becomes necessary to demonstrate such fractures after a serious head injury, it may be easier to invert the skull table, supporting the head with a linen band, in order to make postero-anterior radiographs in the supine position. The same result can be more easily obtained with the 'Orbix' type of apparatus.

The canal may also be involved by erosions of the lesser wing of the sphenoid (*see* page 203).

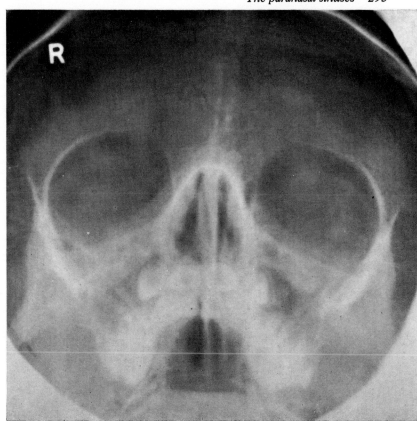

Figure 305. Normal paranasal sinuses in a child aged 4½ years. The antra and ethmoid sinuses are well developed. The frontal sinuses are difficult to see because of their shallowness and relatively thick bony walls

THE PARANASAL SINUSES

A detailed discussion of all the radiological assistance which may be offered to the ear, nose and throat surgeon is outside the scope of this book. What follows is a generalized enumeration of the possible appearances. The frontal sinuses, ethmoids and antra are only mentioned separately where this is essential.

Normal development

THE ANTRA (*Figure 305*)

The antra begin to appear in the fourth or fifth month of fetal life and at birth are generally about half a centimetre in diameter. However, since they may not be pneumatized but tend to remain filled with a jelly-like substance during the first few months of extra-uterine life, opacities of the antra in the neonatal period should be interpreted with caution. At the age of one year the outer walls of the antra are usually still medial to the infra-orbital foramina. The adult size in transverse diameter is reached at about the age of 8 years, and, thereafter, further increase in antero-posterior and vertical measurements proceeds with the growth of the maxilla and the eruption of permanent teeth.

The degree of development of the antra on the two sides is not always symmetrical, particularly as the pneumatization of the alveolar recess depends upon the maxillary dentition, and this may be affected by extraction of teeth. The alveolar recess may fail to pneumatize or may be developed to an unusual degree. There may also be bony or sometimes membranous septa running in a horizontal direction and subdividing the air shadow in the antrum. The septa are not necessarily symmetrical on the two sides.

FRONTAL SINUSES

The frontal sinuses originate as pouches in the lateral nasal walls of the middle meatus. By the end of the first year of life they are still 'ethmoidal' but between the second and third year they reach the frontal bone. Extension of the frontal sinuses much above the nasion is said to depend upon fusion of the metopic suture, but this is erroneous. In general, the frontal sinuses are fully developed at about the time of puberty.

THE SPHENOID SINUS

Pneumatization is not, as a rule, visible on radiographs before the age of 3 years. The sphenoid sinus is paired, but one usually develops at the expense of the other. The sinuses may be very small throughout life or pneumatization may extend to the dorsum sellae, the lesser wing

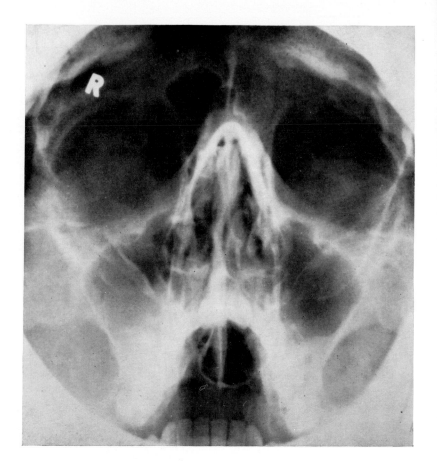

Figure 306. Allergy or infection, or both. The lower part of the right antrum is opaque. The upper surface of this opacity is difficult to see; it is rounded, the mucosa is thickened, the shadow may represent pus or polypoid mucosa. There is also a shadow at the base of the left antrum, but on this side the mucosa is normal

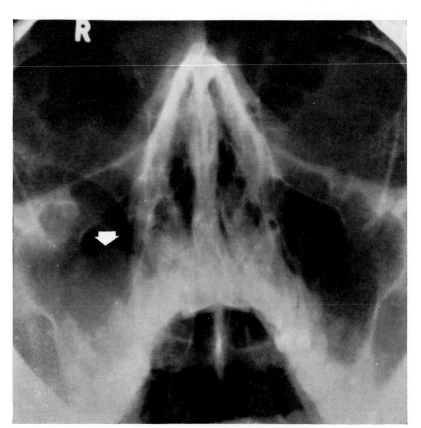

Figure 307. Polyp. A rounded soft-tissue shadow in the antrum may be caused by any one of a number of conditions

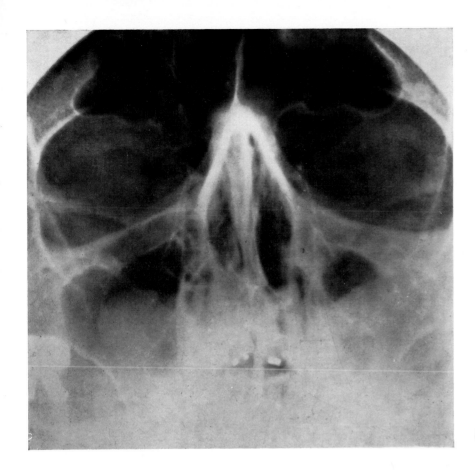

(a)

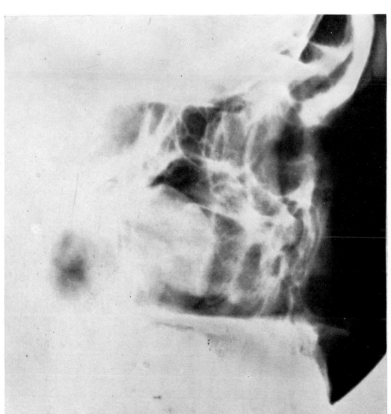

Figure 308. Antral polypi. (a) Occipito-mental view. (b) Lateral view

(b)

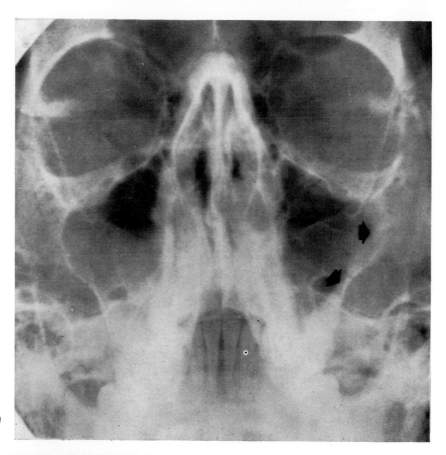

(a)

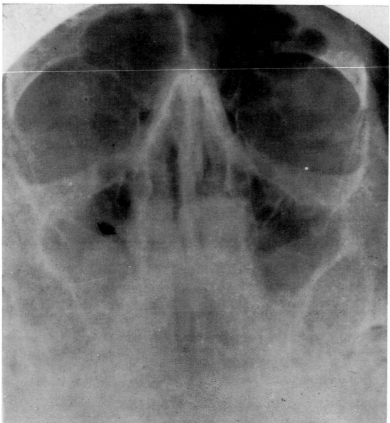

(b)

Figure 309. Polypoid mucosal thickening. Shelving antra. (a) A penetrated occipito-mental view. The appearance is confusing because the normal shelving antral floor on the left gives an outline which is very similar to the opacity in the base of the right antrum. However, close inspection suggests a normal mucosal shadow on the left (closed arrows), but nothing comparable on the right. (b) A less penetrated view confirms the presence of a soft-tissue opacity on the right (closed arrow)

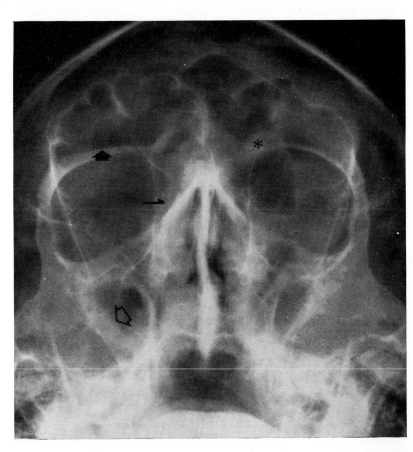

Figure 310. Sinusitis in a man aged 56 years with pain and tenderness over the medial part of the right supra-orbital ridge and photophobia after a minor head injury. There is fluid (closed arrow) in the right frontal sinus and polypoid mucosal thickening (asterisk) in the left. The right maxillary antrum shows generalized swelling of the mucosa (open arrow) and the right ethmoids are opaque due to what were later found to be polypi

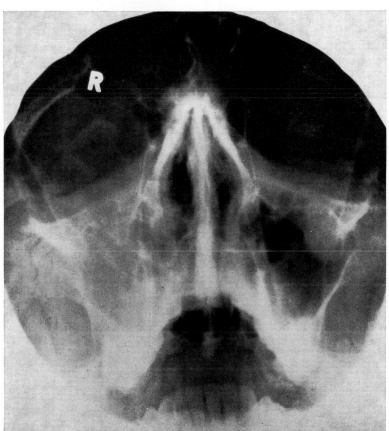

Figure 311. Allergy or infection, or both. An opaque right antrum and a rounded mucosal shadow on the left

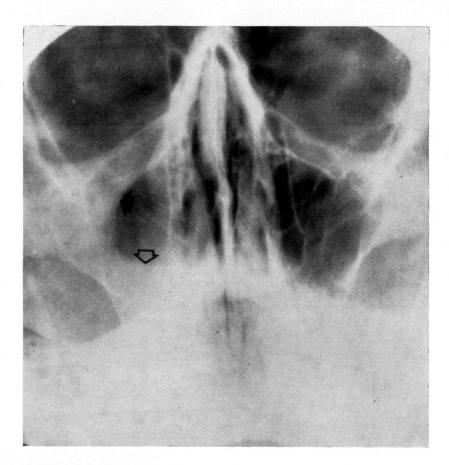

(a)

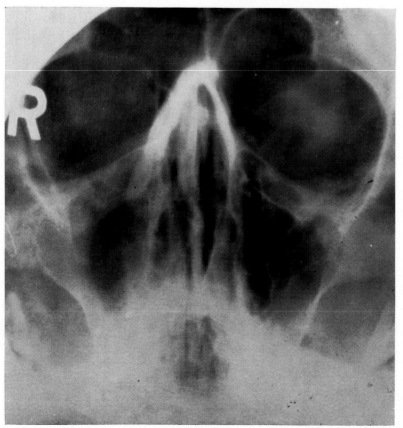

(b)

Figure 312. Acute infection. The patient presented with fever and pain in the face. (a) The occipito-mental view shows a peripheral opacity in the right antrum. This is composed of mucosal thickening (closed arrow) and pus (open arrow). The condition subsided after antral washout and antibiotics, the fluid disappearing quickly and the mucosal thickening much more slowly. (b) Two days later (cont.)

299

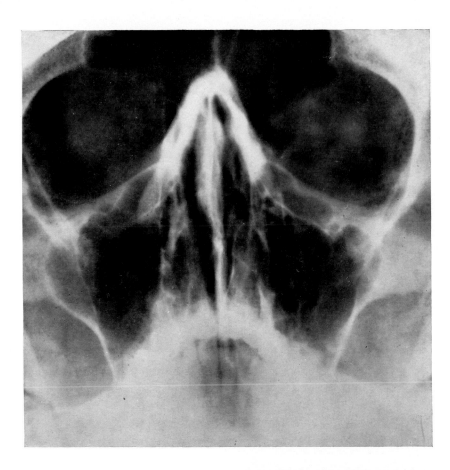

Figure 312 (cont.). (c) Seven weeks later

(c)

Figure 313. Root remnant in the maxillary antrum. The root was left behind after an extraction several weeks before. A fistula persisted. The occipito-mental view shows the root (arrow), upside down, surrounded by swollen mucous membrane and exudate in the base of the right antrum, from which it was removed. The fact that the root is upside down indicates that it had been free in the antrum

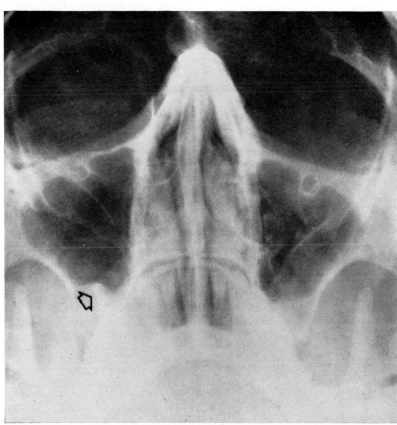

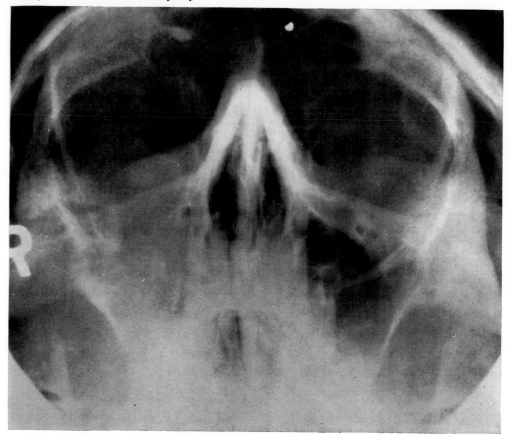

Figure 314. Neurofibrosarcoma of the infra-orbital nerve. There is opacity of the right maxillary antrum and destruction of its bony roof

of the sphenoid, around the optic canal, into the greater wing of the sphenoid or even the pterygoid processes, and this gross pneumatization may be symmetrical or more developed on one side than the other.

THE ETHMOIDAL CELLS

The ethmoidal cells are visible at birth but increase during childhood. They may extend to the medial wall of the antrum or into the sphenoid bone in cases in which the sphenoid sinus fails to develop,

In childhood and in patients in whom the sinuses are poorly developed, their translucency will be relatively diminished because of their thick bony walls.

Abnormal development

The paranasal sinuses may all be small in those conditions in which there is general hypoplasia of the facial bones and skull base. They are described in Chapters 8 and 11.

Over-development sometimes occurs in acromegaly where it particularly affects the frontal sinuses (page 98), and in some cases of cerebral atrophy beginning in infancy in which the distribution of the enlarged frontals and ethmoids suggests a compensatory mechanism (page

126). They are larger on the smaller side of the head. A similar localized over-expansion of sinuses tends to reduce the size of the bony orbit when an eye has been removed in early childhood (page 284).

Excessive development of the frontal sinuses has also been reported below an overlying soft-tissue angioma (Keats and Smith, 1972) and in familial pachydermoperiostosis (Harbison and Nice, 1971) in which the soft-tissue folds of the thick and redundant skin will also be visible on the film.

The condition of pneumosinus dilatans is recognized by some radiologists. A loculus may suddenly begin to expand. Lombardi, Passerini and Cecchini (1968) characterized the condition as follows: It is confined to one or a few air cells with a predilection for the lateral recesses of the frontal sinus, the superior recess of the maxillary sinus, the spheno-ethmoidal region near the sella or the anterior ethmoid near the orbit. The enlarging sinus has a normal mucosa. It contains only air. Pneumosinus dilatans is seen almost exclusively in males and generally in those between 20 and 40 years of age.

Large frontal sinuses are often present in dystrophia myotonica.

In Marfan's syndrome the palate is high, narrow and arched, and the shape of the facial skeleton and thereafter of the paransal sinuses fits with the palatal characteristics.

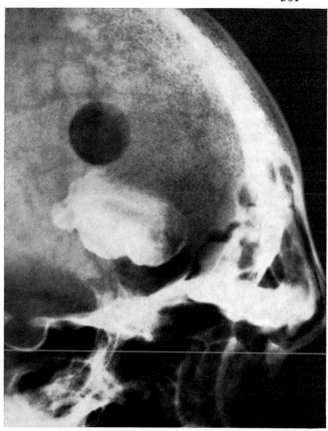

Figure 315. Ossifying fibroma of frontal sinuses. The patient, a man aged 45 years, presented with a frontal lobe abscess following an influenza-like illness. Haemophilus influenzae was cultured from the abscess. The frontal sinus was also infected around the ossifying fibroma. There was no defect in the posterior wall of the sinus, but the bone was inflamed. There was, however, a defect between the floor of the sinus and the orbit. Sections of the mass show a dense cortex of compact bone, and a centre of mutually growing and absorbing fibrous tissue and bone trabeculae. These tumours may also erode the posterior wall of the frontal sinus and lead to direct spread of the infection. (a) Lateral view. The frontal sinus is filled with a tumour, dense on the outside but translucent within. There is a burr-hole and an abscess filled with Thorotrast. (b) Antero-posterior view

(a)

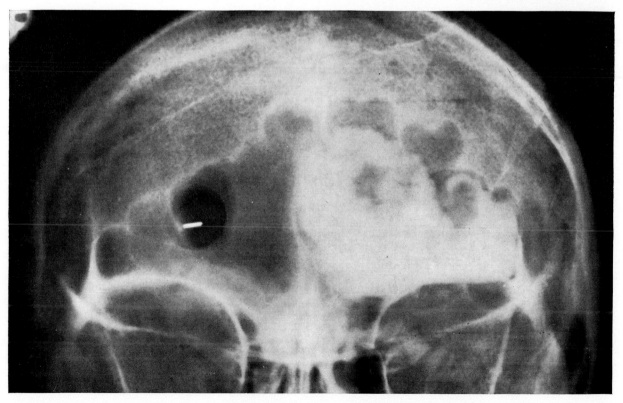

(b)

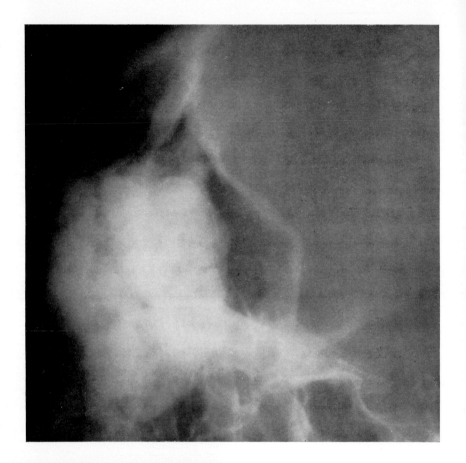

(a)

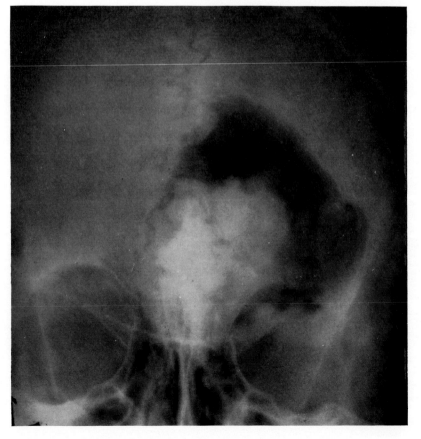

Figure 316. Ossifying fibroma of the frontal sinus. Note the expansion of the frontal sinus and the structure of the lesion. It resembles fibrous dysplasia. In such cases spontaneous fracture of the posterior wall of the frontal sinus may occur and lead to meningitis

(b)

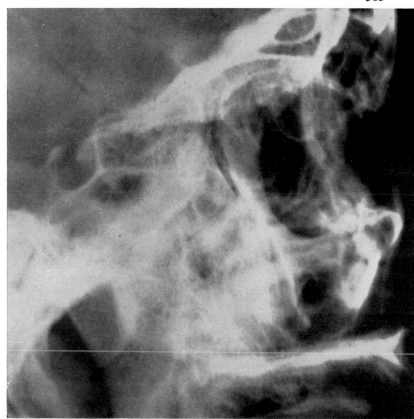

Figure 317. An ossifying chondroma beginning in the pterygoid fossa which has deformed the lateral wall (arrow) of the maxillary antrum. (a) Lateral view. (b) Full axial view

(a)

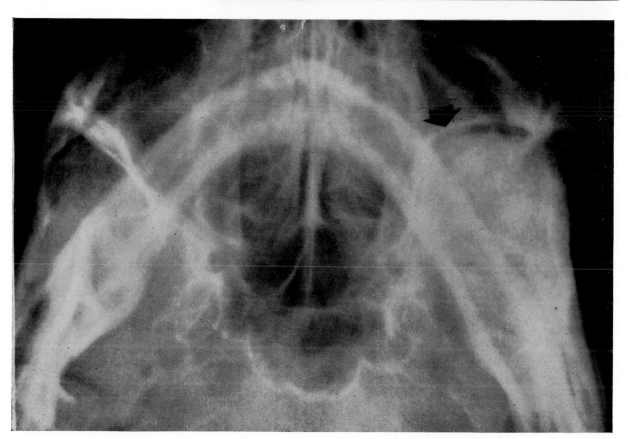

(b)

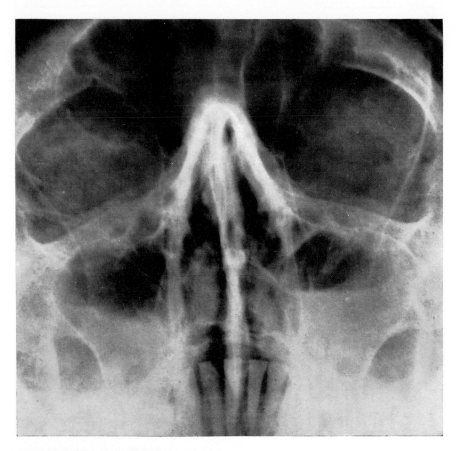

(a)

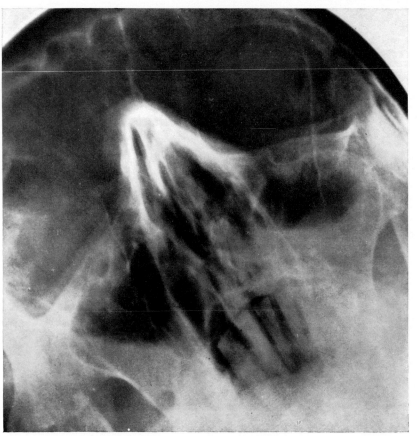

Figure 318. Fluid pus in the antra. (a) Occipito-mental view. (b) Tilted view

(b)

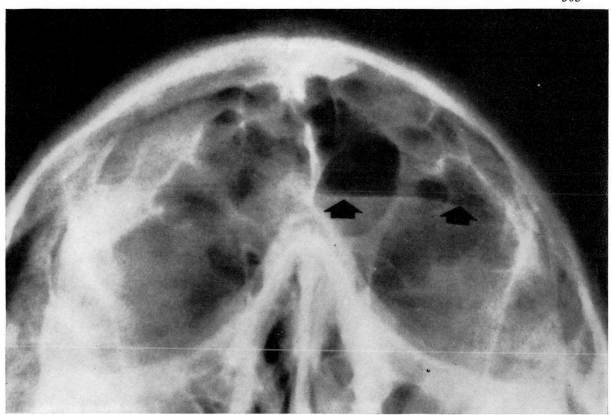

(a)

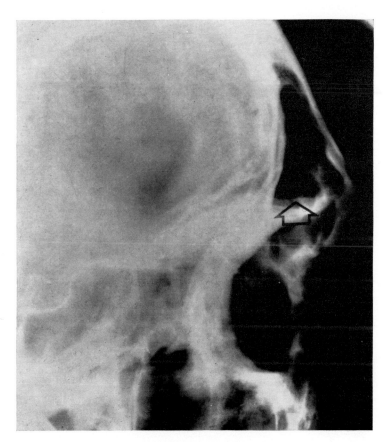

Figure 319. Fluid in the frontal sinus. Infection. It is uncommon to find a fluid level in the frontal sinus. (a) As with fluid in any other cavity, if the x-ray beam is not centred exactly at the surface level, the edge of the shadow may not be straight. It will be curved according to the margin of the cavity. (b) Lateral view

(b)

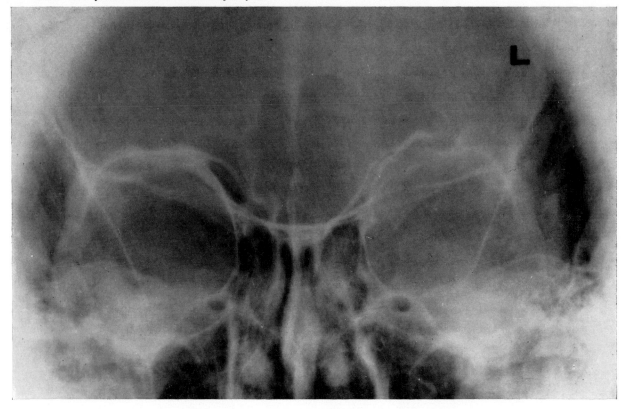

(a)

Figure 320. Mucocoele of the left frontal sinus. (a) The large left frontal sinus is almost as translucent as the small right one. This is because of extreme thinning of its bony walls. There is an actual defect of the orbital plate anteriorly, and there is bulging of the mucocoele into the orbit with proptosis and displacement downwards of the globe. (b) The lateral view demonstrates how thin the walls of the frontal sinus have become

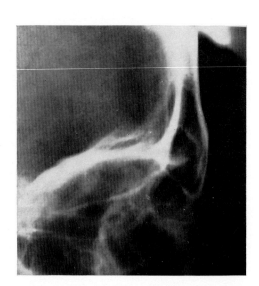

(b)

Opacity

Opacity of antra, frontal, ethmoid or sphenoid sinuses is one of the most frequent of radiological 'reports' and is often given without any attempt at interpretation of the finding. Even the recognition of abnormal opacity is not always a simple matter. Comparison with the translucency of the orbit or of the corresponding sinus on the opposite side may sometimes be of assistance, but there are many pitfalls. The sinus may be absent or poorly developed and have thick bony walls. After injury, or sometimes in association with infection, there may be swelling of the overlying soft tissues.

In the frontal sinuses and in the antra it is often possible by close inspection to discover the shadows thrown by the mocosa lining some part of the wall. Whether the strictly normal mucous membrane can be visualized is uncertain, but if at some point the mucosa

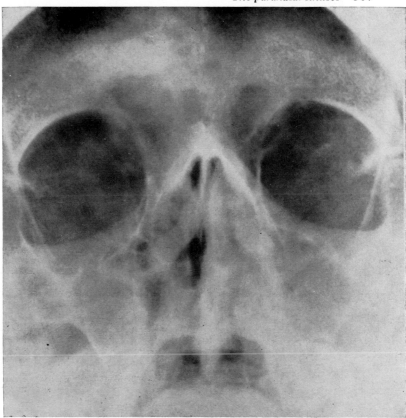

Figure 321. Chronic osteitis in a man aged 66 years with a long history of sinusitis. The sinuses are all opaque. There is increased density of the thickened frontal bone around the sinuses

can be seen and it is 2 mm or less in thickness and the opacity of the sinus is uniform, little significance can be attached to a subjective impression of slight generalized diminution of translucency.

The thickness and visibility of the mucosal shadow is of great importance in the recognition of disease and it should be carefully looked for. However, the exact shape of the shadow is of little help in differential diagnosis.

WIDESPREAD OPACITY (*Figures 306–312*)

Allergy and infection The commonest causes of opacity of any or all of the sinuses are allergy and infection. Both often act together and no firm distinction may be made on radiological grounds. The sinus may show a gross uniform opacity due either to oedematous mucous membrane or to obliteration of the remaining air space by retained secretions or pus.

When a central air space remains, the oedematous mucosa may be seen as a thickened soft-tissue shadow lining the walls. Localized rounded shadows and fluid pus are also seen.

SINUSITIS IN CHILDHOOD

Shapiro and Rossi (1973) have pointed out that although 51 per cent of a large group of children with suspected sinusitis had abnormal soft-tissue or fluid shadows in their sinuses, 57 per cent of children without clinical signs of sinusitis had similar radiological changes, as did 75 per cent of children with upper respiratory infection but without sinusitis. It is suggested that radiographs of the sinuses in upper respiratory infection in childhood are unlikely to be helpful.

ROUNDED OPACITIES

Soft-tissue opacities which do not fill the sinus may have rounded contours.

There are a number of possible causes. Most commonly seen in the maxillary antra, several of them are indistinguishable. These are as follow.

Mucous polyps associated with chronic infection
Retention cysts (which have the same cause)
Localized aggregations of surface exudate
Perhaps localized areas of acute mucosal inflammation
A partly calcified opacity may be a chondroma

Localized rounded opacities invading the sinus from outside and having characteristics likely to indicate the true diagnosis include some dental cysts, dentigerous cysts in the antrum, odontomes and other non-dental developmental cysts arising in the region of the alveolus, as well as ossifying fibromas, osteomas, and (very uncommonly) haemangiomas of bone (*Figure 313–317*).

Cherubism is a rare hereditary condition in which there are hard, painless symmetrical swellings (fibrous dysplasia) of the jaws and, on radiology, sharply defined multilocular areas of translucency in the mandible and often in the maxilla.

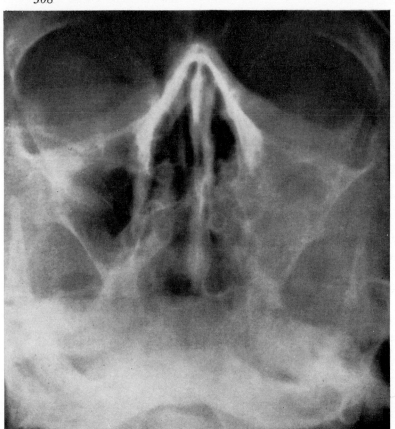

Figure 322. Squamous-cell carcinoma of the left upper jaw. (a) The occipito-mental view shows an opaque left antrum. There may be an erosion of the hard palate, but its limits are difficult to define. (b) Full axial view. The posterior and postero-medial walls of the antrum are not visible, presumably eroded (cont.)

(a)

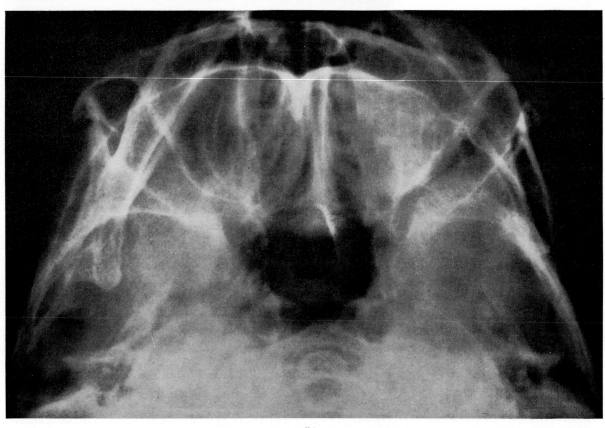

(b)

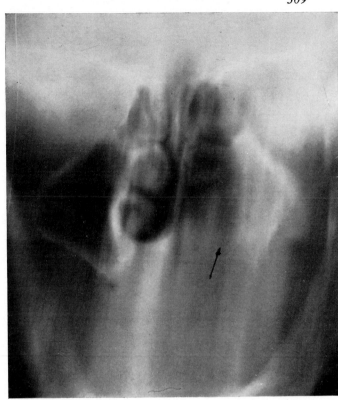

Figure 322 (cont.). (c) Postero-anterior tomogram shows the hard palate erosion (arrow) much more clearly. The inferior turbinate is swollen and there is destruction of the medial wall of the antrum as well

(c)

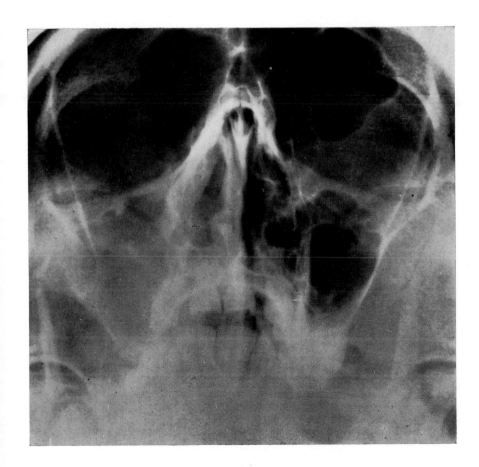

Figure 323. Carcinoma of the maxillary antrum. The right antrum is opaque and there is destruction of the bone of its medial wall. Soft-tissue swelling invades the nose and at operation the middle turbinate was found to be involved

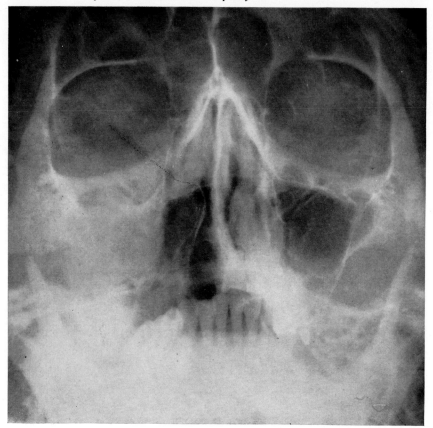

Figure 324. Fibrosarcoma in a man aged 46 years. The tumour was first seen 13 years before in the palate and had gradually spread. There had been several local excisions and he had radiotherapy. The occipito-mental view shows absence of the right half of the hard palate and the right inferior turbinate bone, an opaque antrum, and destruction of the lateral wall of the antrum

Malignant growth usually presents with bone destruction and complete opacity of the affected sinus rather than a localized swelling.

Intrasellar tumours may enlarge into the sphenoid sinus from above or, very rarely, a parasellar tumour such as a meningioma may invade from the side.

FLUID LEVELS (*Figures 318, 319*)

An opacity limited by a *fluid level* which remains horizontal when the head is tilted may be pus or mucopus as a result of infection, or fluid after antral washout or blood following acute injury. Fluid levels in the sphenoid sinus and sometimes in the ethmoids may also be due to a collection of cerebrospinal fluid seeping through a spontaneous traumatic defect in dura and bone.

Opacity of one of the sinuses with expansion of its bony walls may be due to a *mucocoele*, very rarely a *dermoid*, or in the case of the antrum a dental cyst. *Mucocoeles* are commoner in the frontal sinuses, and owing to the thinning of the bony walls, which long-continued pressure may produce, both *mucocoeles* and *dermoids* may sometimes cause expansion with hypertranslucency rather than opacity. *Mucocoele of the sphenoid sinus* may cause destruction and deformity of the pituitary fossa and can be confused radiologically with the changes due to pituitary tumours. Some upward displacement of thin portions of the roof of the sinus should be looked for; this excludes a pituitary mass.

Sclerosis of the surrounding bony walls may be due to fibrous dysplasia, Paget's disease or, rarely, to chronic osteomyelitis. Other causes of sclerosis of bones of the base and face are described in Chapter 7.

Erosion of the walls (*Figures 322–324*)

The walls of the sinuses are usually thin structures and erosions are difficult to see. They may be further masked by soft-tissue opacity. Tomography is of some assistance, but whether plain radiographs or tomography are used the most certain method of recognizing a defect is by visualizing the affected wall edge-on. In tangential views, sudden cessation of the white line of compact bone usually indicates the presence of erosion. In order to examine the complicated shapes of the paranasal sinuses for erosions or defects (the result of trauma, infection or malignant disease) many radiographic views are required.

Osteomyelitis, though it may produce coalescing osteolytic regions (particularly of the frontal bone), does not, as a rule, give rise to complete defects in the walls of the sinuses, except in mycotic infection. Mucor mycosis is more likely if the patient is a diabetic and has been long on antibiotic therapy or immunosuppressant drugs. The presence of such a defect with adjacent soft-tissue swelling, and perhaps opacity of the affected sinus, is however usually evidence of a *malignant primary or secondary tumour*.

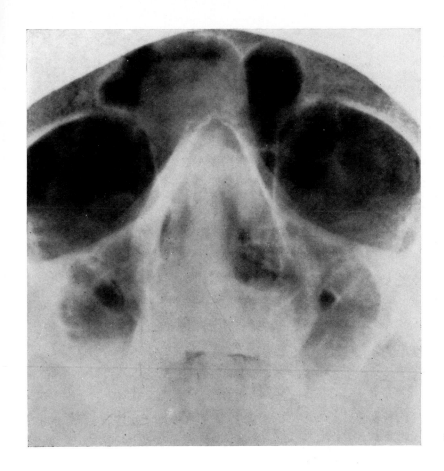

(a)

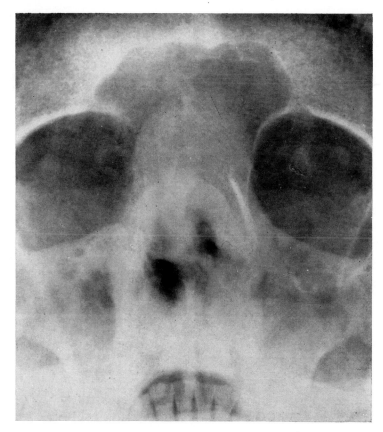

Figure 325. Chordoma in a man aged 51 years with a history of loss of smell for 3 years. He was found to have a mass in the left nasal cavity, extending into the left maxillary antrum and the ethmoid cells. Much of this was removed and found to be a chordoma. (a) Occipito-mental view after partial excision and before radiotherapy, showing erosion of the nasal bones and a mass in the right frontal sinus. (b) Seven years later when a palpable swelling had appeared at the bridge of the nose, there is much more bone erosion

(b)

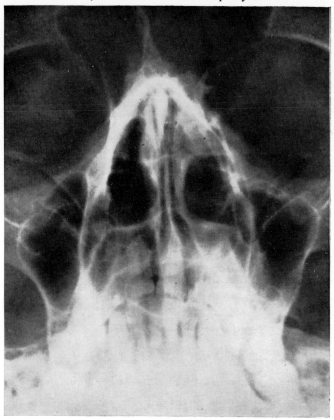

Figure 326. A low-growing malignant tumour of the nasal passage. The left half of the nasal cavity is expanded, and is completely obstructed by tumour tissue

Fractures

Fractures involving the leakage of cerebrospinal fluid are sometimes impossible to demonstrate, even by the most careful technique, but *see* page 340 in Chapter 12 on Head Injuries.

THE NOSE AND NASAL BONES

The nasal bones are best seen in a lateral and in special axial projections, but the cavity of the nose may be examined in the routine postero-anterior and in the full axial views.

The bones may show erosion, deformity or displacement due to congenital abnormality, infection, or benign or malignant tumours. The nasal cavity may show a deformity of shape due to congenital abnormality or sometimes to the presence of tumours, or it may be opaque for a variety of other reasons. In neuroradiological practice, the nasal cavity provides a window through which the floor of the sella may be observed in postero-anterior projection.

Erosion (*Figure 325*)

The nasal bones as seen in the lateral view and occasionally the turbinates and bony septum in the postero-anterior projection may show destruction, sometimes mixed with areas of sclerosis in cases of *lupus vulgaris* and *syphilis* and *goundou* as well as in occasional cases of *chronic infection by other organisms. Leprosy* does not commonly cause severe bone destruction.

Primary carcinoma of the nose or invasion from neighbouring malignant growths may also cause extensive loss of bone.

Because of the complicated structure of the bones and the number of superimposed shadows, tomography is of considerable help in deciding the presence and extent of erosions.

Deformity

The nasal bones may be hypoplastic in several forms of dwarfism and in a variety of other conditions which result in hypoplasia of the base of the skull. A few of these developmental conditions may be given here as examples: *achondroplasia, chondrodystrophia calcificans congenita (Conradi's syndrome), thanatophoric dwarfism, Crouzon's disease*. There is a fuller account of developmental anomalies in Chapter 11.

The upper part of the nasal cavity may be widened and its bones displaced apart, as seen in postero-anterior views, by the presence of a large *encephalo-meningocoele* (*Figure 328*), but small ones which protrude into the upper part of the nose show little or no radiological deformity.

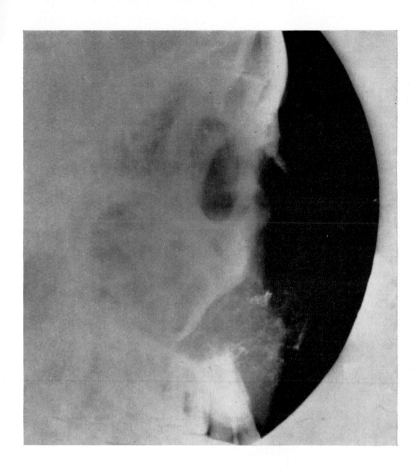

(a)

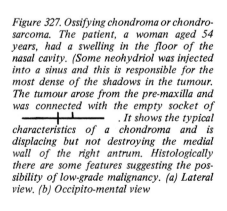

Figure 327. Ossifying chondroma or chondro-sarcoma. The patient, a woman aged 54 years, had a swelling in the floor of the nasal cavity. (Some neohydriol was injected into a sinus and this is responsible for the most dense of the shadows in the tumour. The tumour arose from the pre-maxilla and was connected with the empty socket of ——————————— . It shows the typical characteristics of a chondroma and is displacing but not destroying the medial wall of the right antrum. Histologically there are some features suggesting the possibility of low-grade malignancy. (a) Lateral view. (b) Occipito-mental view

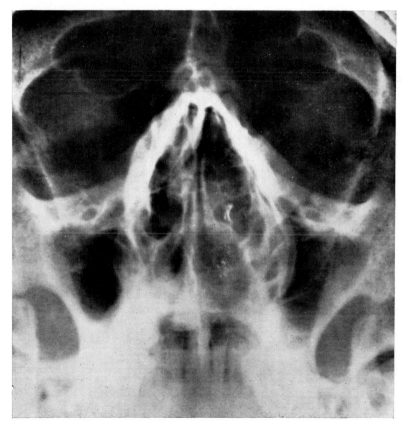

(b)

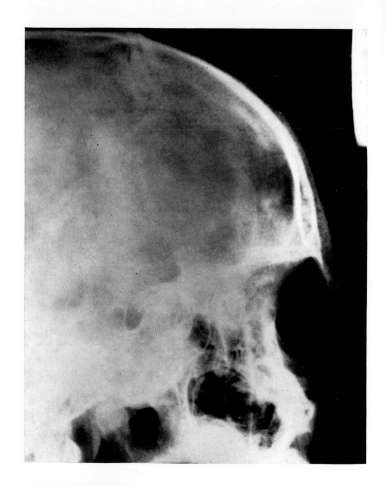

(a)

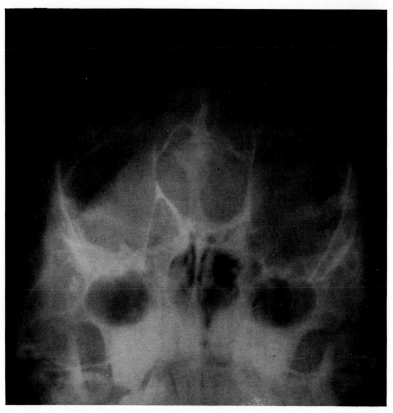

*Figure 328. Nasal meningo-encephalocoele.
The nose was wide and the eyes far apart.
There is a large central bone defect, but in
less severe cases little or no deformity may
be seen on the radiographs*

(b)

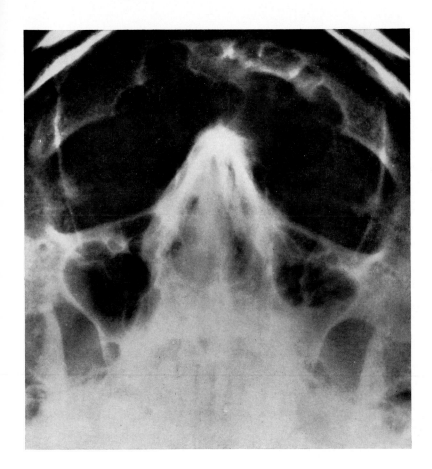

Figure 329. The nasal cavity is obstructed by polypi. There is a shadow in the base of the left antrum which has a straight upper margin. It was not caused by fluid, but probably represented mucosal polypi. A view with the head tilted would have shown that the level did not alter, and since the opacity was not caused by fluid the patient would have been saved an antral puncture and washout

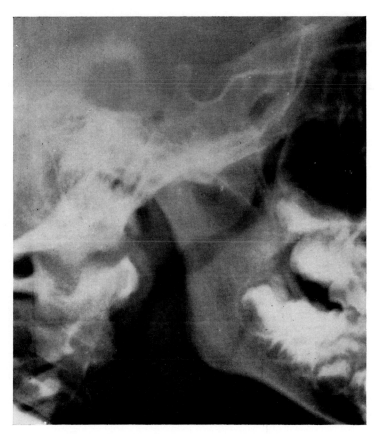

Figure 330. Enlarged adenoids and tonsils in a child aged 5 years. The shadow of the soft palate and uvula blends with that of the enlarged tonsil

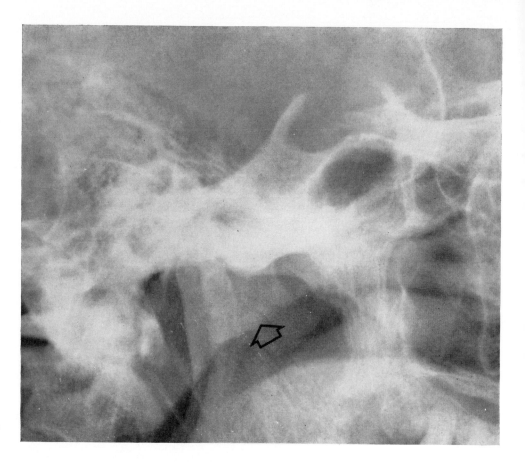

(a)

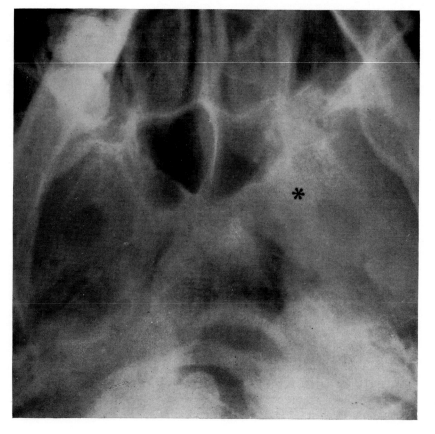

Figure 331. Nasopharyngeal carcinoma.
(a) There is a soft-tissue shadow (arrow)
in the nasopharynx. The basisphenoid
shows a diffuse sclerotic reaction. (b)
This is also apparent in the medial part
of the floor of the left half of the
middle fossa (asterisk). The bone looks
extremely like that affected by a
hyperostosis due to meningioma, but
the size of the nasopharyngeal mass
makes the diagnosis of meningioma
unlikely

(b)

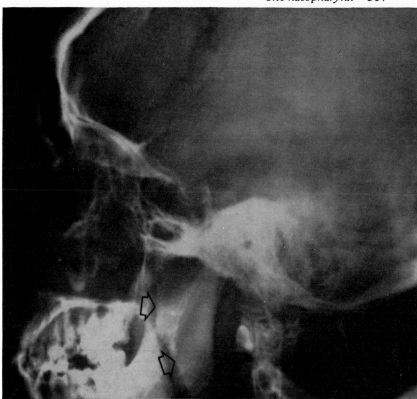

Figure 332. Chordoma. There is a large nasopharyngeal soft-tissue mass. The patient had multiple cranial nerve palsies and the tumour was found to be infiltrating the upper cervical spine and compressing the cervical cord

There are many facial deformities that form parts of more widespread developmental defects, and are mentioned in Chapter 11. It is necessary here to list *cleft palate* and more severe failures of fusion of the bone anlage. *Facial duplication,* a very gross deformity of the whole midline of the face with a transverse slit beneath the nose and two lateral oral stomata, may be, but is not always, associated with developmental abnormalities of the brain.

Benign tumours of the nose are not common, but when they occur they also cause expansion of the nasal cavity with deformity of surrounding bone. Some, such as *dermoids, fibromas* and *neurofibromas,* may be more or less translucent. An *osteoma* may also be found from time to time and this and the *ossifying fibroma* with which it may be confused throw dense shadows of similar nature to those found elsewhere in the body *(Figure 327).*

A *rhinolith* may also enlarge one half of the nasal cavity. Rhinoliths usually result from the long presence of a foreign body, and because they contain calcium salts they are demonstrable as irregular speckled incrustations.

Alterations in translucency of the nasal cavity

It is very common to find the two halves of the nasal cavity of unequal size and translucency as a result of slight *congenital deformities of the bony septum and inequality in size of the turbinates.* Opacity may also be due to *oedematous swelling of the mucosa* to the presence of *polypi, foreign bodies,* any of the *tumours* described above, or to previous trauma *(Figure 329).*

Congenital *atresia* or *stenosis* of one or both choanae also occurs. This may be bony, in which case the deficient development of the nose will result in facial deformity and the diagnosis of atresia may be suggested from the radiograph; or it may be fibrous, in which case plain radiographic examination is of little value. Williams (1971) suggests that atresia is not as rare as might be supposed from the literature because unilateral atresia may be symptomless. Bilateral atresia is, however, of great importance in *neonates.*

The nasal cavity may appear hypertranslucent on one or both sides due to *congenital absence of turbinate bones,* and occasionally in association with deformity as a result of the presence of an *encephalo-meningocoele* or a *dermoid cyst (Figure 328).*

Fractures of the nasal bones

See Chapter 12.

THE NASOPHARYNX

In a general examination of the skull it is important not to overlook possible soft-tissue abnormalities. In the routine lateral skull view the air shadow of the nasopharynx is usually clearly revealed, but if there is some doubt about the possibility of an abnormality in the region a special lateral view should be taken centred over the nasopharynx and the exposure made during full inspiration.

The air shadow may be encroached upon from behind by a smooth soft-tissue mass due to *enlarged adenoids* (*Figure 330*).

A *malignant tumour* of the nasopharynx, the outline of which is sometimes irregular due to the presence of a large ulcer, may also show. However, there are often no radiological changes although a nasopharyngeal carcinoma is discovered later. The inaccessibility of the region to clinical examination and the frequency of negative radiological findings make diagnosis difficult (*Figure 331*).

A *chordoma* involving the base of the skull not infrequently has a massive nasopharyngeal extension. In spite of the presence of such an obvious mass and evidence of an intracranial extension as well, erosion of the intervening bone may be very difficult to see (*Figure 332*).

Very rarely a *large aneurysm* of the intracavernous part of the carotid may so erode the base of the skull that it presents as a soft-tissue swelling through the floor of the middle fossa. Such a mass will very probably contain some calcification. The diagnosis is made by angiography (*Figure 186*).

11 DEVELOPMENTAL ABNORMALITIES

In addition to the better known single or simple abnormalities such as, for example, basilar invagination and occipital dysplasia (Kruyff, 1965), meningo-encephalocoele or congenital parietal foramina, there is now an enormous number of named syndromes of skeletal maldevelopment involving the skull. A chapter is required devoted to the cranial manifestations of the better known of these complex conditions, but it cannot aim to be more than elementary; the material seems inexhaustible and in general there is a lack of theory with which to bind it all together.

To help a radiologist identify an abnormal skull, or at least place it within a limited group, some sort of scheme has to be adopted, though it may not be justifiable on developmental grounds.

The abnormalities to be described briefly in this chapter have been grouped according to six major, usually obvious, characteristics as follows.
(1) The sutures and fontanelles are widely open, thus suggesting, often wrongly, that the intracranial pressure may be raised.
(2) There is premature craniosynostosis.
(3) The vault and/or base are abnormally thick and dense.
(4) The cranial cavity is small. Microcephaly in these cases may be accompanied by facial deformities.
(5) Deformity of the face is the most obvious defect.
(6) The deformity is predominantly determined by a small skull base.

It can be seen at once that several conditions deserve a place in more than one category. To help the reader, but preserve the simplicity of the plan, multiple entries of this sort have been kept to a minimum. Also obvious is the fact that the majority of the conditions are first noticed in early life. Some are incompatible with prolonged survival, but neither the age range of the patients nor the many associated abnormalities outside the skull

have been made a feature of this chapter. References in the text should help those who need to study any particular syndrome more thoroughly. A correct diagnosis may be of great importance because of the genetic implications and the advice to be given to parents of deformed children. Spranger, Langer and Weidemann (1974) is an excellent reference, but the most important advice in this Chapter is that the opinion of an expert should be obtained before counselling the mother or father about the prognosis or likelihood of deformity in subsequent children. Many of the conditions have also already been described in other chapters.

The sutures and fontanelles are widely open, thus suggesting, often wrongly, that the intracranial pressure may be raised

Osteogenesis imperfecta – See Chapter 2 and *Figures 55, 56, 244.*
Cleidocranial dysostosis – See Chapter 2 and *Figures 250, 251.*
Hypophosphatasia – See Chapter 2 and *Figure 50.* During the early stage the bones may be entirely uncalcified and thereafter for a few years their growth delayed so that the sutures are wide and the anterior fontanelle bulges. When ossification catches up craniostenosis may supervene. The vault bones during the stage of ossification may show slight increase in density. The condition may be divided into neonatal, infantile and childhood forms. In the neonate deficiency of bone is the outstanding feature. In the infantile form the condition may go on to craniostenosis. In the childhood form this outcome is rarer and other skeletal changes are usually less severe. The deciduous teeth are affected and often lost prematurely (Ratburn, 1948; Currarino *et al.*, 1957; Fraser, 1957; Bethune and Dent, 1960; James and Moule, 1966).

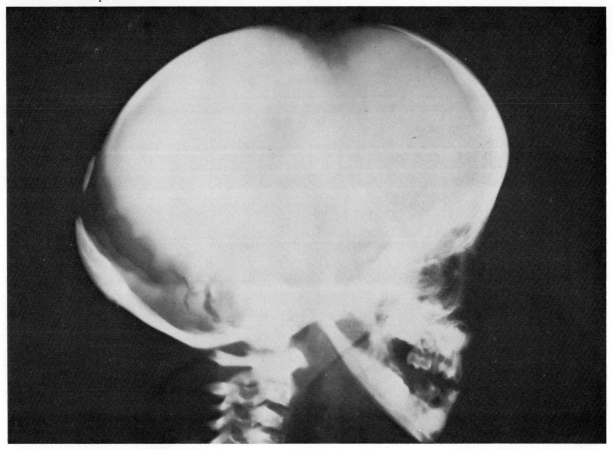

Figure 333. Pyknodysostosis (Toulouse-Lautrec syndrome: osteopetrosis acro-osteolytica). The calvaria is large by comparison with the face. The fontanelles are widely open. The bones are dense

(Reproduced by courtesy of Dr. A. Chrispin, Hospital for Sick Children, Gt. Ormond Street)

PYKNODYSOSTOSIS (TOULOUSE-LAUTREC SYNDROME – *Figure 333*) (Maroteaux and Lamy, 1962)

These individuals of dwarfed stature have bones of increased density with a strong tendency to fracture. The head seems large by comparison with the hypoplastic face and mandible. The sutures are wide and the fontanelles persist, though they eventually partly fill with wormian bones. The vault is thin as well as dense. Short stature results from the short limbs; the terminal phalanges are short and wide.

DYSCEPHALIA MANDIBULO-OCULOFACIALIS (HALLERMANN–STREIFF SYNDROME) (Franconi, 1958)

This syndrome is also characterized by hypoplasia of the mandible and face, but the tubular bones are all of greatly reduced calibre. There is delayed closure of fontanelles and sutures between the thin bones of the calvaria. The skull may show increased convolutional markings and platybasia. The orbits are small with microphthalmia and congenital cataracts. The external genitalia are underdeveloped. There is mental retardation.

There is premature craniosynostosis (craniostenosis)

The appearance of craniostenosis (*Figure 334*) has been described in Chapter 4, where some of its causes and the conditions with which it may be associated are listed. That discussion need not be repeated.

The syndromes with which primary craniostenosis may be associated overlap with one another in a complex way.

CROUZON'S DISEASE

In Crouzon's disease the sutures affected vary, but there is always extreme facial hypoplasia resulting in the grossest deformity, including bilateral proptosis because the orbits are too small and hypertelorism because they are forced apart. The limbs are not affected. It is an autosomal dominant trait (Dodge, Wood and Kennedy, 1959).

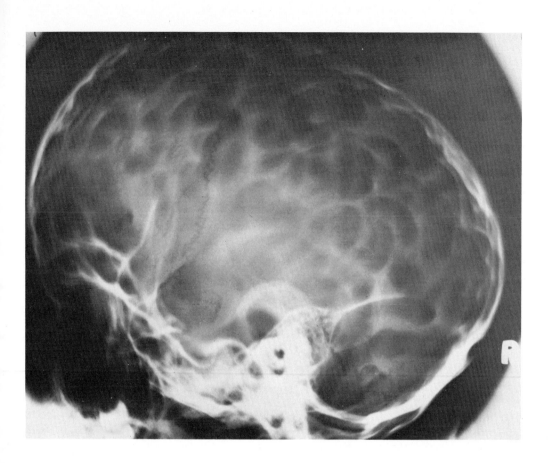

Figure 334. Generalized craniostenosis. By comparison with acrocephaly the skull is a much more normal shape, but this is due to the premature closure of almost all the sutures. Some parts of the coronal suture remain. There has been an extreme attempt by the skull bone to adapt to the growing brain

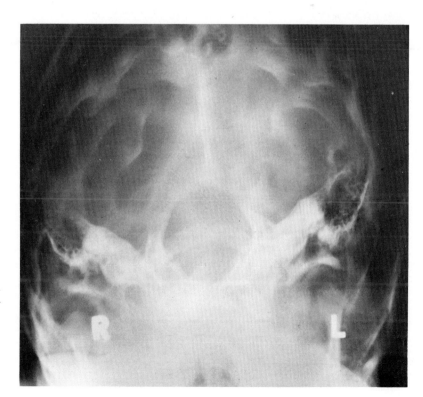

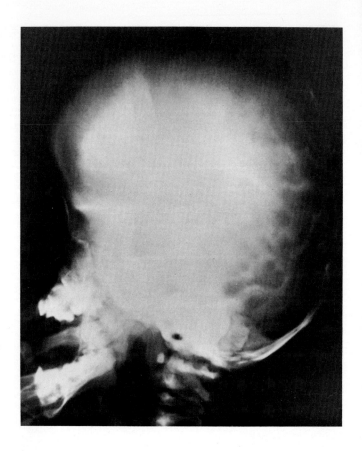

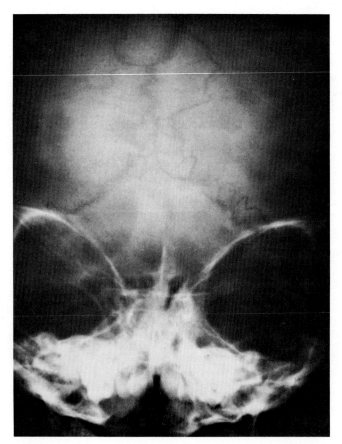

Figure 335. Acrocephaly (Apert's syndrome). (a) The typically shaped head with its steep forehead and short antero-posterior measurement. (b) The lambdoid and sagittal sutures still open, with many wormian bones (cont.)

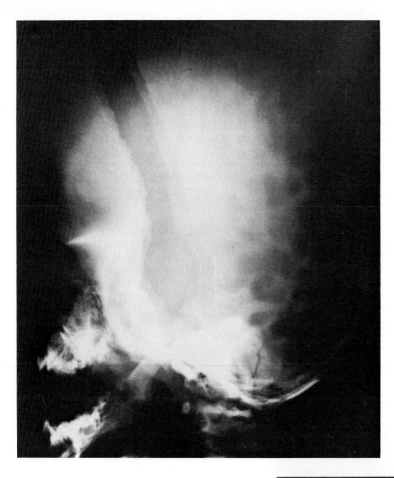

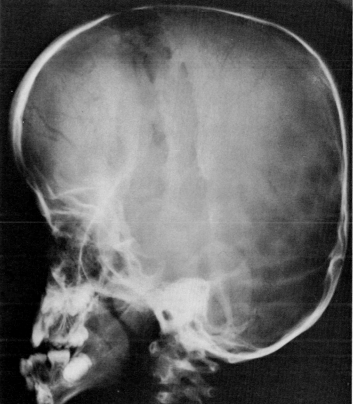

*Figure 335 (cont.) (c) One month after opera-
tion designed to provide a coronal gap. (d) Two
years later. Though bony fusion has occurred
again, antero-posterior growth of the skull must
have taken place in the interval. The skull shows
no abnormal pressure changes*

(Reproduced by courtesy of Dr. R. D. Hoare,
Hospital for Sick Children, Gt. Ormond Street)

ACROCEPHALO-SYNDACTYLY

The association of acrocephaly with fusion of digits is known as Apert's syndrome (*Figure 335*) and is also an autosomal dominant. The forehead is steep and the apex of the skull lies very anteriorly. The face is hypoplastic much as in Crouzon's disease. Bony fusion of fingers and toes is accompanied by other limb deformities such as ankylosis of elbows, hips and shoulders. Familial acrocephalo-syndactyly is also known as Pfeiffer's syndrome (Pfeiffer, 1964). The association of acrocephalo-syndactyly with cardiac disease and ear and skin anomalies has been described by Sakati and Nyhan (1971).

Fishman, Hogan and Dodge (1971) have drawn attention to the occurrence of hydrocephalus in some cases of Apert's syndrome.

THE FRONTO-DIGITAL SYNDROME (Marshall and Smith, 1970)

This appears to be a milder form of sagittal craniostenosis with inconstant syndactyly inherited as an autosomal dominant.

ACROCEPHALO-POLYSYNDACTYLY

This is distinguished from Apert's syndrome and is known as Carpenter's syndrome, inheritable as an autosomal recessive. With the cranial and limb deformities are associated hypogenitalism, abdominal hernias and mental retardation (Temtamy, 1966). The name of Noak is linked with a similar deformity.

THE LAURENCE–MOON–BIEDL–BARDET SYNDROME

This consists of a mild cranial deformity plus mental retardation, hypogenitalism, obesity and retinitis pigmentosa, polydactyly but not syndactyly.

Many of the children suffering from the syndromes mentioned above have some degree of hypertelorism. Unlike them are those in whom premature closure of the metopic suture leads to hypotelorism, the orbits remaining too close together unless synostosis is so widespread that the floor of the anterior fossa is forced down between the eyes by the imprisoned brain. The simple skull deformity resulting from premature fusion of the metopic suture is known as trigonocephaly.

CRANIOTELENCEPHALIC DYSPLASIA

There is premature closure of the metopic, coronal and sagittal sutures with hypotelorism, ear deformities and mental retardation.

CRANIOSYNOSTOSIS AND RADIAL APLASIA

This is another rare but recurrent combination (Greitzer *et al.*, 1974) with other anomalies of the skeleton and soft tissues.

TRIGONOCEPHALY (*Figure 336*) (HYPOTELORISM– ARHINENCEPHALY–TRIGONOCEPHALY COMPLEX: HOLOPROSENCEPHALY)

Craniostenosis may not only cause but also accompany brain deformity. Various degrees of defect may result from an arrest of cleavage of the prosencephalon of the cerebral hemispheres and incomplete development of the prechordal mesoderm between the prosencephalon and the foregut. Alobar holoprosencephaly is the severest form. Semilobar holoprosencephaly is the condition when an interhemispheric fissure has formed but there is, for instance, agenesis of the olfactory bulbs and tracts, or of the corpus callosum. Bony and facial soft-tissue abnormalities include cyclopia (a single orbit), ethmocephaly (in which the orbits are small and the nose vestigial), cebocephaly (a single nostril) and median cleft lip or all the more severe degrees of bilateral cleft lip or palate with defective midline bone development in relation to the nose. Trigonocephaly may be found and severe hypotelorism is the rule (Kurlander *et al.*, 1966).

KLEEBLATTSCHÄDEL (CLOVER-LEAF SKULL – *Figure 337*)

The coronal and lambdoid sutures having closed very early while the sagittal and squamosal sutures remain open, there is extreme bulging of the vertex and temporal regions.

Kleeblattschädel is found in some cases of thanatophoric dwarfism (Iannacone and Gerlini, 1974). Many children with this form of craniostenosis also have hydrocephalus and there is a further common association with skeletal abnormalities resembling achondroplasia (Angle, McIntire and Moore, 1967).

The vault and/or base are abnormally thick and dense

Many of these conditions have also been described in Chapters 3 and 7 and need only be listed here. Thus, for dystrophia myotonica turn to page 99, for Albers–Schönberg to page 219, Englemann's disease to page 219, and Caffey's syndrome to page 109.

In addition to the above mention must be made of the following.

HYPERPHOSPHATASIA OR HYPERPHOSPHATASAEMIA

In childhood this is sometimes known as juvenile Paget's disease. In later life, usually beginning in adolescence, it is known as van Buchem's disease (or hyperostosis corticalis generalisata familiaris). The skull becomes very thick with large, more or less homogeneous areas of density interspersed with translucencies very like severe Paget's disease, in which there is also a tendency to spare the squamous occiput. Cranial nerves may be compressed. In childhood the long bones are thickened but the epiphyses remain relatively normal. In van Buchem's disease the thickening is of the endosteal surface.

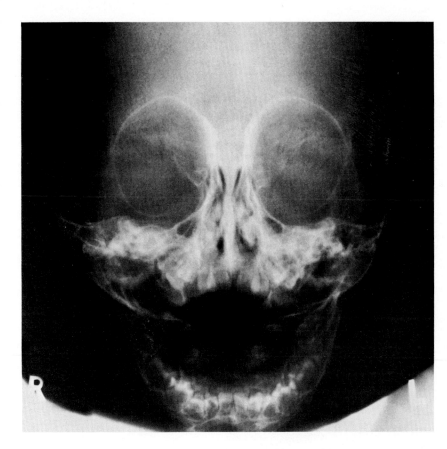

Figure 336. Trigonocephaly. (a) The postero-anterior view shows hypotelorism. (b) A mento-vertical view shows the frontal bone in profile, revealing the pointed forehead

(Reproduced by courtesy of Dr. R. D. Hoare, Hospital for Sick Children, Gt. Ormond Street)

(a)

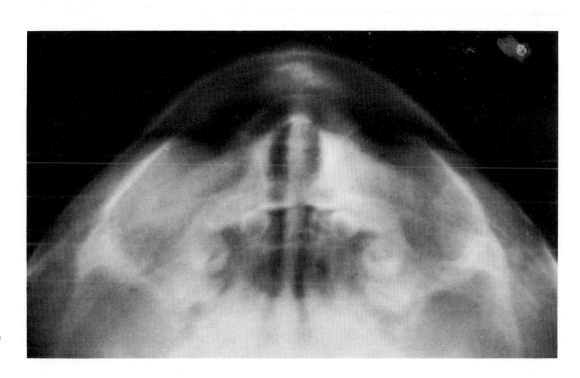

(b)

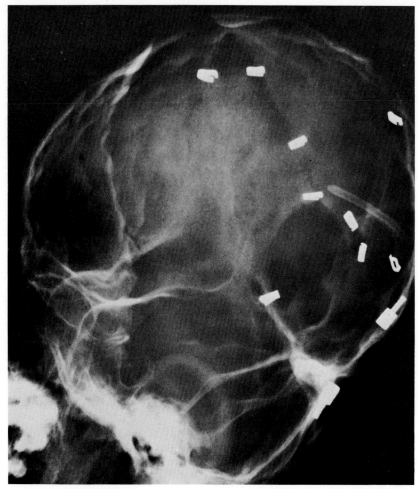

Figure 337. Clover-leaf skull. There has been an attempt to create an artificial suture and a ventricular shunt has been inserted to control the patient's hydrocephalus

(Reproduced by courtesy of Dr. R. D. Hoare, Hospital for Sick Children, Gt. Ormond Street)

At birth the patients are usually normal, but when the disease becomes fully developed after a few years the child is dwarfed, with a large head and saddle nose. The limbs are short and bowed. (Bakwin and Eiger, 1956; van Buchem *et al.*, 1962; Rubin, 1964; Thompson *et al.*, 1969).

CRANIOMETAPHYSEAL DYSPLASIA (*Figure 338*)
(PYLE'S DISEASE) (Pyle, 1931; Gorlin, Koszalka and Spranger, 1970)

It has been suggested that Pyle's disease is one of a group of related syndromes which cannot be exactly separated (Macpherson, 1974). They include familial metaphyseal dysplasia and craniodiaphyseal dysplasia. Perhaps fronto-metaphyseal dysplasia (Gorlin and Cohen, 1969) should be added. There is thickening of the supra-orbital ridge with absence of the frontal sinuses, hypoplasia of the angle and condyloid processes of the mandible, a cervico-occipital abnormality, fusion of carpal bones and undertubulation and sclerosis of the shafts of long bones. In some of the cases there may be hyperostoses of other bones than the frontal.

Other rare syndromes have been described. Caffey (1967) for instance reported congenital stenosis of the medullary spaces in tubular bones and the calvaria in two proportionate dwarfs, but both were liable to attacks of hypocalcaemic tetany.

The cranial cavity is small, with or without facial deformity

Separation of this group from the next is arbitary, but there is some point in distinguishing those children and adults who present most obviously with microcephaly.

Many microcephalics have suffered brain damage at birth or in infancy due to outside influences, metabolic (for instance, maternal phenylketonuria), traumatic, vascular or infective. These are not dealt with here. This section lists a number of hereditary dysplasias and chromosomal abnormalities and one or two conditions that fit with difficulty into any ordered scheme.

PROGERIA (HUTCHINSON-GILFORD SYNDROME)

The skull is small and delicate and of infantile proportions, the face is small by comparison with the cranium. The patients have coxa valga. They do not live to more than 16 years.

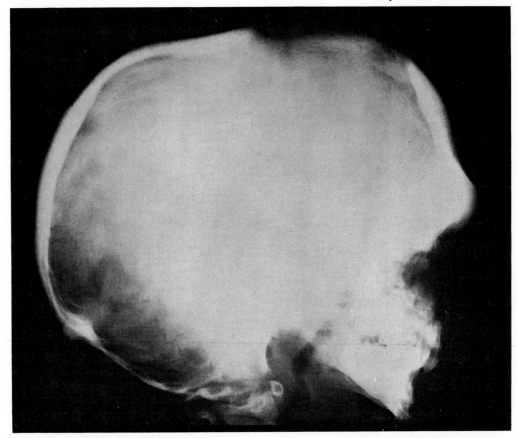

Figure 338. Craniometaphyseal dysplasia. There is hyperostosis of the frontal and parietal bones
(Reproduced by courtesy of Dr. A. Chrispin, Hospital for Sick Children, Gt. Ormond Street)

TRISOMY 13–15 (PATAN'S SYNDROME: TRISOMY D) (James *et al.*, 1969)

Children with this chromosomal translocation die within 4–6 months. They have cebocephaly, hypotelorism and small orbits as well as a small cranium.

TRISOMY 18 (E SYNDROME) (James *et al*, 1969)

Survival is limited to about 6 months. There is scaphocephaly, hypoplasia of the mandible, cleft palate, flexion deformities of fingers and toes, clubbed feet and extensive abdominal abnormalities.

TRISOMY 21 (DOWN'S SYNDROME)

This has already been described.

CRI-DU-CHAT SYNDROME (James *et al.*, 1969)

There is deletion of much of the short arms of No. 5 or sometimes No. 4 chromosome: 46 chromosomes are present. Microcephaly is accompanied by faulty long-bone development. There is either hypertelorism, telecanthus or a prominent epicanthal fold.

4p-SYNDROME (WOLF'S SYNDROME) (Franceschini, Grassi and Marchese, 1971)

This resembles the cri-du-chat syndrome both in its chromosomal origin (partial deletion of short arms of No. 4 chromosome) and in its manifestations—microcephaly, hypertelorism, prominent glabella, cleft palate and clubbed feet.

BRACHMANN–DE LANGE SYNDROME (Lee and Kenny, 1967)

The chromosomal abnormality is inherited as an autosomal recessive trait but many patients die before the age of 15 years. Their eyebrows meet in the middle and they show other evidence of hypertrichosis. The upper lip is long, the nostrils anteverted. They have trigonocephaly and microcephaly and distal limb abnormalities of which the most characteristic are hypoplasia and dorsal dislocation of the radial heads, hypoplasia of the first metacarpal bone and of the middle phalanx of the shortened and incurved fifth finger.

COCKAYNE'S SYNDROME (Cocayne, 1936; Land and Nogrady, 1969)

Microcephaly is accompanied by enophthalmia, prominent maxilla and nose, short trunk, relatively long legs and large feet. There is mental retardation, beginning in the

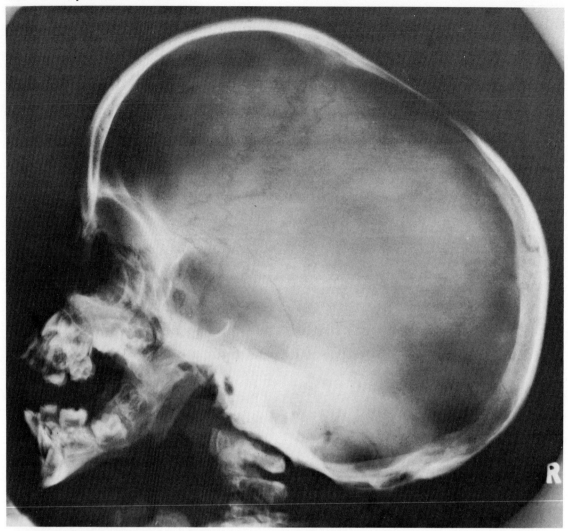

Figure 339. Mucopolysaccharidosis (Type 6). A girl aged 4 years. The head is large but the bones do not show increased convolutional markings. The sella is eroded. The child had hydrocephalus and arachnoid cysts

(Reproduced by courtesy of Dr. R. D. Hoare, Hospital for Sick Children, Gt. Ormond Street)

second year of life, impaired vision and hearing and a scaly eczematous skin. Intracranial calcification is not uncommon.

PRADER-WILLI SYNDROME (Pearson, Steinbach and Bier, 1971)

These mentally retarded children may grow to adult life. They are obese and sexually infantile. The sella may be small. The calvaria shows wormian bones. There are dental abnormalities, hip and limb deformities and vertebral maldevelopment, possibly with scoliosis.

BIRD-HEADED DWARFISM (Fitch, Pinsky and Lachance, 1970)

This dysplasia is inherited as an autosomal recessive. The central part of the face protrudes. The malar bones are hypoplastic as is the mandible. Malocclusion is found. The cranium is small and mentality severely retarded. There are vertebral, sternal and limb abnormalities, notably joint dislocation and absent patellae.

KINKY-HAIR SYNDROME (Wesenberg, Gwinn and Barnes, 1969)

The skull is small with extra wormian bones in the lambdoid suture.

Deformity of the face is the most striking observation

Deformity of the face may be the presenting sign in a few of the conditions in the previous groups, particularly holoprosencephaly (which has been described in relation to trigonocephaly) and Trisomy 13—15. In

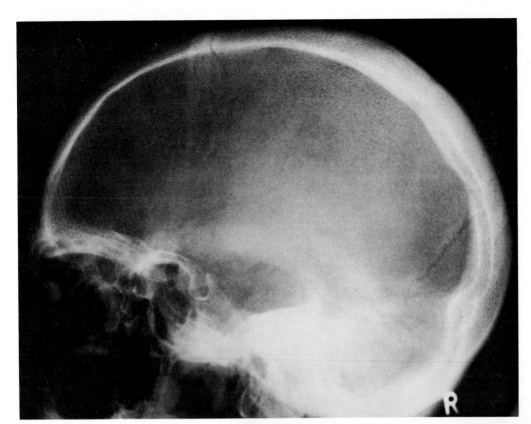

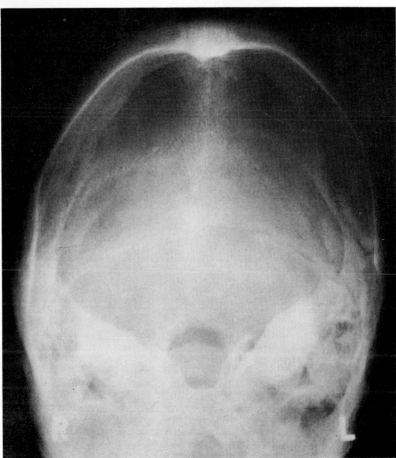

(a)

(b)

Figure 340. Mucopolysaccharidosis: Sanfilippo syndrome. (a) Lateral view: (b) Towne's view: A small, very thick skull

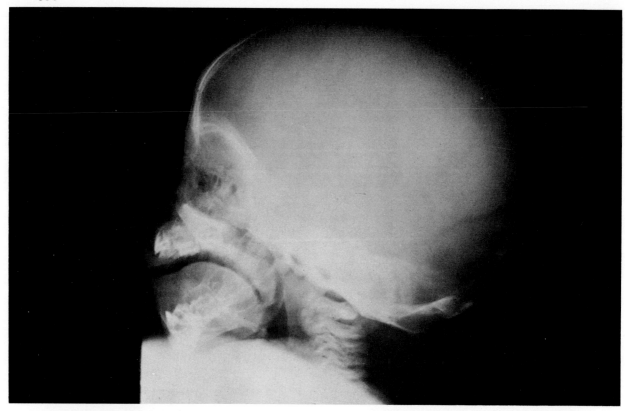

(a)

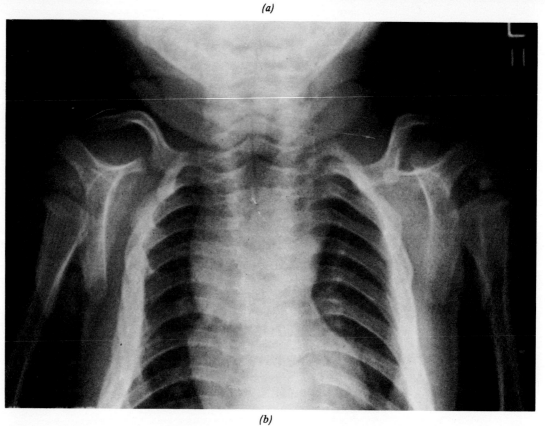

(b)

Figure 341. Mucolipidosis II: Leroy's I-cell disease. (a) A very thin vault but with rather thick orbital plates, thought at one time to be Pyle's disease. (b) Wide and deformed ribs. Diaphyseal expansion of the humeri too, as well as periosteal new bone formation

addition to these there are many syndromes mentioned elsewhere in this book and again placed here for comparison with one another.

MEDIAN CLEFT FACE SYNDROME (FACIAL DUPLICATION)

Malformations result from the failure of medial migration of the embryonal structures destined to make up the midline of the face. Kurlander, DeMyer and Campbell (1967) have divided the manifestations into four types of decreasing severity. These are as follows.

Type I   Orbital hypertelorism
          Complete cleft nose
          Absence or marked hypoplasia of cleft pro-
          labium and maxilla
          Cranium bifidum occultum frontalis
          Widely separated palatine process of maxilla
Type II   Orbital hypertelorism
          Median cleft nose
          Cranium bifidum occultum frontalis
Type III Orbital hypertelorism
          Median cleft nose
          Median cleft prolabium
Type IV   Orbital hypertelorism
          Median cleft nose

There may additionally be, as in two of Kurlander's type II cases, a frontal lipoma (which did not penetrate the skull in his cases) or a dermoid or teratoma.

The frontal defect may eventually be filled by a plate of bone.

Few patients with median cleft face are mentally retarded.

HYPERTELORISM-HYPOSPADIAS SYNDROME

This is one of many associations of developmental abnormalities described in the literature.

NOONAN'S SYNDROME (PSEUDO-TURNER'S SYNDROME) (Noonan, 1968)

Hypertelorism accompanies the Turner phenotype with the addition of congenital heart disease.

TURNER'S SYNDROME

The XO chromosome is absent. Most are females and are mildly retarded. The mandible is hypoplastic, the neck webbed. Other skeletal changes include hypoplasia of the medial condyle of the knee.

KLEINEFELTER'S SYNDROME

This is discussed in Chapter 8.

ORODIGITOFACIAL DYSOSTOSIS (PAPILLON–LEAGE SYNDROME)

These female children have telecanthus, a median pseudo-cleft upper lip and many thick, fibrous bands dividing the tongue (amongst other soft-tissue abnormalities).

There is a lateral cleft palate. The basal angle of the skull is increased by elevation of the cribriform plate. The mandible is hypoplastic. There are abnormalities of the fingers (Gorlin and Psaume, 1962).

OTOPALATODIGITAL SYNDROME (Taybi and Linden, 1967)

The abnormality appears during the first two years. The face is described as that of a battered prize fighter. Supra-orbital ridges are prominent with thickening extending through the orbital plates to the sphenoid and temporal bones. Pneumatization is decreased. The facial bones are small. The foramen magnum is stenotic and the odontoid lies more anteriorly than normal in relation to the clivus. There are deficiencies of ossification of the neural arches, especially of the lower spine. There are characteristic abnormalities of the elbows, wrists and hands.

OCULODENTODIGITAL DYSPLASIA (MICROPHTHALMOS SYNDROME) (Gorlin, Meskin and St. Geme, 1963)

The orbits are small, often with hypotelorism. In the base view it can be seen that the mandible is wider than normal, as are all the tubular bones. Hypoplasia of one or more of the middle phalanges of the fingers or toes is usual.

DYSCEPHALIA MANDIBULO-OCULOFACIALIS (HALLERMAN–STREIFF SYNDROME)

This syndrome, characterized by hypoplasia of mandible and face, has been described under the heading of conditions associated with widened sutures.

PIERRE-ROBIN SYNDROME (Robin, 1934)

This syndrome consists of severe hypoplasia of the mandible leading to glossoptosis and cleft palate, with congenital heart lesions, deformed external ears and sometimes microphthalmos

FAMILIAL OSTEODYSPLASIA (Buchignani, Cook and Anderson, 1972

The face is flat due to maxillary hypoplasia and hypoplasia of the zygomata. There is also hypoplasia of the mandible, which may fracture spontaneously. The calvaria is thin and brachycephalic. The petrous bones are hypoplastic and the mastoids pointed.

LARSEN's SYNDROME (Larsen, Schottstaedt and Bost, 1950)

The flattened face is found with multiple congenital dislocations. There is hypertelorism, hypoplasia of the malar bones and depressed, thickened nasal bones.

BECKWITH–WIEDEMANN SYNDROME (Beckwith *et al*, 1964; Wiedemann, 1968)

The syndrome presents a combination of exomphalos, macroglossia, gigantism and mild microcephaly.

TREACHER–COLLINS SYNDROME (MANDIBULO-FACIAL DYSOSTOSIS) (Stovin *et al*, 1960)

Treacher–Collins syndrome is inherited as an autosomal dominant. In the fully developed syndrome the children and young adults have severe hypoplasia of the malar bones with non-fusion of the zygomatic sutures, hypoplasia of the mastoids, absent ossicles in the ear and a cleft secondary palate. The supra-orbital ridges are poorly developed. The anti-mongoloid features are most striking. The mandible is hypoplastic.

RUBINSTEIN-TAYBI SYNDROME (Rubinstein and Taybi, 1963)

Cranio-mandibulo-facial dysplasia with exotropia or exophoria and ptosis, and characteristically short, broad terminal phalanges. An enlarged foramen magnum has been described.

CEREBRO-HEPATO-RENAL SYNDROME (ZWELLEGER'S SYNDROME) (Poznauski *et al.,* 1970)

These children are sometimes mistaken for mongols with their high foreheads, high arched palate, flaccid muscles and epicanthal folds. They have Brushfield spots.

GOLDENHAR'S SYNDROME (OCULO-AURICULO-VERTEBRAL DYSPLASIA) (Darling *et al*, 1968)

The malar deformity is like that of Treacher–Collins. There is also unilateral mandibular hypoplasia and maxillary hypoplasia. The eyes are affected by epibulbar dermoids and/or lipodermoids. There are auricular appendices and pre-tagal blind-end fistulae. There are gross vertebral anomalies.

HEMIFACIAL MICROSOMIA

This resembles the Treacher–Collins syndrome, but is unilateral.

OVERGROWTH SYNDROME

There is accelerated skeletal maturation, with hypertelorism and camptodactyly.

CONGENITAL HEMIFACIAL HYPERTROPHY

Half the face, jaw and teeth hypertrophy. There may be a similar overgrowth of one arm and leg. Some of the children are retarded.

FAMILIAL PACHYDERMOPERIOSTOSIS

Thickened facial soft tissues overlie enlarged frontal sinuses. The condition may be compared with the enlarged frontal sinuses underlying a soft-tissue angioma described by Keats and Smith in 1972.

HURLER'S SYNDROME

The mucopolysaccharidoses present in more than six different forms (McKusick, 1966) (*Figures 247* and *339*). Hurler's syndrome is a very severe form in which an excess of chondroitin sulphate B and heparitin sulphate are excreted. These gargoyles have large scaphocephalic heads. The sella is elongated when the head is large. Some are hydrocephalic or have arachnoid cysts. The facial bones are thickened. There are corneal opacities. The dorso-lumbar spine has a characteristic kyphus.

The mucolipidoses present with similar bone changes but excrete only normal amounts of acid mucopolysaccharide.

HUNTER'S SYNDROME

The appearance is similar to Hurler's syndrome, but there may be less gross deformity.

SANFILIPPO SYNDROME (Harris–Sanfilippo) (*Figure 340*)

The severe central nervous system signs are accompanied by mild skull thickening and other slight somatic changes. Heparitin sulphate is excreted.

MORQUIO–ULLRICH SYNDROME (*Figure 249*)

Excessive amounts of kerato-sulphate are excreted. The face is coarse but the skull normal. Corneal opacities are found and the teeth have thin enamel layers. There are severe spinal and epiphyseal anomalies.

MORQUIO–BRAILSFORD SYNDROME (*Figure 249*)

This is probably a mixed group of conditions and is also known as adult dysplasia spondylo-epiphysealis, pseudo-achondroplasia or juvenile osteochondrosis.

SCHEIE SYNDROME

Chondroitin sulphate is excreted. Skull changes may be minimal, though the face is deformed and there are corneal opacities. Most patients are dwarfs.

MAROTEAUX–LAMY SYNDROME (Maroteaux and Lamy, 1968)

Only chondroitin sulphate B is excreted. The head may be large and the general appearance similar to Hurler's syndrome, but intelligence is normal.

OTHER MUCOPOLYSACCHARIDOSES

A considerable number of other syndromes associated with similar metabolic and storage diseases has been described. Some have skull changes resembling gargoyles of the Hurler—Hunter type.

PARASTREMMATIC DWARFISM (Langer, Peterson and Spranger, 1970

This name was suggested for an unusual, severe bone dysplasia resembling Morquio's syndrome, inherited as a dominant trait.

The abnormality is predominantly determined by the smallness of the skull base

Within this group lie the following: achondroplasia, thanatophoric dwarfism, achondrogenesis and hypochondrogenesis. All have been described in Chapter 8.

There is also a very lage number of skeletal dysplasias in which the skull is generally normal. Some resemble achondroplasia, namely: metaphyseal dysostosis; cartilage-hair hypoplasia; chondro-ectodermal dysplasia (Ellis van Creveld syndrome); diastrophic dwarfism; mesomelic dwarfism of the hypoplastic ulnar, fibular, mandibular type; lymphopenic agammaglobulinaemia—short limb dwarfism syndrome; and congenital hyperuricosuria.

12 HEAD INJURIES

The indications for radiological examination are complicated by a fear of legal action after even a mild blow, and at the same time a reluctance to allow patients with serious head injuries to be taken to the radiological department. Many patients with such injuries are drunk and more or less disorderly, while head injury itself often causes confusion and irritability which undermine the patient's powers of co-operation with the radiographer. Computerized axial tomography is of great value and although it does not outdate plain x-ray examination, it may precede it.

Some principles about the radiology of head injuries may, therefore, help to decide when and how they should be examined.

(1) Failure to demonstrate a fracture of the base, even after careful and adequate radiography, by no means excludes the presence of such an injury.

(2) A patient who has been concussed requires treatment. The demonstration of a linear fracture does not affect this, but may alert the clinician to the possibility of an extradural haematoma developing later – within the first few hours of the injury.

(3) Only good radiographs are useful. These cannot be obtained in bed in the ward. The patient must be taken to the radiological department because apparatus available for ward radiography is not capable of producing the definition required, nor is it possible, in most cases, to position the patient satisfactorily in bed. If the patient is moved carefully there is no danger, and perhaps less discomfort, in being taken to the radiological department.

(4) If it becomes necessary to obtain radiographs of an intoxicated or confused patient, particularly at night, the radiographer needs the help of a doctor, a student, or an experienced porter in addition to the nurse with the patient.

After head injuries relatively few abnormalities may be demonstrated on the radiographs. The possibilities include: (*a*) displacement of the calcified pineal as a result of haematoma or cerebral oedema; (*b*) linear fractures; (*c*) depressed fractures; (*d*) air in the cranial cavity as a result of fractures involving the paranasal sinuses, the cribriform plate, or the mastoid air cells and middle ear; (*e*) cerebrospinal fluid in the sphenoid and ethmoid sinuses.

There are also certain late effects of previous head injury.

Consideration of these facts suggests possible courses of action in different circumstances.

(1) The patient has had a trivial blow on the head not resulting in unconsciousness. He has no evidence of cerebral damage, bruising is only moderate, there is no laceration and there is no suggestion on palpation of a depressed fracture. The chance of finding an unsuspected abnormality is remote and the treatment of the patient will almost certainly be unaffected by the result of radiological examination.

(2) The patient has had a blow on the head, about the severity of which there is genuine doubt perhaps because he is intoxicated. For the same reason a neurological examination and an assessment of the conscious level is difficult. A negative radiological examination provides no answer to the problem of his management but a positive finding is useful. It may well be that the patient should be admitted for observation, and radiography postponed until the clinical condition becomes clearer or the patient more co-operative, when CT scanning will also be easier.

(3) The patient has had a head injury and on palpation or, because of its known severity or the presence of a laceration, a depressed fracture is suspected. This patient undoubtedly requires a full routine set of skull radiographs since a depressed fracture may be overlooked when only one or two pictures are taken. Whether the examination should be made before the patient is taken to the ward or a few hours is at the discretion of the surgeon.

(4) The patient is unconscious, has an alteration in the level of consciousness, or has neurological signs of cerebral damage. He requires immediate skull radiography, particularly if his condition is deteriorating, but even more urgently he will require a CT scan. The plain x-ray examination may consist of a full series of pictures if it is thought that the patient has a depressed fracture. If a CT scanner is not available and there is no clinical suspicion of a depressed fracture, it may be sufficient to perform simply those views which will demonstrate the position of a calcified pineal.

(6) The patient has had a head injury of sufficient severity to make a fracture likely, and it seems probable from clinical evidence that the injury also involves the paranasal sinuses or the structures of the middle ear. A radiological examination is required either at once, with a repeat lateral view after about 12 hours, or the initial examination may be postponed. The pictures should include a horizontal ray, lateral in order to demonstrate the presence of any intracranial air, and thus the presence of a fistula and the possibility of subsequent meningitis.

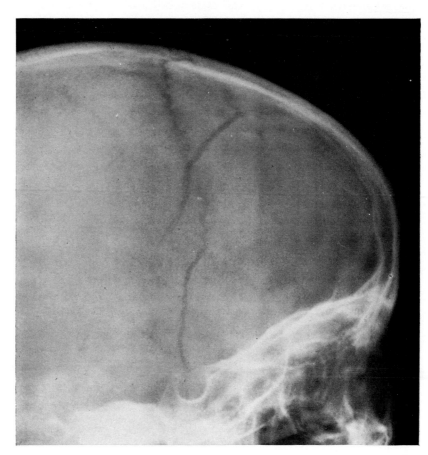

Figure 342. Linear fracture and suture diastasis. There is a bilateral frontal fracture which runs into the coronal suture

The two most useful views for the demonstration of the calcified pineal may be made with little disturbance to the patient. They are a lateral (which should be made with the patient lying flat on his back and the beam horizontal for reasons given below), and an antero-posterior view in which the x-ray beam is centred a little above the nasion and parallel to the radiographic base line.

If the pineal is calcified and displaced, a haematoma is probably present and burr holes may be required. If the pineal is calcified and not displaced, subsequent deterioration in the patient's condition indicates the necessity for another radiological examination so that the onset of pineal displacement may be detected.

(5) The patient's condition may deteriorate too rapidly for any radiological examination to be made with safety, and the decision whether or not to operate must then be made on clinical grounds alone.

APPEARANCES

Displacement of the calcified pineal

Confirmation of the presence of an intracranial haematoma, if C.A.T. scanning is not possible, may be obtained when the calcified pineal is shown to be displaced, and this may sometimes be of the greatest importance when clinical evidence is dubious (*see* Chapter 9) (*Figures 253–255*).

Linear fractures of the vault (*Figure 342*)

A linear fracture of the vault shows as a black line which will have sharp edges, particularly if the injured side is close to the film. The line crosses vascular markings, and when it changes direction it tends to do so with a sharp angle. At the edge of a bone the fracture may be diverted into the suture, which will show localized diastasis, and the fracture then tends to pass out of the suture into another bone, perhaps at some distance from its entry.

Linear fractures have to be distinguished from vascular channels on the inner table, which are usually wider and less translucent, which tend to taper as they branch and which may, in places, be seen to have a white line representing the inner table of the skull along their edges. They must also be distinguished from vascular channels of the outer table – the supra-orbital and middle temporal arteries – which may be much more difficult since these straight, narrow grooves resemble fractures very closely. However, they too may sometimes be seen to have a bony cortex and their anatomical position is fairly constant.

In some skulls, interdigitation at the sutures is confined largely to the outer table, the inner table edges being merely butted together. Such a straight black line along the course of the suture is easily mistaken for traumatic diastasis. Careful inspection reveals the intact, normal, close interdigitation of the outer table, thus excluding an injury.

Diploic veins may sometimes produce a superficial resemblance to fracture lines, but on good radiographs the continuous wall of trabeculae which confines them may be seen forming a white edge to the translucent channels.

Depressed fractures of the vault (*Figures 343–345*)

A typical depressed fracture of the vault when viewed *en face* is seen as an irregular ring comminuted with radiating lines; but sometimes a single piece of bone is driven in as a detached fragment without comminution. In tangential views, if the area is large enough, loss of the contour of the vault is recognizable. If the area is small, the white lines representing the inner and outer tables of the fragment appear discontinuous with the rest of the vault. The fragment may lie deep within the cranial cavity.

If the defect lies in the parasagittal region it may be difficult to see and the radiologist should be aware of this danger. Sometimes, at a cursory examination, the only abnormality noted may be the single white line of inner or outer table of a small fragment of bone driven in for some distance and seen edge-on.

Difficulties also arise when the depressed fracture is not either truly *en face* or truly tangential in any view. It lies perhaps somewhere toward the periphery of one frontal bone, and if the depressed fragment has hinged inwards along one border most of the radiographs may show neither the translucency of a defect nor the obvious white line of depressed inner table. In such cases a rather irregular white area due to superimposition of the edges of the depressed fragment and the bone around its original position give a clue to the possibility. Careful examination and, if necessary, oblique view will always provide a diagnosis.

A depressed fracture in the temporal region may be particularly difficult to demonstrate because in lateral projection the shadow of the base and of the petrous bone are so dense that they obscure all detail, while the squamous temporal may be so thin that a linear fracture is difficult to pick up. In the postero-anterior or Towne's view some idea of a general flattening of that side of the head may be suggested, but it is rarely possible to confirm the presence of depression without the full axial view.

Fractures in infancy and childhood

It is sometimes difficult to see fractures running through the thin bones in infancy and early childhood.

The relative flexibility of these bones may also allow a small dent in the vault of the infant with very little to show in the way of an actual crack; such areas may only be recognizable in tangential views. Subsequently, a small depressed or comminuted piece of bone may become completely absorbed and for a while there will be a translucent, circumscribed area which should not be confused with the appearance of cephalhydrocoele.

A history of injury may not be obtained, particularly when it is non-accidental.

Williams *et al.* (1972) drew attention to the many soft-tissue changes that may be found after repeated, minor, self-inflicted head injury in the 'head-bangers'. These include soft-tissue haematomas, cauliflower ears and calcification of the eye.

In neonates where fractures of thin bones are so difficult to see, the clue to injury may be an overlying soft-tissue swelling.

Fractures of the base of the skull

Fractures of the skull base are always difficult and may be impossible to demonstrate. Moreover, tomography has not proved of as much help as might be expected, perhaps because of the difficulty of immobilizing a restless patient. The four routine radiographic projections are usually considered sufficient.

It is important that the lateral should be made with a horizontal ray because cerebrospinal fluid rhinorrhoea is not always obvious, and air in the head, indicating as it does a dural tear, must not be overlooked. It may show as a small bubble in the subarachnoid space over the frontal lobe, in the region of the chiasmatic cistern, or much more extensive shadows over the cerebrum and between the hemispheres. Sometimes the presence of dural adhesions encourages the local collection of air and an aerocoele invades the brain. When there is also cerebral laceration a spontaneous ventriculogram may be found.

The presence of a fistula between the sphenoid or ethmoid sinuses and the subarachnoid space may also be revealed by a fluid level shown in one of these sinuses in the horizontal ray lateral radiograph. Although in theory such a fluid level might be the result of an effusion of blood, in practice the majority are due to cerebrospinal fluid. The situation of the fluid is of some importance in a pre-operative search for the position of the fistula. For instance, if the ethmoid sinuses remain clear and the fluid level is seen in the sphenoid, then the fracture and dural tear probably involve the sella turcica.

Fractures of the base of the skull are commonly, but not always, accompanied by one or more fracture line extending upwards into the bones of the vault from the petrous temporal or diagonally across the orbital plate

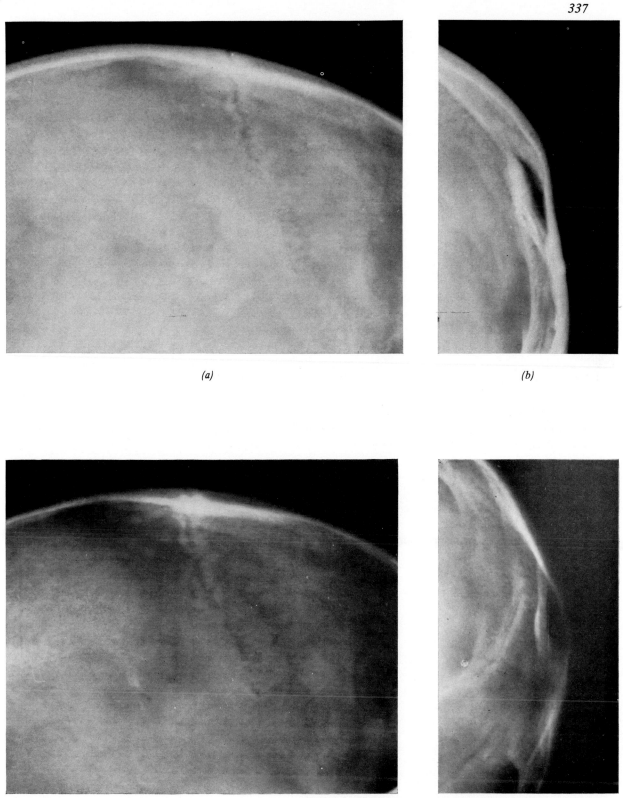

(a)   *(b)*

(c)   *(d)*

Figure 343. Depressed fracture and union. A depressed fracture in a child aged 12 years. (a) The lateral view shows stones in the scalp. The depressed fracture is not very easy to see, but has the typical circumferential crack. (b) It is obvious in a tangential view. (c) and (d) Two months later union has occurred in the depressed position. If such a fracture were left without surgical intervention in an infant and no cerebral complication occurred, growth and remoulding would probably obliterate all trace of it

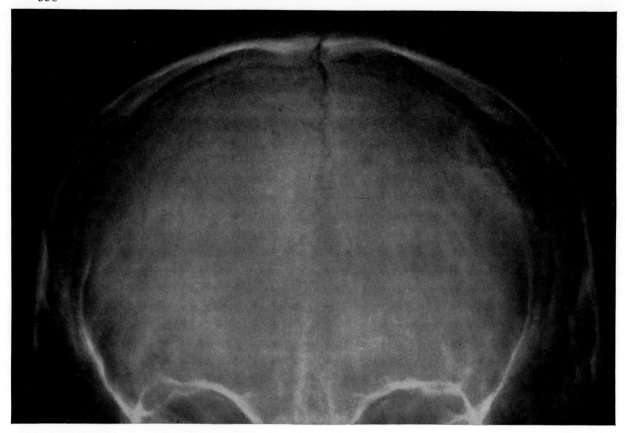

(a)

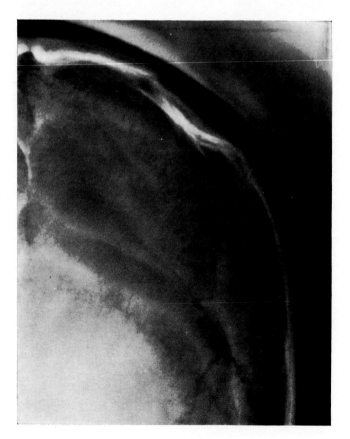

Figure 344. A depressed fracture in the parietal bone of a boy aged 7 years. (a) In the postero-anterior view where it is neither en face nor tangential it is quite difficult to see. Notice the area of translucency bounded on one side by the added shadow of a double thickness of vault. (b) Tangential view

(b)

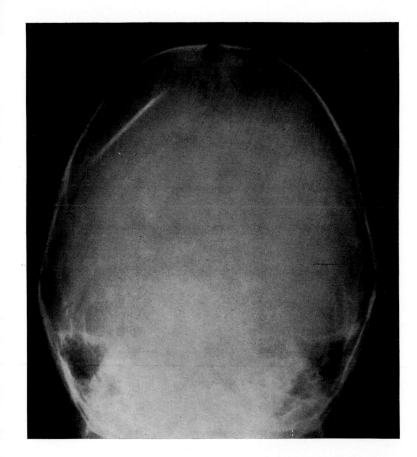

(a)

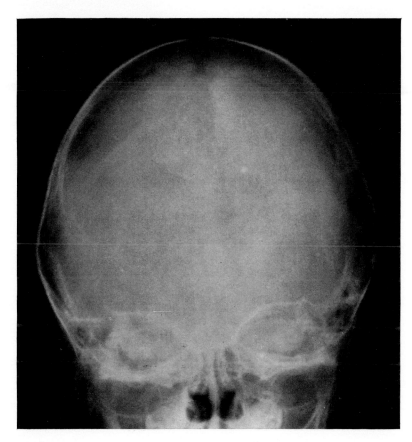

Figure 345. A depressed fracture in a child aged 2 years. (a) It is easy to see where a fragment is tangential to the x-ray beam, but (b) very much harder in other views

(b)

and into the frontal bone. This may give a clue to the position of a basal fracture which is otherwise difficult to see.

THE FLOOR OF THE ANTERIOR FOSSA (*Figures 346–349*)

A fracture of the floor of the anterior fossa is often an extension from a large fracture of the base of the skull and may continue upwards across the orbital plate (involving the roof of the ethmoids or the posterior wall of the frontal sinus) to be more easily seen in the squamous part of the frontal bone.

Fractures in these regions tend to run round, rather than through, the thicker areas of bone between convolutional impressions and the ridges at the edge of the ethmoidal plate, and if these thicker ridges are displaced they are a frequent source of dural laceration. Isolated fractures of the cribriform plate or the roof of the ethmoids without extensive fissuring also occur occasionally.

It is of considerable advantage before surgery to know the exact situation of fractures in the floor of the anterior fossa, and yet the routine radiographs are very difficult to interpret. Tomography in the coronal and lateral planes is valuable here. Oblique and stereoscopic views are rather less helpful but the projection devised by Johnson and Dutt may show fractures of the ethmoid plate which are not otherwise visible.

THE SPHENOID (*Figure 350*)

Fractures confined to the base of the skull and not spreading into the bones of the vault usually involve the sphenoid bone, and extension of fracture lines across the lesser wings or the walls of the optic canal are an important source of visual disturbance. The postero-anterior view in such cases may be supplemented by oblique radiographs of the optic canals. If suitable radiographic apparatus is available, it is not difficult to obtain postero-anterior views without the necessity of turning the patient over. This will be appreciated particularly if the patient has limb, rib or facial injuries.

Fractures of the sphenoid, resulting from deceleration accidents and from falls on the feet or on the vertex, are likely to be followed by cerebrospinal rhinorrhoea because the superior or lateral walls of the sphenoid sinus have buckled. There may also be displacement of the dorsum sellae due to sudden traumatic tension on the tentorium.

THE PETROUS BONE (*Figure 351, 352*)

Routine views often fail to demonstrate a fracture line running through the petrous bone. Many of these fractures involve the bony labyrinth and cause deafness. Unless treatment depends upon the result, elaborate radiographic studies are wasted, but operative improvement of a damaged ossicular chain may be possible, so partial deafness after head injury is an indication for detailed high quality tomographic studies.

THE BASI-OCCIPUT

Fractures of the basi-occiput around the occipital condyles should be looked for in the postero-anterior view.

Fractures of the facial bones

Fractures of the base of the skull may be accompanied by fractures of the facial bones and by fractures of the mandible. (Fractures of the mandible are not dealt with in this volume.)

Fractures of the facial bones are nearly always the result of direct violence. In their radiological examination the main points of importance to be remembered are as follows.

Severe displacement may be masked by oedema and bruising or swelling of the soft tissues, and may give a false impression of deformity of the underlying bones. Correction of deformity may be more easily carried out at an early stage than when the fractures have had time to consolidate.

Full demonstration of displacement, particularly depression of the anterior wall of the frontal sinus, the nasal bones, the malar bone or perhaps the whole of the middle third of the face, may be very difficult. It will require a true lateral and probably a basal and an occlusal view, perhaps also tomography and a projection in which the area under suspicion is tangenitally visualized. A 60 degree occipito-mental view, however, will usually show any fracture line.

There may be an accompanying injury to the anterior or middle fossa, perhaps with a dural laceration.

The more common fractures which will be discussed are those of the anterior wall of the frontal sinus, the middle third of the face, and the orbit.

THE ANTERIOR WALL OF FRONTAL SINUSES

Fractures of this region are usually due to direct violence, and may be depressed. Owing to the amount of bruising and oedema, depression is difficult to assess from clinical examination. The basal view is useful but a radiograph at a tangent to the broken bone is of the greatest value.

THE MIDDLE THIRD OF THE FACE, NOT INVOLVING TEETH AND ALVEOLI (*Figures 353, 354*)

Central region: fractures of the nasal bones — The nasal bones are best demonstrated by a soft lateral, an occlusal and a postero-anterior view. Sub-classification of the types of fractures may be attempted as follows.

In *greenstick fractures* there are virtually no radiographic signs.

Linear fractures may result in a mild degree of displacement, probably best seen in the lateral view. The groove for the anterior ethmoidal nerve should not be confused with a fracture line.

Lateral and frontal fractures are the commonest serious injuries to the nose. There is a depression of one or both nasal bones under the ascending rami of the maxilla. There is probably also separation of the nasal bones and the one on the side opposite to the blow

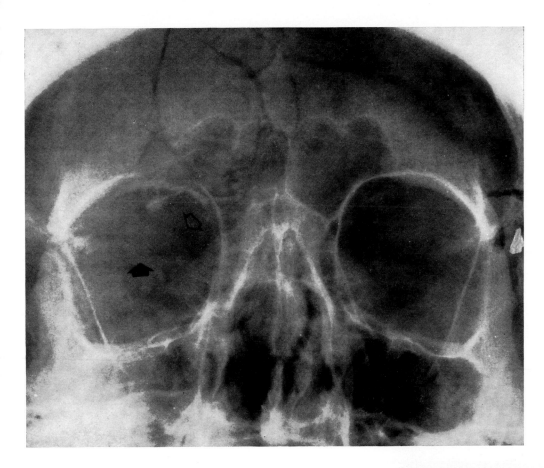

(a)

Figure 346. Fracture of the frontal sinus. There are a number of linear fractures of the frontal bone and of the anterior and inferior walls of the frontal sinus due to direct violence. A flake of the superior orbital wall is displaced downwards. There is air in the soft tissues of the orbit (open arrow). The eyelids are swollen and the palpebral fissure flattened and narrowed (closed arrow). (a) Occipito-frontal view. (b) Lateral view

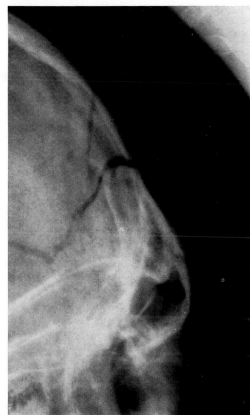

(b)

342

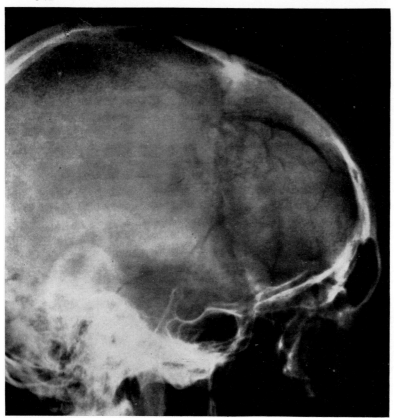

Figure 347. Cerebrospinal fluid rhinorrhoea. The patient had a head injury 8 weeks before. There is a slightly depressed fracture of the left frontal bone with fissures extending over a wide area. Two of these run across the right frontal sinus, a third runs into the left orbital plate. (a) The lateral view was made with the head brow-up, but there is no fluid level in the sinuses, suggesting that the fistula involves neither the sphenoid nor the ethmoids. (b) The postero-anterior view also shows a small air shadow behind the left frontal sinus (arrow). This is the situation of the fistula, where there was a fairly wide defect at the medial end of a fissure fracture. The air lies in an extradural pocket

(a)

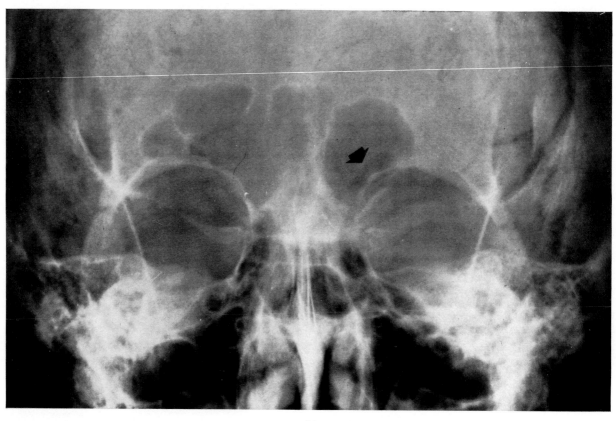

(b)

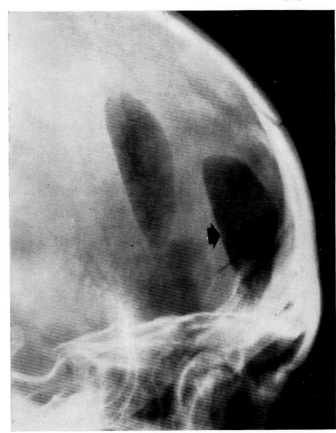

Figure 348. Spontaneous ventriculogram and aerocoele. The patient suffered a head injury 6 weeks before developing transient cerebrospinal fluid rhinorrhoea. There is a slightly depressed fracture of most of the frontal bone, and a gaping linear fracture (open arrow) running across the posterior wall of the left frontal sinus to the region of the ethmoid plate. (a) In the lateral view there is air in a frontal horn and in a frontal aerocoele (closed arrow). (b) In the postero-anterior view air is visible in the posterior parts of the lateral ventricles (asterisks)

(a)

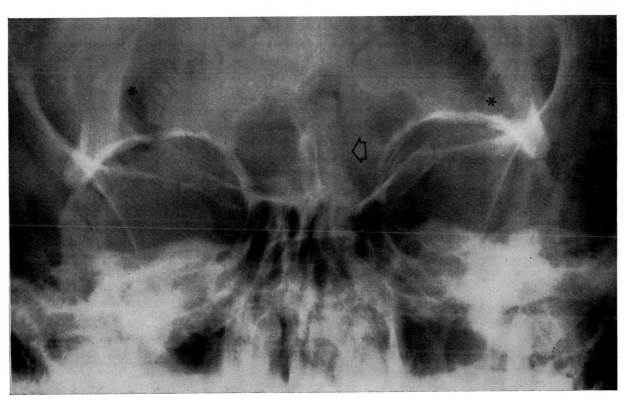

(b)

may also be out of alignment with the maxilla. The septum may be concerntina'd.

In *fractures from below* the nasal bones override the maxillary bones on both sides and are displaced apart.

The importance of radiology in fractures of the nasal bones is in the early detection or exclusion of gross deformity, which may be masked by the amount of bruising.

The more severe fractures of the nasal bones may be accompanied by injury of the frontal process of the maxilla. If there is sufficient violence in the blow the break may extend into the ethmoid bone.

Lateral region: triple fracture of the malar bone (*Figures 355, 356*) — This is one of the commonest of facial injuries. It results from a direct blow upon the cheek. The fractures occur through the fronto-zygomatic suture or in its vicinity, through the zygomatic process of the malar bone and through the floor of the orbit as well as the lateral wall of the maxillary antrum. The alteration in the fronto-zygomatic suture is easy to compare with the appearance on the opposite side in an occipito-mental or an 'overtilted' occipito-mental view. The latter, as well as the full axial view, demonstrates the extent of depression or comminution of the zygomatic arch.

The fracture through the antrum is often more difficult to see, although a clue to its presence may be obtained by clouding of the antrum or an isolated swelling resulting from haematoma. The fracture line commonly runs medial to the infra-orbital canal but may sometimes cross it. It tends to involve the lower half of the lateral wall of the antrum. (There is a groove in the lateral wall of the antrum caused by branches of the posterior dental vessels. This should not be mistaken for a fracture as it is usually present in a symmetrical position in the opposite antrum.)

The following are the three degrees of this type of fracture.

First degree: the zygomatic arch of the zygomatic bone is fractured without interference with mandibular movement or with minimal displacement.

Second degree; there is a fracture of the zygomatic bone with or without involvement of the zygomatic arch. There is interference with mandibular movement or some alteration in facial contour and a fracture of the lateral wall of the maxillary antrum is apparent.

Third degree: in addition to the fractures and displacement of the second degree fracture, there is comminution of the orbital floor or gross separation of the zygomatico-frontal suture with depression of the orbital level.

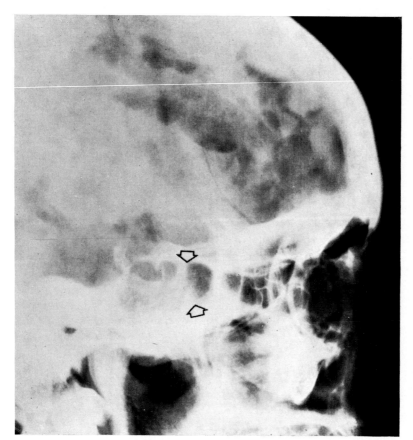

Figure 349. Cerebrospinal fluid rhinorrhoea. The patient was injured by sudden deceleration in a motor car collision. She had cerebrospinal fluid rhinorrhoea. There is a fracture of the floor of the sella and of the dorsum sellae. (a) Horizontal ray lateral radiograph shows a fluid level (arrows) in the sphenoid sinus, indicating the site of the cerebrospinal fluid fistula. There is a considerable amount of air in the subarachnoid space, and possibly some in the ventricles (cont.)

(a)

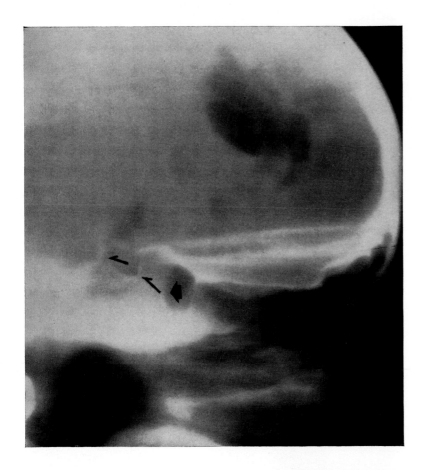

(b)

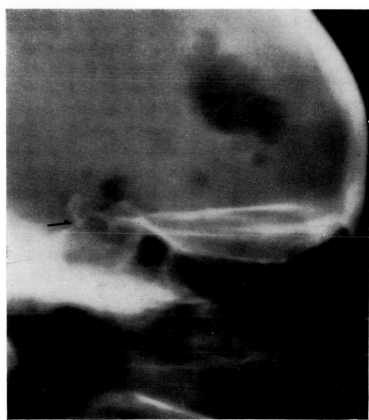

Figure 349 (cont.). (b) and (c) Brow-up tomograms show the fracture lines (half arrows) and, incidentally, the fluid level (closed arrow). The clinical problem was to decide whether the fistula could be closed surgically. Radiology indicated that the fistula must lie at the base of the dorsum sellae. No other fracture was found, and the fluid level showed that it ran into the sphenoid sinus. Because of the difficulty of a surgical approach to this region, the sphenoid sinus was packed

(c)

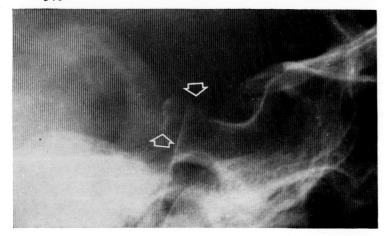

Figure 350. Fracture of the dorsum sellae which resulted from indirect violence. Presumably torsion of the head has resulted in a pull exerted on the tentorial attachment to the dorsum sellae

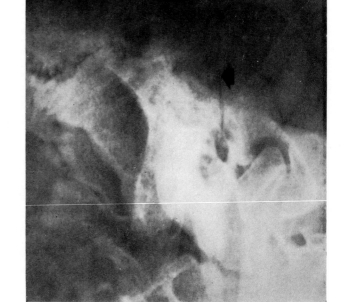

Figure 351. A linear fracture through the squamous temporal, the external auditory meatus, and probably the middle ear. Such a radiographic finding is quite uncommon, even when there is clear clinical evidence of a fracture of the petrous bone

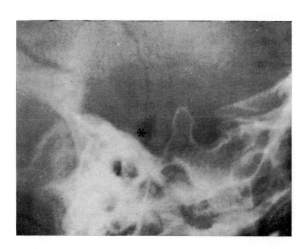

Figure 352. Head injury (aerocoele). This child had linear fractures in the vault. There is a collection of air (asterisk) behind the clivus, presumably as a result of a fracture involving the middle ear

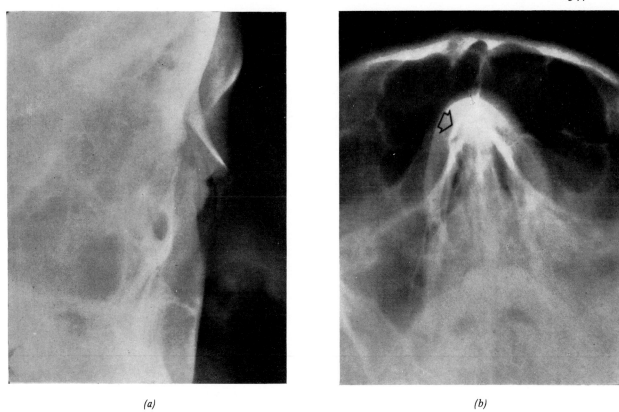

(a)   (b)

Figure 353. Fractured nasal bones. (a) In the lateral view the nasal bones appear normal, but there is slight displacement of the nasal spine of the maxilla. (b) The occipito-mental view shows lateral displacement

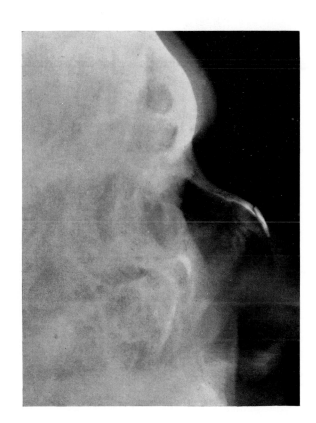

Figure 354. Slight depressed fracture of the nasal bones

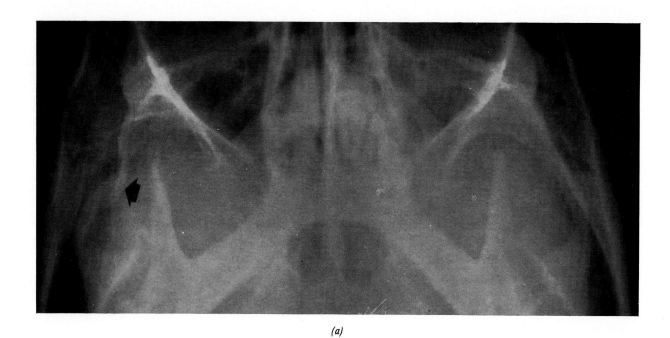

(a)

(b)

Figure 355. A fracture of the right zygomatic arch caused by direct violence demonstrated (a) by an over-tilted occipito-mental view. In (b) a slight 'wrinkle' is shown in the lateral wall of the maxillary antrum

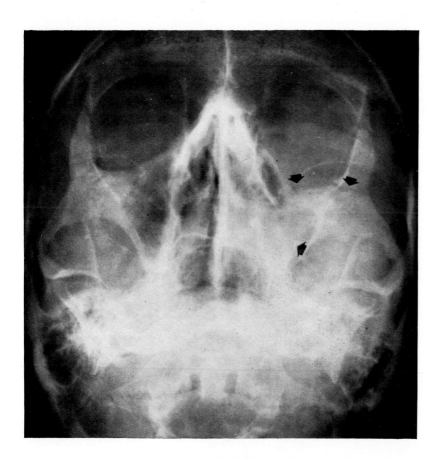

Figure 356. Triple fracture of the malar bone. The zygomatic arch is intact. The frontal process of the zygoma often fractures higher than this or through the fronto-zygomatic synchrondrosis

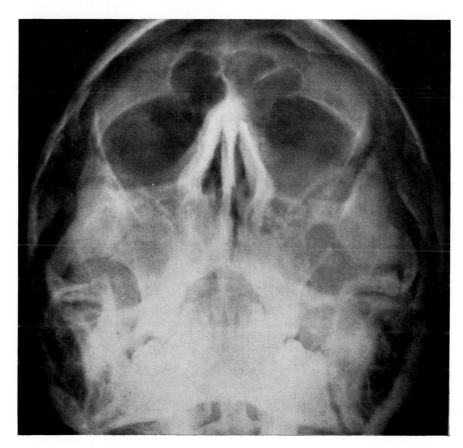

Figure 357. Le Fort type II and III fractures. On the right side the patient has a Le Fort type II fracture, on the left where violence has been greater the fracture is of the Le Fort type III; in addition there are fractures of the zygomatic arch and of the mandible

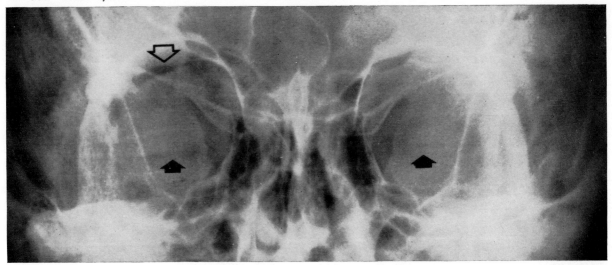

Figure 358. Orbital emphysema. The patient had been kicked in the region of the orbit. The first radiographs showed no fracture. Orbital emphysema (open arrow) appeared 2 days later. It indicates that there must be a fracture into the ethmoids, the frontal sinus or, perhaps, the maxillary antrum. Observe also the soft-tissue shadow of the swollen eyelids (closed arrow) and the normal palpebral fissure on the opposite side (closed arrow)

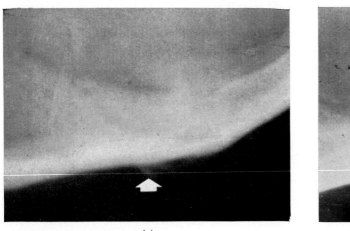

(a)

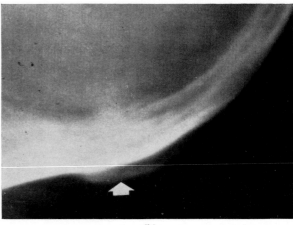

(b)

Figure 359. (a) Cephal-haematoma in a 1-week-old baby. (b) Fourteen days later. The calcified shell has increased and now gives the false impressions of a cyst

FRACTURES INVOLVING THE TEETH AND ALVEOLUS (*Figure 357*)

Aveolar fractures — The alveolus may be fractured around a single tooth, or if the blow is more violent and distributed over a wide area a block of alveolus containing a number of teeth may be displaced.

Low level, sub-zygomatic fractures (Le Fort type 1 or Guérin) — More violent force still, applied over an extensive area, may result in a fracture not confined to one section of the alveolar bone. The maxilla breaks horizontally above the apices of the teeth on one side or both and is displaced in a direction depending upon the direction of the force.

Pyramidal, sub-zygomatic fractures (Le Fort type 2) — A violent force applied between the glabella and the alveolar margin may result in a fracture known as Le Fort type 2. The break occurs transversly through the

nasal bones and runs out more or less symmetrically across the frontal processes of the maxillae, the lacrimal bones and then downwards through the anterior part of the inferior orbital wall, through, or close to, the infra-orbital foramen. From this point the fracture runs round the lateral wall of the antrum, the pterygo-maxillary fissure and the pterygoid laminae. There is backward, or backward and sideways displacement of the detached portion of the middle third of the face.

These fractures involving the alveolus may also be unilateral and may sometimes be associated with fractures of the zygomatic bone.

High level, supra-zygomatic (Le Fort type 3) This fracture occurs at a slightly higher level than the Le Fort type 2. There is usually a greater degree of posterior displacement and the zygomatic bones are liable to be splayed apart.

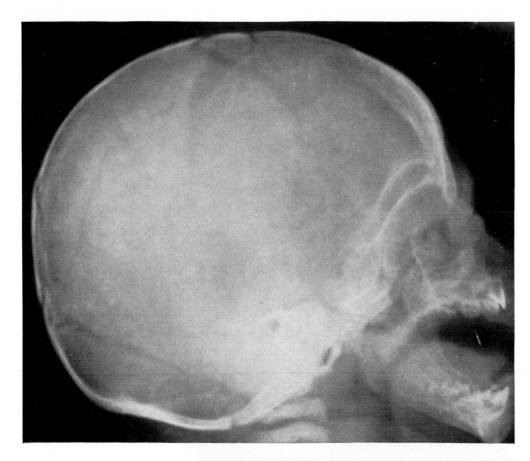

(a)

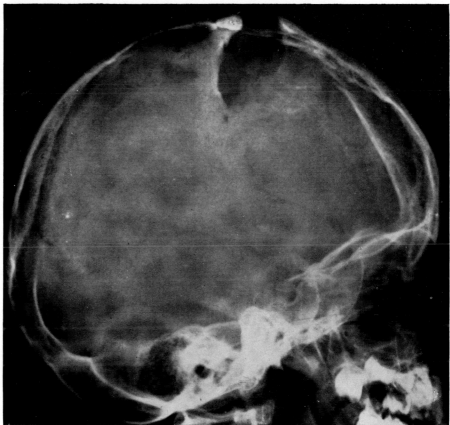

Figure 360. Cephal-hydrocoele (leptomeningeal cyst; growing fracture). (a) An infant with a gaping parietal fracture. A cephal-hydrocoele developed. (b) Three years later. The fracture gapes more widely due to bone absorption at its edges, but the condition is static at this stage and a subsequent radiograph (6 years later) showed no advance (cont.)

(b)

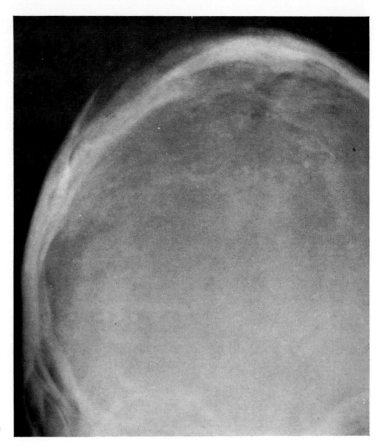

Figure 360 (cont.). (c) Antero-posterior view 9 years after the injury showing how the vault near the fracture has been thinned by pressure from within the skull

(c)

On the fronto-nasal junction, the fracture extends backwards causing disruption of the cribriform plate. There may, therefore, be cerebrospinal fluid rhinorrhoea. It crosses the frontal process of the maxilla and the upper limit of the lacrimal bones, breaks the orbital plates of the ethmoids and runs into the medial aspect of the posterior limit of the inferior orbital fissure. Passing through the upper pterygo-maxillary fissure, it reaches the roots of the pterygoid laminae. In addition, fractures run from the antero-lateral ends of each infra-orbital fissure across the lateral walls of the orbits, adjacent to the junction of the zygomatic bone and greater wing of the sphenoid. The fronto-zygomatic suture is opened or fractured and the line runs on downwards across the infra-temporal surface.

Displacement of this large central fragment depends upon the direction of force.

Midline separation of maxillae This may be found with the Le Fort type 3 fracture as well as the Le Fort type 2. Occasionally, midline separation is seen with less severe maxillary fractures.

FRACTURES OF THE ORBIT (*Figures 346-348, 358*)

In addition to the 'triple fractures' of the malar bone described above which may cause displacement of the globe, a bursting type of fracture also occurs due to direct trauma to the eye. Pressure is transmitted downwards to depress the floor of the orbit. It may be disastrous for the patient to overlook such a 'blow-out' of the orbital floor which, in healing, can trap the inferior rectus muscle, causing diplopia. When in doubt, because of an unclear orbital floor shadow, P.A. tomography is decisive.

Puncture wounds may pass from the orbit, through the orbital plate of the frontal bone with very little radiographic evidence.

Injuries of the adjacent air cells provide a pathway by which air may enter the orbit, and this orbital emphysema (often showing as a semi-circular collection of air bubbles conforming to the general shape of the globe) is definite evidence of the presence of such a fracture.

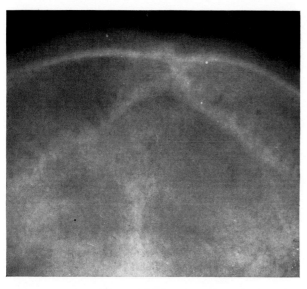

(a)

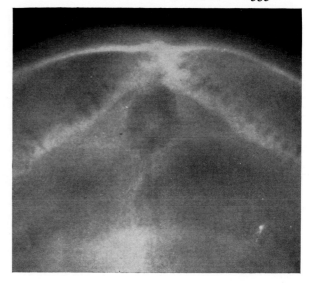

(b)

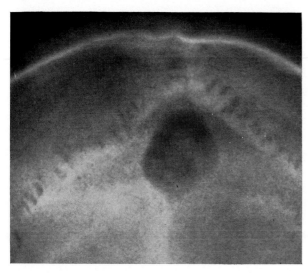

(c)

Figure 361. Post-traumatic fibroma. (a) Immediately after localized injury to the occiput. (b) Three years later. There had been pain at the site since the injury. (c) One month after (b). A nodule could now be felt beneath the scalp. At operation a mass of fibrous tissue and giant cells was found

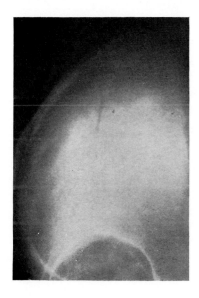

(a)

Figure 362. Bone absorption after fracture. In childhood, particularly, small areas of depressed bone may be spontaneously absorbed. (a) At the time of injury. (b) Four months later

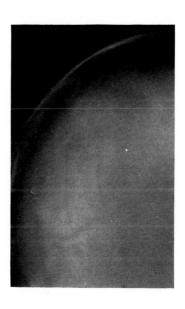

(b)

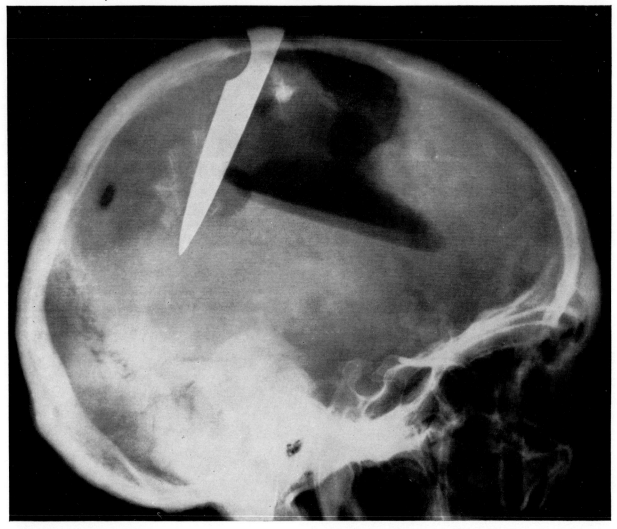

Figure 363. Spontaneous ventriculogram. A self-inflicted wound by a determined would-be suicide whose legs were in plaster as a result of a fall from a window. The nail file was worked through an old craniotomy wound; The patient made a satisfactory recovery

THE LATER EFFECTS OF HEAD INJURY

Calcification in subdural or extradural haematomas (*Figure 262*)

Calcification is very uncommon in either subdural or extradural haematomas but is found from time to time. In subdural haematoma the calcification is usually an incomplete shell conforming to the general shape of the collection of fluid. It is evidence of a very long-standing condition.

Calcification in extradural haematoma is also known as internal cephal-haematoma. It usually appears as a complete shell continuous with the inner table (rarely of any great volume). It also indicates a long-standing haematoma.

Cephal-haematoma (*Figure 359*)

In infancy, particularly at birth, an injury to the head is liable to produce a cephal-haematoma; that is, a haematoma between the outer table and the pericranium. Ossification commonly occurs in the haematoma at the edge of the area where the pericranium is lifted free from the underlying bone, and may be seen on radiographs within 14 days.

Occasionally, a complete shell of bone may develop over the surface of the haematoma. In tangential view the effect may be that of an intradiplöic expanding lesion except that, in addition to the new shell of bone, the true outer table is recognizable, conforming in shape to the adjacent skull or depressed as a result of the injury.

Subsequently the original vault at the site of injury may diminish in thickness by absorption of the outer table, and the appearance comes closer still to that of an expanding cyst.

The subsequent history of these lesions is obscure, but it is probable that they are obliterated by active growth and remoulding.

Cephal-hydrocoele (acute leptomeningeal cyst; growing fracture) (*Figure 360*)

When, particularly in childhood, a fracture of the vault is accompanied by extensive dural tearing, a cephal-hydrocoele may form. It is more likely if the fracture is a gaping one.

The injury is followed by very great swelling of the tissues of the scalp which become distended with cerebrospinal fluid. Then, over the course of a few weeks, the fracture line begins to widen by thinning and erosion of bone along its borders, and in due course a large defect may be seen.

Fibrosing osteitis (post-traumatic fibroma) (*Figure 361*)

From time to time, in both children and adults, cases are seen in which a translucent area appears in the vault at the site of, but some months after, an injury. The translucency affects the middle table most obviously, but the outer table may also be involved. The translucency becomes larger under observation, and microscopic examination of its contents shows fibrous tissue, blood and giant cells at the periphery.

There is great confusion in the literature, and it has been suggested that these lesions are a form of fibrous dysplasia.

It is clear, however, that a distinction must be made on the grounds of natural history between fibrous dysplasia (in which a clear history of trauma is rarely obtained and which progresses very slowly) and the condition described above which has its definite onset after injury and a relatively rapid growth. Moreover, fibrous dysplasia is always associated with or surrounded by some sclerosis, while fibrosing osteitis may be purely lytic, except for a central area of bony density. The appearance suggests an American doughnut. 'Doughnut lesion' is a descriptive term for any process producing a similar shadow (Keats and Holt, 1969).

Intradiplöic haematoma

Another condition in which bone may disappear after injury in adults and in late childhood is believed to be due to intradiopöic bleeding. The process does not affect the whole thickness of the skull and the translucent area in the diploë appears within a week or two of the injury.

Intradiplöic haematoma and fibrosing osteitis are also confused in the literature, in which intradiplöic haematoma has been suggested as the cause of fibrosing osteitis.

Post-traumatic blistering of the planum sphenoidale

Bonneville *et al* (1978) have reported an appearance resembling the pneumatized enostosis of a meningioma, following some long time after a fracture through the roof of the sphenoid sinus.

HEALING OF FRACTURES

The healing of linear fractures of the skull is usually complicated so that even in adults no trace will remain visible on the radiographs 2–3 years after injury. Depressed fractures, when they occur in infancy, tend to disappear as the skull remoulds with growth, but a defect may persist when a portion of dura has been removed with the overlying bone. If the bone alone is missing, some re-ossification may take place, and if the area of bone loss is extensive (as after craniotomy or decompression) a bulging shell may be formed (*Figure 362*).

FOREIGN BODIES

The chief importance of the demonstration of foreign bodies in the head is not that they should be removed, as this is rarely possible, but that their presence may lead to a more careful search for a puncture wound which might otherwise have been overlooked, and may help the surgeon in a decision as to the extent of exploration prior to suturing (*Figure 363*).

It is important to remember the general shape of the head. Stereoscopic or tangenital views may be necessary before it may be said with confidence that a particular foreign body lies within the cranium rather than buried in the scalp.

The problem of localizing foreign bodies in the orbit is complex and may be of great importance — it is not discussed in this book.

13 RADIOGRAPHY

There are four features of skull radiography which, to some extent, set it apart from radiography of other regions. They are as follows.

(1) Abnormalities, particularly of the sella turcica and of intracranial calcification, may be overlooked except on films of the highest definition.

(2) Some important points of diagnosis depend upon a comparison of the two halves of the head. It is thus essential that the sagittal plane should be at right-angles to the film and the centring exactly correct in axial radiographs.

(3) A wide range of contrast is essential in order that small flecks of calcification should not be overlooked; but the skull shows so much variation in translucency that, even if the correct kilo-voltage is used, some areas must be viewed with extra strong illumination.

(4) Limitation of the amount of radiation which falls on the patient's head is less important than, for instance, limitation in abdominal examinations. The gonad dose will, in any case, be less, and many of the conditions for which skull radiography is indicated are potentially so serious that the radiation dose is of secondary importance.

INTENSIFYING SCREENS

Even the smallest visible specks of calcification within the head may be of diagnostic importance. It is therefore essential that the intensifying screens used should be clean and undamaged. The easiest way to do this is to clean all screens at frequent and regular intervals. Even when this precaution is taken it may sometimes be necessary to repeat a radiograph and to identify the cassette from which the first film was taken so that the screens in it may be attended to out of turn.

There is no doubt that useful bone detail may be lost if high definition screens are not employed. However, high definition screens require a greater exposure. If the available x-ray apparatus will give tube currents in the region of 200 mA or above the exposure may be kept short, and in such circumstances high definition screens used for all views. Where the generator will only provide a low output, some compromise is probably necessary, and it is suggested that high definition screens should then be reserved for the lateral view.

Choice of screens is sometimes influenced by the kilo-voltage employed in routine radiography. High kilo-voltage skull radiography has not proved to be of value. The kilo-voltage usually employed is in the 50—90 range.

Rare earth screens are very sensitive indeed and greatly reduce the radiation exposure, but they do not improve resolution or contrast.

FILM

Except for taking some pictures of the nasal bones and the maxilla, non-screen film has no place in skull radiography.

The modern tendency is towards faster film emulsion. This increase in speed is nearly always obtained at the expense of resolving power, and as definition is of paramount importance in skull radiography fast film should not be used unless the most careful comparative trials have shown that detail in the radiographs is not lost by its employment.

Some rapid emulsions which are just acceptable when newly supplied show a tendency to deteriorate in storage more than less sensitive film.

STATIONARY GRIDS

Stationary grids are employed very widely in skull radiography, particularly for horizontal ray pictures. Modern grids with 24 or more lines to the centimetre cause very little interference with the bone detail on the radiograph. Grids with more than 40 lines to the centimetre are almost invisible without a magnifying glass.

No one grid is adequate for the many purposes of different projections. The following principles are worth remembering.
(1) For the kilo-voltage range recommended, grids of ratio greater than 8/1 or 10/1 are probably not required.
(2) The higher the ratio the more essential does it become to place the grid exactly normal to the centre of the incident beam and to use a grid focused for the appropriate tube distance.
(3) Other things being equal, the higher the grid ratio and the more exact its focusing, the greater will be its efficiency and the better the resulting radiography.

A 24 or 48 line, 8/1, 25 × 30 cm grid focused to the appropriate tube distance is ideal for lateral radiographs of the skull, but virtually useless if a slightly different focus-film distance has to be employed or where it is difficult to keep the x-ray beam precisely at right-angles to the grid. It is therefore suggested that, in addition to this most efficient grid, at least one much lower ratio grid should be available, and this may well be of the parallel rather than focused type, and perhaps a smaller size.

These grids should, as far as possible, be reserved for their own special purpose and not used in angiography or borrowed by other radiographic rooms, because they are easily damaged and, when damaged, throw confusing shadows.

Grid-cassettes are more satisfactory. The grid is protected from damage and cannot fall out of its correct positioning relative to the film.

PROCESSING

Since the first edition of this book was published automatic processing has become almost univeral and x-ray film emulsions have been designed to suit it, but for those who still have to use hand development the following quotation is still appropriate. 'There is no alternative to full development by time and temperature. Processing by inspection is not permissible with skull work and if the film has been over-exposed or under-exposed it should be repeated. The most acceptable radiographs are usually those which have received a moderately 'fine grain' development at ordinary temperatures for a time between 2½ and 4 minutes, depending upon the exact composition of the developer.'

Where the film, screen or processing fall short of the above recommendations, it is not possible to attach much significance to a loss of definition of the cortical edge of the sella turcica.

X-RAY TUBE

For skull radiography a tube focus of 1 millimetre square or less is required. If a skull table is in use the most satisfactory tube has two foci, one in the region of 0.6 millimetre square and the other 0.3 millimetre square (for very high definition studies).

X-RAY GENERATOR (TRANSFORMER)

There are considerable advantages in being able to use a high tube current (400 mA and above). One has already been mentioned: it enables high definition screens to be used for all views. Another advantage arises from the fact that many patients with diseases of the head are restless and good radiographs are therefore much more easily obtained with very short exposures.

THE X-RAY TABLE

Some patients prefer to be in a sitting position for radiography of the skull, but many are unable to support themselves and must be radiographed lying down. It is better wherever possible to employ one position and become proficient at it. The author strongly recommends that all patients should be radiographed lying down except when, for very special reasons, an erect view is required (for example, the demonstration of fluid levels in the maxillary antra).

It is difficult but not impossible, with care and time, to obtain good radiographs using an ordinary x-ray table or an upright Potter-Bucky diaphragm.

Properly designed apparatus for radiography of the head makes it far easier to obtain satisfactory radiographs of every patient. Since skull work forms a fair proportion of the general examinations of any department, a skull table is usually well worth the expense, while a proper table with a floating top saves a good deal of heavy lifting and may make the constant employment of a porter unnecessary. Whichever skull table is used, a period of training in its use is necessary before the best results can be obtained.

Skull tables have a variety of attachments for different purposes, and although these are of great importance in choosing the type of apparatus a discussion is out of place in this volume.

The focus-film distance of the skull table is relevant to the visibility of different structures. Early skull tables were made with the focus-film distance in the region of 27 inches, with the deliberate purpose of blurring, by enlargement, the structures on that side of the head furthest from the film, thus providing a clear and relatively unimpeded picture of the near side of the vault. There is no doubt that with the 1 mm focus at 27 inches the vault on the near side of the head is shown with great clarity. Longer focus-film distances and smaller foci produce radiographs in which superimposition of the shadows of both sides of the vault may lead to some confusion.

The longer focus-film distance (in the region of 90 cm) now employed is more effective in demonstrating small areas of calcification in the head, including the calcified pineal. It probably produces a clearer picture of the sella turcica and the petrous bones.

Attention should be drawn to the possibility of making good postero-anterior views of all kinds in patients who are unable to turn over, particularly those with fractured limbs. It is relatively easy to invert the skull table and support the head by means of a linen band.

In positioning using stands derived from Lysholm's original design, it is, of course, essential that the angulations to the base line and centring points be carefully

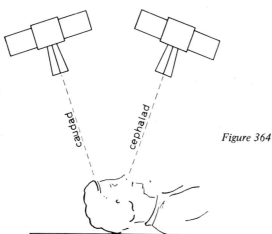

Figure 364

Figure 365. (1) Infra-orbital point. (2) Nasion. (3) Bregma. (4) Vertex. (5) Lambda. (6) Inion. (7a) Centre of the external auditory canal or axis of the external auditory meatus. (7b) Superior border of the meatus. (8) Superior border of the orbit. (9) Centre of the orbit. (10) Pterion. (11) Asterion. (12) Lowest point of the occiput. (13) Mastoid tip. (14) Glabella. (A) The anthropological basal line on lateral view; the infra-orbital line on antero-posterior view. (B) The inter-orbital or inter-pupillary line. (C) The superior horizontal line. (D) The orbito-meatal basal line. (E) The median-sagittal plane

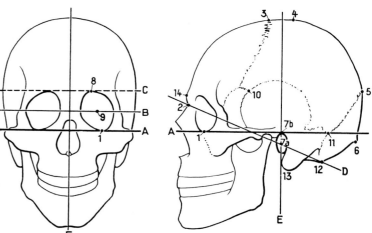

projection is only truly lateral at one point, and in the other the natural asymmetry of the skull makes the sagittal plane more or less a matter of choice. There is, however, a real purpose in attempting more exact definition. What follows applies to the author's work; but is not universally adopted.

Lateral The structures of the sella, its shape and, in particular, the cortex of the bone around it are seen most clearly when the radiograph is made with the point of centring precisely over the sella. In the vast majority of correctly centred and correctly positioned lateral radiographs made in this way the posterior clinoid processes are superimposed, the anterior clinoid processes are superimposed and the two orbital plates of the frontal bones are seen as a single line. Very occasionally the skull is so asymmetrical in its shape that such a view is difficult to obtain. However, in most such cases inspection of the postero-anterior radiograph will show by how much a line joining the lesser wings of the sphenoid falls out of parallel with a line joining the superior margins of the orbits; appropriate allowance

followed. However, a slight tilt of the table (and therefore the film) may make the patient very much more comfortable and is permissible if by this means an adequate radiograph is obtained.

Supine radiography of the skull has been made even easier and much more accurate as a result of the work of Thibaut, Delvaux and Radberg (Radberg and Thibaut, 1971) based upon the earlier efforts of Dulac. There is now a satisfactory apparatus capable of making all routine projections without turning the patient over. A fine focus tube and a long object-film distance give good magnified pictures of foramina.

POSITIONING

IS THE HEAD STRAIGHT?

The terms 'lateral' and 'axial projection' do not, as a rule, have a precise meaning because in the one case divergence of the rays of the incident beam ensures that the

can then be made in order to obtain a radiograph which is lateral to the sella. *The author's definition of a lateral view of the skull is a view lateral to the sella.*

Axial From the neurological point of view the most important sagittal plane is that of the falx. The two halves of the cranial cavity divided by the plane of the falx should be of equal volume, and it is the displacement of the pineal and other midline structures away from this plane which is of significance. However, the falx is not always visible on the radiographs. The surface markings by which its position may usually be gauged are the nasion and the lambda. The nasion is easily seen; the lambda may be felt after a little experience. The author's definition of the straight axial view is therefore one in which the lambda and the midpoint between the orbits lie in the same vertical plane. This definition is adhered to regardless of the amount of asymmetry of the vault.

For practical purposes it is often quicker and usually successful to gauge the posterior end of this sagittal plane by the middle of the ligamentum nucha, and only when this technique fails to produce a straight radiograph is it necessary to feel for the exact position of the lambda.

Nomenclature

The exact directions for obtaining different radiographic projections have varied from author to author. In 1961 a Commission under the auspices of the World Federation of Neurology made recommendations for standardization of technique. They have not been superceded.

The extensive quotations in the following pages are taken from the report of the Commission, and where the author's practice has not entirely coincided with these recommendations a note is made.

The meaning of the phrases 'angulation towards the head', or 'towards the feet' varies in different countries.

The English practice is followed here, and 'angulation towards the head' means that the x-ray tube is tilted so that the rays travel in that direction (*see* diagram). Angulation 'cephalad' is used synonymously (*Figure 364*).

The synonym for 'angulation to the feet' is 'angulation caudad'.

In the report of The Commission on Neuroradiology, the phrase 'the central ray is directed cranio-caudally' has the same meaning as 'angulation caudad'.

The Commission chose the following three lines which appear to them to be fundamental for skull radiology.

LINES (*Figure 365*)

Basal line Two base lines as follows are used by most neuroradiologists.
(1) The basal line accepted at the Munich Congress in 1877. Also known as the line of Frankfurt, or Reid's base line, it is the line which joins the infra-orbital point to the superior border of the external auditory meatus and is also known as the anthropological base line.
(2) The orbito-meatal line which joins the outer canthus of the eye to the central point of the external auditory meatus.

To avoid any confusion in the nomenclature and to eliminate proper names, Dr. Bull suggested that the following names should be used.
(1) The anthropological basal line
(2) The orbito-meatal basal line
These two lines are at an angle of 10 degrees.

Auricular line This line is perpendicular to the anthropological base line and passes through the external auditory meatus.

Inter-orbital or inter-pupillary line It is this line which joins the centre of the two orbits or the two pupils. It is perpendicular to the median-sagittal plane.

The infra-orbital line (which joins the two infra-orbital points), and the superior horizontal line which passes through the upper borders of the orbits), were considered to be used less frequently.

The commission considered that the lines and the angles of the base of the skull described by anthropologists and used in the study of semeiology could not be included.

PLANES

The Commission suggested the following four planes.
(1) *The median-sagittal plane* — This is the plane which divides the skull symmetrically in half.
(2) *The horizontal plane of Frankfurt* — This plane contains both anthropological base lines (anthropological plane).
(3) *The frontal bi-auricular plane* — This plane is perpendicular to the horizontal plane of Frankfurt and passes through the centre of the two external auditory meatuses.
(4) *Orbital-meatus plane* — This plane contains both basal orbito-meatal lines.

The first three planes are anthropometric and perpendicular to each other. The fourth is a radiological plane.

It will be seen that the definition of the median-sagittal plane as shown in *Figure 365* is incomplete as no landmark is provided for its posterior limits. The normal asymmetry of the skull and the necessity to make and recognize good axial projections require something more in the way of practical help, and suggestions have already been made earlier in this chapter.

The author has found the superior horizontal line of great value as it is easily recognized both on the routine postero-anterior radiograph and on the patient, and therefore provides a convenient means of making and, if necessary, correcting the lateral projection.

PROJECTIONS

Four routine projections are often used. These are the lateral projection, the basal or axial projection which is also frequently known as the submento-vertical view, the postero-anterior projection (inclined) and the antero-posterior half axial projection often known as Towne's view. In some departments left and right laterals are made of every patient, but the usual practice is to place that side of the head which is more likely to show abnormality next to the film and rely on a single lateral for routine use. It has been shown that one good lateral view, if examined with care by experts, will reveal nearly all the abnormalities present. This should be supplemented by a straight antero-posterior picture if the pineal is calcified, and by other views as dictated by clinical signs or by the abnormalities seen.

Lateral projection The Commission recommended the following.

'The median-sagittal plane is parallel to the film. The central ray is perpendicular to the median-sagittal plane and centred on the auricular line 3 or 4 cm above the external auditory meatus.'

The centring point coincides approximately with the centre of the head.

This differs considerably from the author's practice. Although the Commission's recommendation is ideal for ventriculography and angiography, it does not in many patients provide a true lateral view of the sella turcica which is of paramount importance. In order to avoid the necessity for special projections of the sella, the author makes all lateral skull radiographs with the centring point 2.5 cm anterior to the centre of the external auditory meatus and 1 cm above the orbito-meatal line.

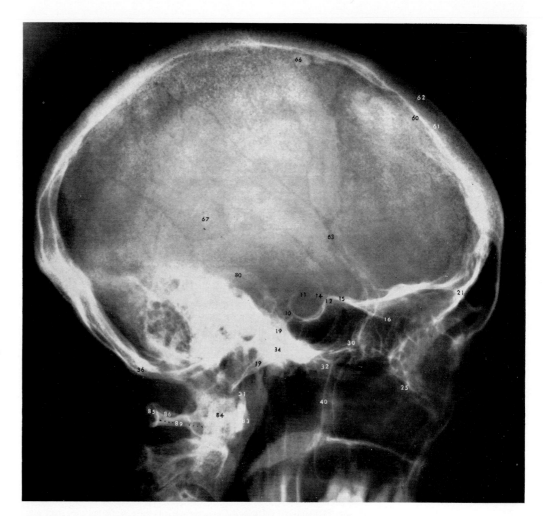

Figure 366. Lateral projection. (For the convenience of the reader, the numerals on Figures 343–360 are fully described on the insert facing page 372)

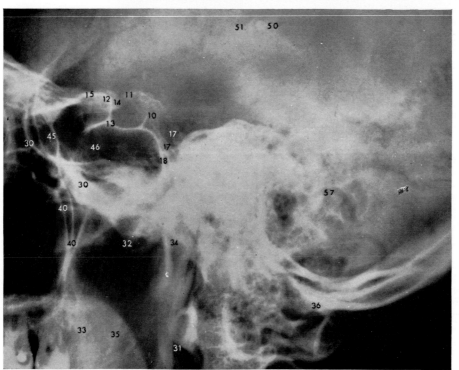

Figure 367. Lateral projection

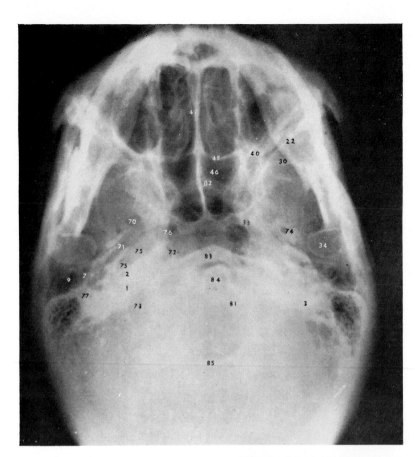

Figure 368. Full axial projection. (Basal view; submento-vertical view)

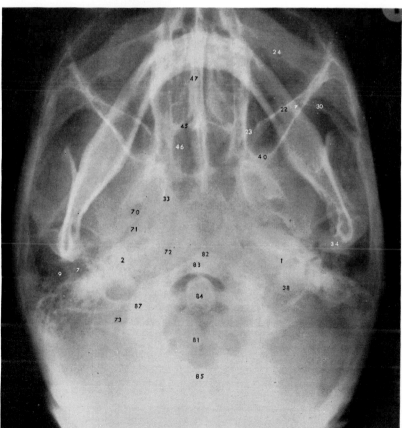

Figure 369. Full axial projection. (Basal view; submento-vertical view)

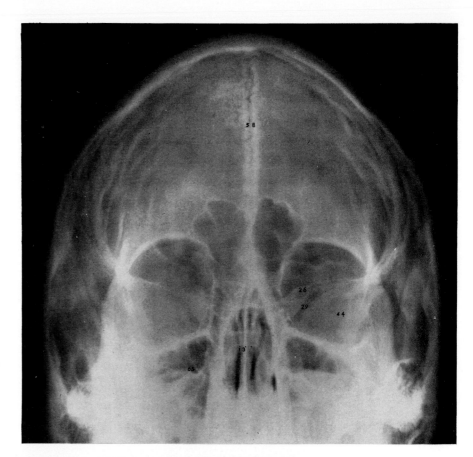

Figure 370. Postero-anterior view (inclined 20 degrees)

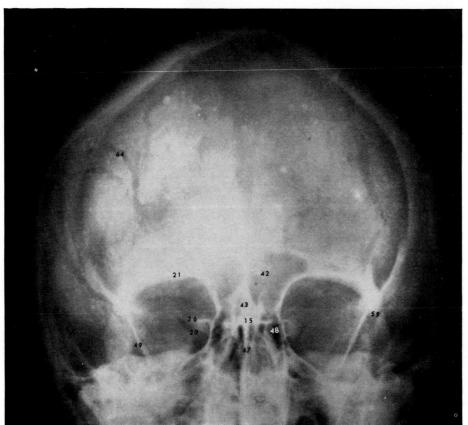

Figure 371. Postero-anterior view (inclined 25 degrees)

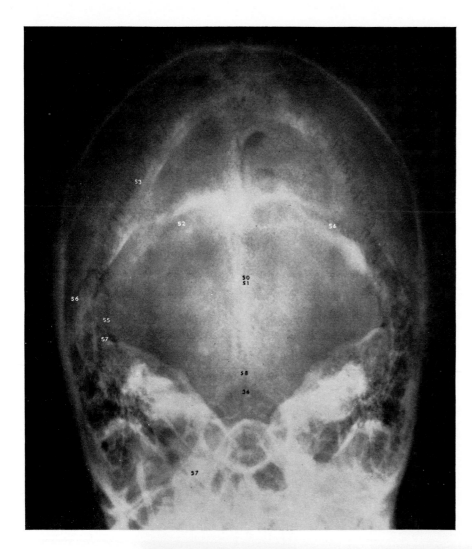

Figure 372. Antero-posterior view (inclined 33 degrees) (Towne's view)

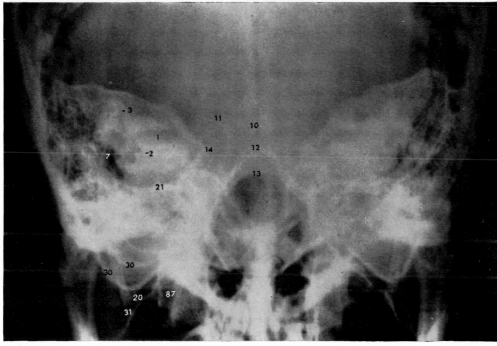

Figure 373. Antero-posterior view (inclined 28 degrees)

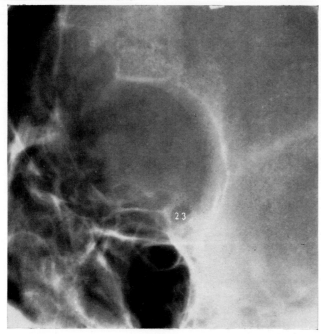

Figure 374. Optic canal view

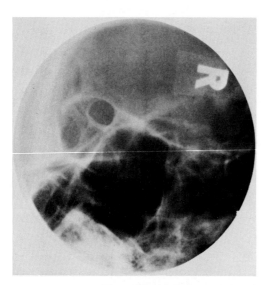
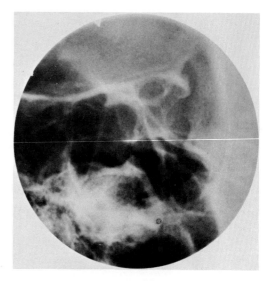

Figure 375. (a) Optic canal view. (b) The view of the apex of the orbit (same patient)

If, due to gross asymmetry of the base, this projection does not provide a true lateral of the sella turcica, correction may be made after looking at the postero-anterior view and noting by what angle the superior horizontal line is out of parallel with the line joining the anterior clinoid processes (*Figures 131, 366, 367*).

Basal or full axial projection Many radiologists know this as the submento-vertical view.

The Commission's report reads as follows. 'The head is placed in hyperextension and the anthropological plane should be parallel to the film. The central ray is perpendicular to the anthropological plane and passes along the bi-auricular plane. This is the true axial projection.

If the central ray is perpendicular to the orbito-meatal plane, the projection may be called sub-axial.'

The author now adopts this definition but many of the radiographs reproduced in this book have been made with the orbito-meatal plane parallel to the film, the beam angled 5 degrees cephalad and centred on the mid-point of a line joining the angles of the mandible (*Figures 368, 369*).

The postero-anterior projection (inclined) This is widely known as the occipito-frontal view. Directions for this projection given by the Commission are as follows.

'The forehead and nose touch the film, the median-sagittal plane being perpendicular to the film. The orbito-

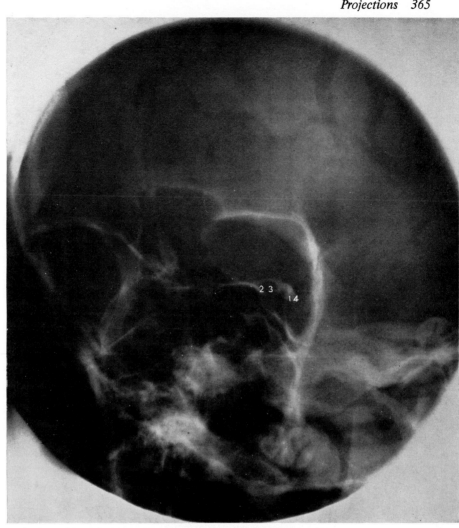

Figure 376. Orbital view (25 degrees rotation)

meatal plane is also perpendicular to the film. The central ray is directed cranio-caudally to form an angle 15 degrees with this plane (or about 20 degrees to the anthropological plane).

The point of exit of the central ray is the nasion. However, the Commission noted that if the point of exit is on the infra-orbital line it coincides with the centre of the radiograph.'

Most of the radiographs illustrated have been made according to directions which differ from these. The centring point used is 6 cm above the external occipital protruberance and the centre of the beam is angled either 20 or 25 degrees caudad. There seems no particular point in recommending the exact degree of inclination which should be used. Lesser degrees of tilt tend to show the sella floor in profile a little better than greater degrees of tilt. The sphenoid fissures and lesser wings of the sphenoid are satisfactorily demonstrated with the 20 degrees angulation (*Figures 370, 371*).

Antero-posterior, half axial projection This projection is known as Towne's view. 'The head rests on the occiput. The median-sagittal plane is perpendicular to the film. If

the orbito-meatal plane is perpendicular to the film, the central ray makes an angle of 25–35 degrees cranio-caudally to the plane. If the anthropological plane is perpendicular to the film, the central ray makes an angle of 35–45 degrees cranio-caudally. The true half axial projection will by definition be obtained by using an angle of 45 degrees. The central ray which coincides with the medial-sagittal plane passes through the midpoint of the line which joins two external auditory meatuses.'

The directions by which these radiographs have been made are very similar to the recommendations of the Commission of Neuroradiology (*Figures 372, 373*).

Special projections

APEX OF THE ORBIT

'The Commission differentiated the projection of the optic canal, which is important in lesions of the structures within the canal, from the projection of the

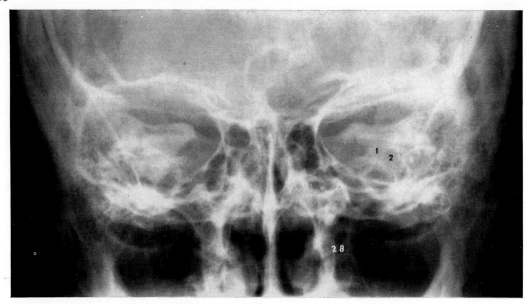

Figure 377. Symmetrical per-orbital view of petrous bones (antero-posterior)

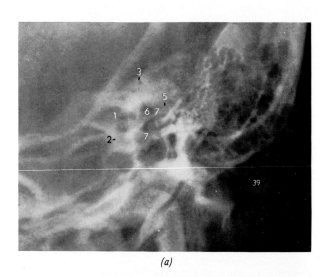

(a)

Figure 378. (a) Stenver's view (12 degrees). (b) Stenver's view (8 degrees). (c) Stockholm 'C' view

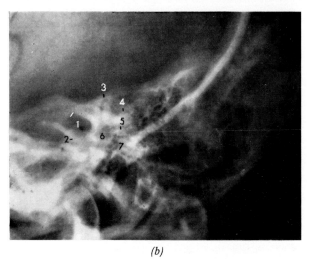

(b)

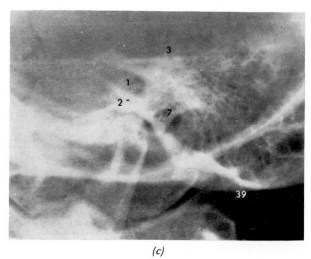

(c)

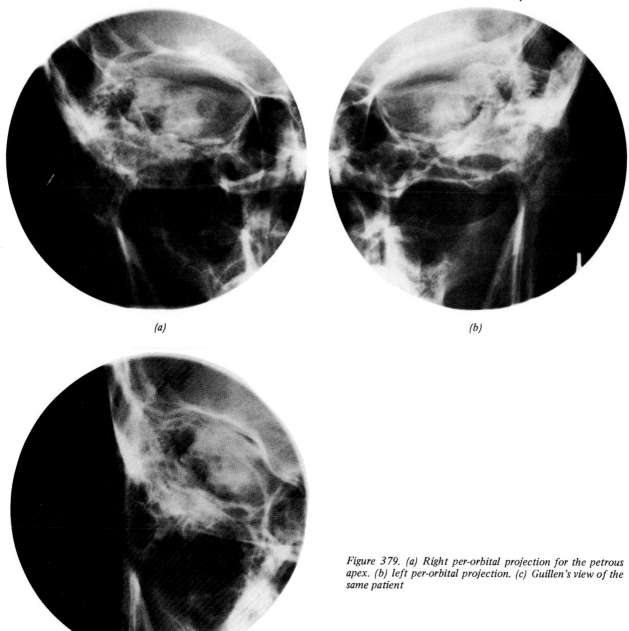

(a)

(b)

(c)

Figure 379. (a) Right per-orbital projection for the petrous apex. (b) left per-orbital projection. (c) Guillen's view of the same patient

apex of the orbit, which is also important in lesions situated outside the canal.

(1) The projection of the *optic canal* is obtained when the central ray coincides with the central axis of the canal. Under these conditions the canal is projected in its usual shape, without distortion, into the infero-lateral quadrant of the orbit' (*Figure 374*).

Directions for obtaining this view are as follow.

From the occipito-frontal position raise the chin until the orbito-meatal line is at 30 degrees to the film. Rotate the head 39 degrees away from the affected side. Centre on the midpoint of the line joining the

external occipital protruberance and the external auditory meatus most remote from the film.

(2) 'If the optic canal is projected into the centre of the orbit, the surrounding structures such as sphenoid fissure, anterior clinoid process, *jugum and sphenoid sinus* are projected with the minimum of distortion at the expense of the optic foramen, which then appears oval in its vertical axis. The edges of the sphenoidal fissure can be seen in the postero-anterior projection of the skull.'

To obtain this projection, from the occipito-frontal position, raise the chin until the orbito-meatal line is at

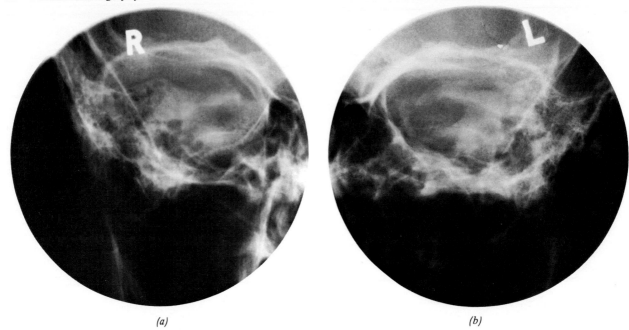

(a)   (b)

Figure 380. (a) Right per-orbital projection of another patient. (b) Left per-orbital projection

25 degrees to the film. Rotate the head 39 degrees away from the affected side and centre on the midpoint of a line joining the external occipital protruberance and the external auditory meatus most remote from the film (*Figure 376*).

Other views essential to a proper examination of the orbit are: a *lateral,* in which the median-saggital plane lies a few degrees out of parallel with the film; a *postero-anterior projection (inclined);* a *full axial projection;* and an *occipito-mental projection (see* below).

THE SELLA TURCICA (*Figure 367*)

'The Commission decided to radiograph this area in the lateral and *en face* projection.

The sella turcica appears with great detail in profile on the routine lateral projection. Depending on clinical demands, however, it may be necessary to take a special lateral view. It is usually achieved by directing the central ray, which is perpendicular to the median-saggital plane, on to a point situated about 2 cm above and 2 cm in front of the external auditory meatus.

To study the sella turcica *en face,* the two following methods can be used (*Figures 372, 373*).
(1) The first projects the dorsum sellae within or behind the foramen magnum.
(2) The second projects the cortex of the sella floor in the superimposed translucency of the ethmoid sinuses, sphenoid sinuses and nasal cavities (*Figure 370*). However, more exact visualization will be obtained from frontal tomography'.

It will be seen that the routine *lateral* projection used by the author more or less corresponds to the special lateral suggested for the sella turcica.

The views suggested for *en face* visualization of the sella at (1) above is the *half axial projection,* and at (2) the *postero-anterior projection (inclined).*

THE PETROUS BONES

'In neuroradiology, examination of the petrous bones must be separated from the rest of the temporal bone. The petrous bone has already been seen in the routine basal and antero-posterior half axial projections, which may sometimes need to be modified in certain cases (tilt of the ray, penetration). To these two general projections, two more can be added.
(1) *Per-orbital* projections — the antero-posterior view of the petrous bones (*Figures 379, 380*).
(2) The projection devised by Stenver in which the long axis of the petrous bone becomes parallel to the plane of the film and perpendicular to the central ray' (*Figure 378*).

The first paragraph of the Commission's recommendations suggest that the half axial and basal views should be modified in certain cases. Perhaps the most valuable way is to make a stereoscopic pair for each view, using at the same time a rectangular cone or diaphragm (slits) just large enough to include both petrous bones on the film.

The *per-orbital symmetrical projection* provides an excellent method of comparing the internal auditory meatuses of the two sides. It should be made in the antero-posterior position and, depending upon the shape of the particular head, may require up to 5 degrees angulation to the orbito-meatal line either caudad or cephalad.

Stenver's view is made with the patient prone. Begin with the orbito-meatal line at right-angles to the film. Rotate the head 45 degrees towards the unaffected side.

Angle the beam 12 degrees cephalad and centre midway between the external auditory meatus remote from the film and the external occipital protruberance. The author believes that in the majority of patients an angulation of 8 degrees rather than 12 degrees is more satisfactory for the clear visualization of the internal auditory meatus.

The *reverse Stenver's view* is also a good one. The patient lies supine with base line at right-angles to the film. The head is then rotated 45 degrees away from the affected side and the beam angled 12 degrees (or 8 degrees) caudad. The centring point for this view is half an inch posterior to the outer canthus of the eye remote from the film along the orbito-meatal line.

Stockholm 'C' position This projection corresponds closely to Stenver's view; but it is very convenient when a skull table is used. 'The patient lies prone with the head lateral. The head is positioned so that the cross is seen in the mirror at a point 2 cm in front of the external auditory meatus and 1 cm above the orbito-meatal line. The pointer should be directed to the corresponding point on the other side of the head, the position of the head accordingly being true lateral.' The tube is angled to point the rays 10 degrees cephalad and 30 degrees towards the face.

MASTOIDS

The mastoids and the air cells in the more lateral parts of the petrous bone are shown well in the full axial view and in the Stenver's and reverse Stenver's projection. The antero-posterior half axial (Towne's) projection is widely used, but can cause a great deal of confusion because of superimposition of the groove for the sigmoid sinus upon the antrum. The following additional views are recommended.

Lateral oblique With the head in the lateral position and the external auditory meatus at the centre of the film, angle the beam 30 degrees caudad, centring about 6 cm above the external auditory meatus remote from the film. A lateral oblique view may also be made with 15 degress angulation (*Figures 381, 382*).

Stockholm 'A' and 'B' projections These correspond closely to a 15 degrees and to a 35 degrees lateral oblique. The cross in the mirror of the skull table should be seen just behind the external auditory meatus in one case and 1 cm lower in the other.

Per-orbital projection This is sometimes called Guillen's view. With the patient supine and the orbito-meatal line perpendicular to the film, the face is rotated 5–10 degrees towards the affected side. The beam is angled 0–5 degrees caudally, centring through the middle of the orbit on the affected side (*Figures 379c and 383*).

THE JUGULAR FORAMEN

'The commission agreed that, apart from tomography, the problem of demonstrating the jugular foramen and the condylar canal has not yet been settled satisfactorily, especially in view of the great anatomical variation and asymmetry of that region. Indeed, the unilateral and bilateral projections recommended do not satisfy all the criteria mentioned above.'

In order to show the jugular foramina the author uses a *sub-axial view* (in which the head is hyperextended). The central ray makes an angle of about 70 degrees to the orbito-meatal plane. An occipito-mental view in which the orbito-meatal line is at 60 degrees is also valuable, the centring point being adjusted to show the jugular foramen through the open mouth (*Figures 384, 385*).

THE FORAMEN MAGNUM AND ATLANTO-OCCIPITAL JOINT

'As with the petrous bone, the foramen magnum will be seen in the routine survey of the skull, the *lateral,* the *basal* and the *antero-posterior half axial*. They show the structures as follows.
(1) On the lateral projection – the clivus and nasion anteriorly, the squamous portion of the occipital bone with the opisthion posteriorly, the odontoid process in its relation to the clivus, together with the two mastoid processes and the arch of the atlas (*Figure 366*).
(2) In the basal view – the whole of the foramen magnum with reasonable accuracy (*Figure 368, 369*).
(3) In the half axial – the posterior half of the foramen magnum more or less completely (*Figures 372, 373*).

Apart from tomography, the clinical problems may require special projections. These may be carried out in two ways: (*a*) the central ray coinciding with the longitudinal axis of the foramen magnum, the head in flexion or extension; and (*b*) the central ray perpendicular to the long axis of the foramen magnum through the open mouth.'

PARANASAL SINUSES

The views recommended for the paransal sinuses are as follow.

The *occipito-mental* The orbito-meatal line is at 45 degrees to the film. The central ray at right-angles to the film passes 7.5 cm above the external occipital protuberance (*Figures 386, 387*).

The *postero-anterior projection (inclined)* (*Figures 370, 371*).

The *lateral view* It is necessary to centre over the outer canthus of the eye remote from the film (*Figure 320*).

The *full axial view* (*Figures 368, 369*).

Lateral of the post-nasal space (*Figure 330*) With the body and skull in lateral position, the beam is centred below the lobe of the ear remote from the film, and the view is taken on inspiration.

It is better, if possible, to make radiographs of the sinuses with the patient erect in order to demonstrate any fluid levels which may be present.

THE NASAL BONES AND MIDDLE THIRD OF FACE (FOR FRACTURES)

Lateral view Non-screened film is used here. With the skull in the lateral position, the beam is centred 1 cm below the nasion (*Figure 353*).

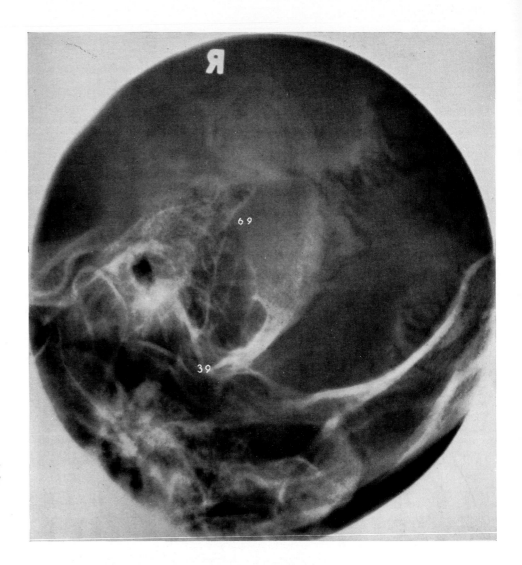

Figure 381. Lateral oblique view of mastoid

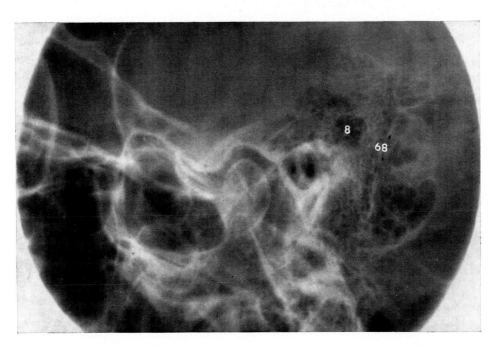

Figure 382. Lateral oblique view of mastoid

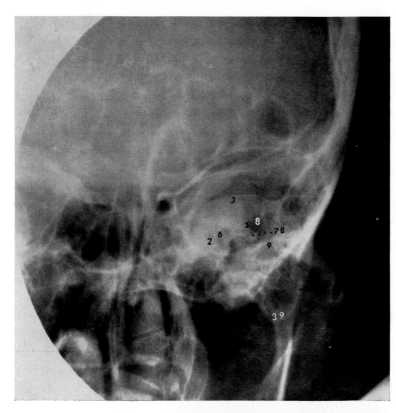

Figure 383. Per-orbital view of middle and inner ear

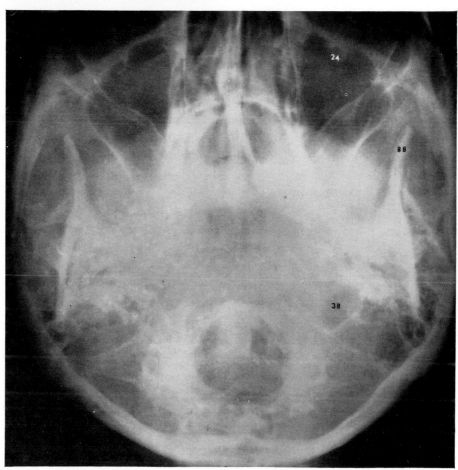

Figure 384. Sub-axial view

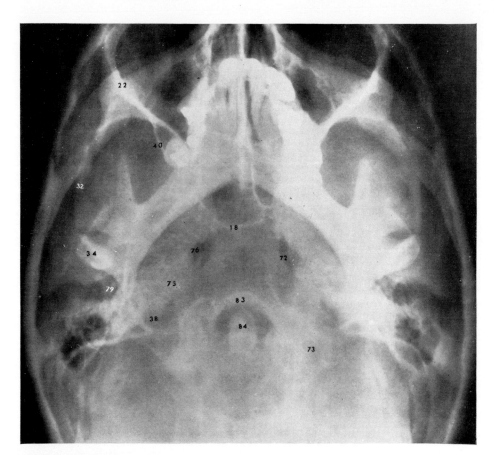

Figure 385. Vertico-sub-mental view

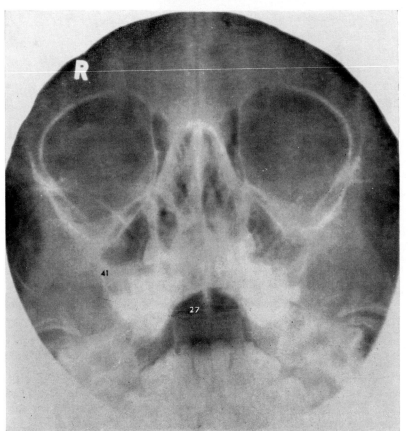

*Figure 386. Occipito-mental projection.
A child aged 6½ years*

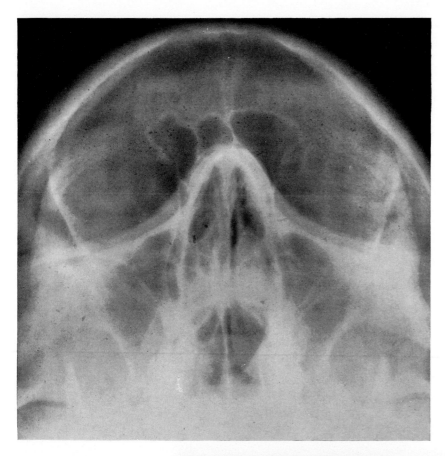

Figure 387. Occipito-mental pro-jection

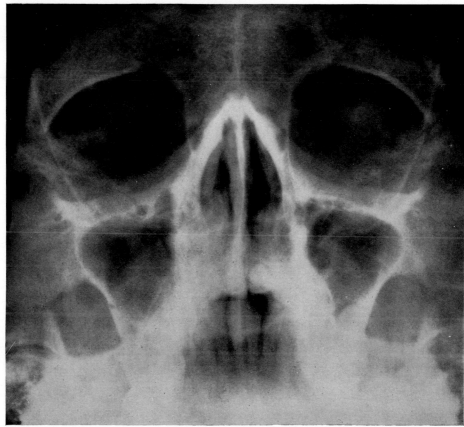

Figure 388. Occipito-mental view for the antra and sinuses

374

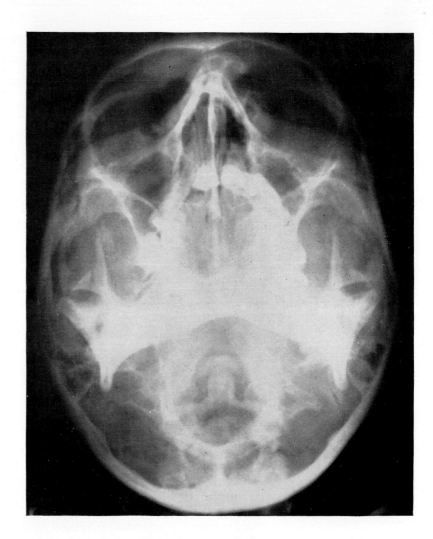

Figure 389. Occipito-mental view (60 degrees)

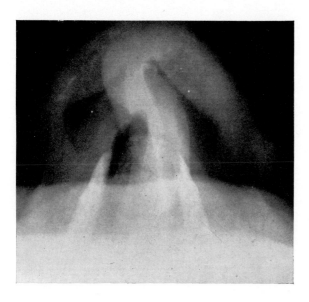

Figure 390. Supero-inferior view of the nasal bones

Occipito-mental view These are often known as the 'over-tilted' occipito-mental views. The orbito-meatal line is at 60 or 70 degrees to the film. The central ray at right-angles to the film is arranged to emerge through the nose (*Figure 388*).

Fronto-dental An occlusal film is placed in the mouth, tube side upwards, as far back as possible. The mouth is gently closed to hold it in place. The axis of the beam passes through the nasion at right-angles to the film (*Figure 390*).

Johnson and Dutt's view The head is positioned as for an examination of the optic canal. The tube is then angled 10 degrees so that the central ray is inclined towards the feet. The beam shows half the cribriform plate edge-on through the opposite orbit.

Tomography

Tomography is of great value in examination of the skull. Only a few practical directions are given here.

(1) The best radiographs will be obtained when the area to be examined is projected with as little super-imposed shadowing as possible. For this reason it is often useful to have an apparatus capable of moving the tube through a linear arc with its centre not necessarily at 90 degrees to the film. It should be possible, for instance, to carry out tomography in the half axial position.

(2) Where it is not possible to project the area free from dense superimposed shadows, it is important that the direction of the arc should not coincide with dense linear markings such as, for instance, the nasal septum. Circular and figure-of-eight motion of the tube and film are often advantageous.

(3) Multisection techniques with one exposure are ideal during air studies or for a general survey, and may require an arc as small as 15 degrees, but for a detailed examination of the bones 30–50 degrees linear arcs are required at a focus-film distance of 90 cm, and the multisection technique should be replaced by one in which single radiographs are made at the predetermined levels.

Stereoscopic views

Stereoscopic radiography is of great value in the location of small areas of calcification, and in detailed examination of the petrous bones. A stereoscopic pair may be obtained with any slight difference in angle at which the two radiographs are made, but ideally the tube shift should bear the same proportion to the observer's interpupillary distance as the focus-film measurement does to the viewing distance.

$$\frac{\text{Tube shift}}{\text{Interpupillary distance}} = \frac{\text{Focus-film distance}}{\text{Viewing distance}}$$

For example, at 90 cm focus-film distance a total shift of 8 cm is satisfactory. It is usually best to make the shift symmetrically 4 cm on either side of the appropriate centring line.

The direction in which the tube is offset is also of importance. For instance, angulation is altered in the sagittal plane for the half axial radiographs of the petrous bones. For examination of the sella turcica antero-posterior shift may be required if, in the supra-inferior shift, the dense structures of the base are thrown over the floor of the sella.

Magnification

Magnification greater than × 1.5 is now rarely used for pictures of the plain skull. It requires a tube focus of 0.3 mm, or less. The 'Orbix' skull table, however, using a 0.6 mm tube focus and the technique of Thibaut, Delvaux and Radberg, makes excellent localized views of structures such as the optic canals and internal auditory meatuses with a magnification of about × 1.4.

BIBLIOGRAPHY

KEY TO BIBLIOGRAPHY INDEX LETTERS

A. Anatomical
C. Calcification
D. Developmental abnormality
E. Diseases of the ear
G. General
I. Infection and infestation
K. Generalized skeletal diseases

M. Metabolic and endocrine
N. Neoplasm; brain and meningeal tumours, bone tumours
O. Orbital lesions
P. Pituitary tumour
R. Raised intracranial pressure
S. Sinuses
T. Trauma
W. Brain parenchymal diseases

ABRAHAM, J. M. and RUSSELL, A. (1968). 'de Lange syndrome. A study of nine examples.' *Acta paediat. scand.*, 57, 339–353. (D)

ABRAHAM, J. M. and SNODGRASS, G. J. A. I. (1969). 'Soto's syndrome and cerebral gigantism.' *Archs Dis. Childh.*, 44, 203–210 (D)

ABRAMS, H. S. (1957). 'Choroid plexus calcification in an unusual location and mobile.' *Am. J. Roentg.*, 78, 95 (C)

ACHENBACH, W. and BÖHM, A. (1953). 'Skelettveränderungen bei Parathyrogenen Tetanien.' *Fortschr. Röntg.*, 79, 95 (M)

ACHESON, R. M. (1958). 'Bony changes in the skull in tuberculous meningitis.' *Br. J. Radiol.*, 31, 81 (I)

ADLER, H. and KAPLAN, G. (1956). 'Improvement of osseous changes in the sella turcica following irradiation of a pituitary tumour.' A case report. *Radiology*, 66, 856 (P)

AGRAWAL, G. N., NATA, N. K. and TANDON, P. N. (1966). 'Sellar changes in cases of increased intracranial pressure.' *J. Indian med. Ass.*, 47, 420–425 (R)

ALBRECHT, K. L. (1929). 'Gefässzeichnung am Roentgenbild des Schädels.' *Zentbl. ges. Neurol. Psychiat.*, 53, 670 (G)

ALBRIGHT, F. and REIFENSTEIN, E. C. (1948). *The Parathyroid Glands and Metabolic Bone Disease, Selected Studies.* Baltimore; Williams and Wilkins (M)

ALBRIGHT, F., SCOVILLE, B. and SULKOWITCH, H. W. (1938). 'Syndrome characterized by osteitis fibrosa disseminata, areas of pigmentation and a gonadal dysfunction: further observations including the report of two more cases.' *Endocrinology*, 22, 41 (D)

ALBRIGHT, F., BUTLER, A. M., HAMPTON, A. O. and SMITH, P. (1937). 'Syndrome characterized by osteitis fibrosa disseminata, areas of pigmentation and endocrine dysfunction with precocious puberty in females, report of five cases.' *New Engl. J. Med.*, 216, 727 (D)

ALLEN, E. P. (1940). 'Pineal localization: a rapid direct method.' *Br. J. Radiol.*, 13, 102 (C)

ALLEN, J. H. and RILEY, H. D. (1958). 'Generalized cystomegalic inclusion disease with emphasis on roentgen diagnosis.' *Radiology*, 71, 257 (I)

ALPERS, B. J. (1935). 'Cerebral osteochondroma of dural origin.' *Ann. Surg.*, 101, 27–37 (N)

ALTON, D. J., McDONALD, P. and REILLY, B. J. (1972). 'Cockayne's syndrome. A report of three cases.' *Radiology*, 102, 403–406 (D)

ALVERDES, C. (1957). *Untersuchungen über die A Meningica Media des Erwachsenen Menschen.* Leipzig; Diss (G)

ANDERSON, L. G., COOK, A. J., COCCARO, P. J., CORO, C. J. and BOSMA, J. F. (1972). 'Familial osteodysplasia.' *J. Am. med. Ass.,* **220,** 1687–1693 (D)

ANDERSON, P. E. (1953). 'The radiological diagnosis of lipoma of the corpus callosum.' *Radiologia. clin.,* **22,** 211 (N)

ANDERSON, R., KIEFFER, S. A., WOLFSON, J. J., LONG, D. and PETERSON, H. O. (1970). 'Thickening of the skull in surgically treated hydrocephalus.' *Am. J. Roentg.,* **110,** 96–101 (R)

ANDERSSON, H. (1966). 'Craniosynostosis as a complication after operation for hydrocephalus.' *Acta paediat., scand.,* **55,** 192–196 (R)

ANDERSSON, H. and GOMES, S. P. (1968). 'Clinocephaly: consideration on the pathophysiology of craniosynostosis.' *Acta paediat., scand.,* **57,** 294–296 (D ; R)

ANDREW, J. (1956) 'Osteoma of the paranasal sinuses.' *Br. J. Surg.,* **43,** 489 (S)

ANGELL, J., PENRY, J. B. and ROSS, F. G. M. (1964). 'Tomography in atresia of the external auditory meatus.' *Br. J. Radiol.,* **37,** 511 (D)

ANGLE, C. R., McINTIRE, M. S. and MOORE, R. C. (1967). 'Cloverleaf skull: Kleeblattschädel-deformity syndrome.' *Am. J. Dis. Child.,* **114,** 198–202 (D)

ANSPACH, W. E. (1937). 'Sunray hemangioma of bone with special reference to roentgen signs.' *J. Am. med. Ass.,* **108,** 617 (N)

ANTOINE, M. and de KERSAUSON, M. C. (1958). Images radiologiques de céphal-hématomes.' *J. Radiol. electrol.,* **39,** 163 (T)

APLEY, J. (1944). 'Familial tuberose sclerosis with calcification. Report of two cases.' *Brain,* **67,** 258 (W ; C)

APPELMAN, H. B. and MOEHLIG, R. C. (1954). 'Metabolic craniopathy. Report of two cases associated with osteopokilosis.' *Am. J. Roentg.,* **71,** 420 (M)

APPELT, H. (1952). 'Fenestrae Frontales Symmetricae.' *Mschr. Kinderheilk,* **100,** 335 (D)

APPELBY, A., FOSTER, J. B., HANKINSON, J. and HUDGSON, P. (1968). 'The diagnosis and management of the Chiari Anomalies in adult life.' *Brain,* **91,** (Pt. I), 131–140 (D)

ARGER, P. H., MISHKIN, M. M. and NENNINGER, R. H. (1972). 'An approach to orbital lesions.' *Am. J. Roentg.,* **115,** 595–606 (O)

ARSENI, C., SIMIONESCU, M. and MIHAILESCU, N. (1960). 'Röntgenbefunde bei Hernzystizerkose.' *Zentb. Neurochir.,* **20,** 279 (I)

ASENJO, A., VALLARDES, H. and FIERRO, J. (1951). 'Tuberculomas of the brain.' Report of 150 cases.' *Archs Neurol. Psychiat.,* **65,** 146 (I)

ASENJO, A., PERINE, F. R., GARCIA, E. and GALLO, H. (1947). 'Cien cases de Tuberculomas del Sistema Nervioso central.' *Revta. méd. Chile,* **75,** 1 (I)

AZAR-KIA, B., SCHECHTER, M. M., LIEBESKIND, A. and MARC, J. A. (1973). 'The enlarged foramen ovale.' *Am. J. Roentg.,* **118,** 420–425 (G)

BABBITT, D. P., TANG, T., DOBBS, J. and BERK, R. (1969). 'Idiopathic familial cerebrovascular ferrocalcinosis (Fahr's disease) and review of differential diagnosis of intracranial calcification in children.' *Am. J. Roentg.,* **105,** 352–358 (D ;C)

BADE, H. (1939). 'Zur Diagnostik der Schädeltumoren: (Xanthom and Cholesteatom des Schädeldaches)' *Röntgenpraxis,* **11,** 223 (N)

BAKWIN, H. and EIGER, M. S. (1956). 'Fragile bones and macrocranium.' *J. Pediat.,* **49,** 558–564 (D)

BALESTRY, G. L. (1939). 'Sulle calcificasione della falce cerebral.' *Archo Radiol.,* **6,** 731 (C)

BARNETT, D. J. (1959). 'Radiologic aspects of craniopharyngiomas.' *Radiology,* **72,** 14 (N)

BARTLETT, J. E. and KISHORE, P. R. E. (1976). 'Familial "doughnut" lesions of the skull: a benign hereditary dysplasia.' *Radiology,* **119,** 385–387 (D)

BARTON, C. J. (1961). 'Tuberculosis of the vault of the skull.' *Br. J. Radiol.,* **34,** 286 (I)

BATSON, R., SHAPIRO, J., CHRISTIE, A. and RILEY, H. D. (1955). 'Acute non-lipid disseminated reticuloendotheliosis.' *Am. J. Dis. Child.,* **90,** 323 (D)

BEBIN, J. and TYTUS, J. S. (1955). 'Ossification in gliomas.' *J. Neurosurg.,* **12,** 577 (N)

BECKER, M. H. and WALLIN, J. K. (1968). 'Congenital hyperuricosuria. Associated radiological features.' *Radiol. Clin. N. Am.,* **6,** 239–243 (M ; D)

BECKER, M. H., NGO, N. and BERANBAUM, S. L. (1968). 'Mycotic infection of the paranasal sinuses.' *Radiology,* **90,** 49–51 (I)

BECKWITH, J. B. (1969). 'Macroglossia, omphalocele, adrenal cytomegaly, gigantism and hyperplastic visceromegaly.' *Article Series,* **5,** 188–196 (D)

BECKWITH, J. B., WANG, C., DONNELL, G. N. and GWINN, J. C. (1964). 'Hyperplastic fetal visceromegaly with macroglossia, omphalocele, cytomegaly of the adrenal cortex, postnatal somatic gigantism, and other abnormalities: a newly recognized syndrome.' Presented at the Annual Meeting of American Pediatric Society, June 16–18, 1964, Seattle, Washington (D)

BEGG, A. C. and ROBINSON, R. G. (1955). 'Radiological calcification in posterior fossa tumours.' *Br. J. Radiol.,* **28,** 470 (N ;C)

BEK, V. S. (1952). 'Chranicema Koncentrická osteoatrofie lebni Klenby.' *Cas. Lék cesk.,* **91,** 242 (G)

BELLINI, M. A. and NEVES, I. (1956). 'The skull in childhood myxedema, its roentgen appearance.' *Am. J. Roentg.,* **76,** 495 (M)

BERGERHOFF, W. (1960). *Beitr. Neurochir,* Heft 2: Die Sella turcica im Röntgenbild Leipzig. Barth; Ambrosius (G)

BERGERHOFF, W. (1961). *Atlas normaler Roentgenbilder des Schädels.* Berlin; Göttingen (G)

BERKMEN, Y. M. and BLATT, E. S. (1968). 'Cranial and intracranial cartilaginous tumours.' *Clin. Radiol.,* **19,** 327–333 (N)

BERNSTEIN, C. and PITEGOFF, G. I. (1951). 'Tuberose sclerosis. Two cases of sub-tentorial calcification.' *Conn. St. med. J.,* **15,** 1051 (W ;C)

BERRETT, A., BRÜNNER, S., COOK, A. J. and ANDERSON, L. G. (1967). 'Thin-section tomography in diagnosis of cholesteatoma of temporal bone in children.' *Acta Radiol.* **6,** 33–40 (E)

BETHUNE, J. E. and DENT, C. E. (1960). 'Hypophosphatasia in the adult.' *Am. J. Med.,* **28,** 615–622 (D ;M)

BEVERIDGE, B., VAUGHAN, B. F. and WALTERS, M. N. I. (1959). Primary hyperparathyroidism and secondary renal failure with osteosclerosis.' *J. Fac. Radiol.,* **10,** 197 (M)

BICKEL, W. H., GHORMLEY, R. K. and CAMP, J. D. (1943). 'Osteogenesis imperfecta.' *Radiology,* **40,** 145 (D)

BICKERSTAFF, E. R., SMALL, J. M. and WOOLF, A. L. (1956). 'Cysticercosis of the posterior fossa.' *Brain,* **79,** 622 (I)

BINET, E. F. (1974). 'The base of the adult skull.' *Semin. Roentg.,* **9,** 137–150 (G)

BINET, E. F., KIEFFER, S. A., MARGIN, S. H. and PETERSON, H. O. (1969). 'Orbital dysplasia in neurofibromatosis.' *Radiology,* **93,** 829–833 (O)

BISHOP, P. A. (1936). 'Bone changes in chronic fluorine intoxication; a roentgenographic study.' *Am. J. Roentg.,* **35,** 577 (M)

BITTER, T., MUIR, H., MITTWOCH, U. and SCOTT, J. D. (1966). 'A contribution to the differential diagnosis of Hurler's disease and forms of Morquio's syndrome.' *J. Bone Jt. Surg.,* **48B,** 637–645 (D)

BLEES, O. (1941). *Enstehung der Sellavergrösserungen nicht-hypophysären Ursprungs.* Münster; Diss (G)

BLIGH, A. S. and LAURENCE, K. M. (1967). 'The radiological appearances in arrhinencephaly.' *Clin. Radiol.,* **18,** 383–393 (D)

BLOOM, D. L. and KEOHANE, M. F. (1965). 'Epidermoid tumor of the skull and brain.' *Radiology,* **95,** 485–493 (N)

BLOOMFIELD, J. A. (1970). 'Cloverleaf skull and thanatophoric dwarfism.' *Australas. Radiol.,* **14,** 429–434 (D)

BOHE, A. (1928). 'Schädelmessungen, Lumbaldruck bestimmungen am Rachitiker.' *Jb. Kinderheilk, phys. Erzieh.*, **118**, 340 (M)

BOKELMANN, O. (1934). 'Die spezielle Anatomie Sella Turcica und ihre klinische Bedeutung für die Erkennung der Hypophysengrösse zugleich ein Beitrag zur Frage der Beiziehung der Hypophysengrösse sowie Grösse und Form der Sella zum anatomischen und funktionellen Hypogenitalismus.' *Fortschr. Röntgenstr.*, **49**, 364 (M)

BONAKDARPOUR, A. (1967). 'Echinococcus disease: Report of 112 cases from Iran and a review of 611 cases from the United States.' *Am. J. Roentg.*, **99**, 660–667 (I)

BONGIOVANNI, A. M., EBESLEIN, W. R. and JONES, I. T. (1957). 'Idiopathic hypercalcemia of infancy with failure to thrive.' *New. Engl. J. Med.*, **257**, 951 (M)

BONNET, P. and BRET, P. Y. (1954). 'Tomographie de la carotide intracranienne.' *Archs Ophthal., Paris*, **14**, 775 (G)

BONNEVILLE, J. F., TUETEY, J. B., VERNIER, F., JACQUET, G. and STEINEL, R. (1978). 'Post-traumatic blistering of the planum sphenoidale.' *J. Neuroradiol.* (In press) (T)

BOOGARD, J. A. (1865). 'Basilar impression: its causes and consequences.' *Ned. Tÿdschr. Geneesk.*, **2**, 81 (G)

BORCK, W. F. and TÖNNIS, W. (1955). 'Zur Differentialdiagnose infratentorieller Geschwütze.' *Fortschr. Neurol. Psychiat.* **23**, 125 (N)

BORNS, P. F. and RANCIER, L. F. (1974). 'Cerebral calcification in childhood. Leukaemia mimicking Sturge-Weber syndrome. Report of two cases.' *Am. J. Roentg.*, **122**, 52–55 (C ; N)

BOWEN, P., LEE, C. S. N., ZELLWEGER, H. and LINDENBERG, R. (1964). 'A familial syndrome of multiple congenital defects.' *Bull. Johns Hopkins Hosp.*, **114**, 412–414 (M)

BOYD, D. A. and MERRELL, P. (1943). 'Calcified subdural haematoma.' *J. nerv. ment. Dis.*, **98**, 609 (C ; T)

BRAILSFORD, J. S. (1953). *The Radiology of Bones and Joints*, 5th ed. London; Churchill (G)

BRAUTE, G. (1952). Gargoylism: a muco-polysaccharidosis.' *Scand. J. clin. Lab. Invest.*, **4**, 43 (D)

BRITTON, H. A., CANBY, J. P. and KOHLER, C. M. (1960). 'Iron deficiency anemia producing evidence of marrow hyperplasia in the calvarium.' *Pediatrics*, **25**, 621–628 (M)

BROMER, R. S. (1933). 'Osteogenesis imperfecta.' *Am. J. Roentg.*, **30**, 631 (D)

BRONNER, H. (1927). 'Die Verkalkung des Corpus pineale im Rötgenbild.' *Fortschr. Röntgenstr.*, **35**, 277 (A)

BROWN, A. and KEMP HARPER, R. (1946). 'Craniofacial dysostosis: the significance of ocular hypertelorism.' *J. Med., (N.S.)* **15**, 171 (D)

BROWN, O. L., LONGACRE, J. J., deSTEFANO, G. A., WOOD, R. W. and KAUL, J. B. (1965). 'Roentgen manifestations of blow-cut fracture of the orbit.' *Radiology*, **85**, 908–913 (T)

BRUCH, G., BUSHE, K. A. and GREGL., A. (1965). 'Die nichtpathologischen intrakraniellen Verkalkungen.' *Fortschr. Geb. RöntgStrahl.*, **103**, 444–449 (C)

BRÜNNER, S. and PEDERSEN, C. B. (1970). 'Roentgen examination of the facial canal.' *Acta Radiol.*, **10**, 545–552 (A)

BRÜNNER, S. and PEDERSEN, C. B. (1971). 'Experimental roentgen examination of the vestibular aqueduct.' *Acta Radiol.*, **11**, 434–448 (A)

BRÜNNER, S., ROVSING, H. and JENSEN, J. (1966). 'Tomographic changes in otosclerosis.' *Acta Radiol.*, **4**, 632–638 (E)

BUCHIGNANI, J. S., COOK, A. L. and ANDERSON, L. G. (1972). 'Roentgenographic findings in familial osteodysplasia.' *Am. J. Roentg.*, **116**, 602–608 (D)

BUCY, P. C. and CAPP, C. S. (1930). 'Primary hemangioma of bone with special reference to roentgenologic diagnosis.' *Am. J. Roentg.*, **23**, 1 (N)

BULL, J. W. D. (1940). 'The radiological diagnosis of chronic subdural haematoma.' *Proc. R. Soc. Med.*, **33**, 203–225 (T)

BULL, J. W. D. (1946). 'Paget's disease of the skull with platybasia.' *Proc. R. Soc. Med.*, **40**, 85–87 (K)

BULL, J. W. D. (1949). 'The diagnosis of chronic subdural haematoma in children and adolescents.' *Br. J. Radiol.*, **22**, 68–80 (T)

BULL, J. W. D. (1953). 'The radiological diagnosis of intracranial tumours in children.' *J. Fac. Radiol.*, **4**, 149–170 (N)

BULL, J. W. D. (1953). 'The radiological differential diagnosis of lesions of the posterior fossa.' *Proc. R. Soc. Med.*, **46**, 729–735 (G)

BULL, J. W. D., NIXON, W. L. B. and PRATT, R. T. C. (1955). 'The radiological criteria and familial occurrence of primary basilar impression.' *Brain*, **78**, 229–247 (D)

BULLOCK, L. J. and REEVES, R. J. (1959). 'Unilateral exophthalmos: roentgenographic aspects.' *Am. J. Roentg.*, **82**, 290–299 (O)

BURROWS, E. H. (1963). 'Bone changes in orbital neurofibromatosis.' *Br. J. Radiol.*, **36**, 549 (O)

BURROWS, E. H. (1964). 'The so-called j-sella.' *Br. J. Radiol.*, **37**, 661 (P)

BURWOOD, R. J., GORDON, I. R. S. and TAFT, R. D. (1973). 'The skull in mongolism.' *Clin. Radiol.*, **24**, 475–480 (D)

BYNUM, G. A. (1952). 'Eosinophilic granuloma of the skull: report of six cases.' *Am. Surg.*, **18**, 793 (N ; K)

CAFFEY, J. (1952). 'Chondro-ectodermal dysplasia (Ellis-van Creveld disease). Report of three cases.' *Am. J. Roentg.*, **68**, 875 (D)

CAFFEY, J. (1952). 'Gargoylism (Hunter–Hurler disease; dysostosis multiplex-lipochondrodystrophy), prenatal and neonatal bone lesions and their early postnatal evolution.' *Am. J. Roentg.*, **67**, 715 (D)

CAFFEY, J. (1956). *Pediatric X-ray Diagnosis*, 3rd ed. Chicago; Year Book Publishers (G)

CAFFEY, J. (1967). 'Congenital stenosis of medullary spaces in tubular bones and calvaria in two proportionate dwarfs – mother and son; coupled with transitory hypocalcemic tetany.' *Am. J. Roentg.*, **100**, 1–11 (D)

CAFFEY, J. (1967). *Pediatric X-ray Diagnosis*, 5th ed., pp 81–89. Chicago; Year Book Publishers (G)

CAMP, J. D. (1924). 'The normal and pathological anatomy of the sella turcica as revealed by roentgenograms.' *Am. J. Roentg.*, **12**, 143 (A ; G)

CAMP, J. D. (1929). 'Roentgenologic manifestations of intracranial disease.' *Radiology*, **13**, 484 (G)

CAMP, J. D. (1930). 'Intracranial calcification and its roentgenologic significance.' *Am. J. Roentg.*, **23**, 615, 628 (C)

CAMP, J. D. (1931). 'Roentgenologic observations in meningiomas of the olfactory groove and meningiomas arising from the tuberculum sellae.' *Proc. Mayo Clin.*, **6**, 221 (N)

CAMP, J. D. (1932). 'Osseous changes in hyperparathyroidism: a roentgenologic study.' *J. Am. med. Ass.*, **99**, 1913 (M)

CAMP, J. D. (1947). 'Symmetrical calcification of the cerebral basal ganglia – its roentgenologic significance in the diagnosis of parathyroid insufficiency.' *Radiology*, **49**, 568 (M ; C)

CAMP, J. D. (1948). 'Pathologic non-neoplastic intracranial calcification.' *J. Am. med. Ass.*, **137**, 1022 (C)

CAMP, J. D. (1949). 'Roentgenologic observations concerning erosion of the sella turcica.' *Radiology*, **53**, 666 (P)

CAMP, J. D. (1950). 'Significance of intracranial calcification in the roentgenologic diagnosis of intracranial neoplasms.' *Radiology*, **55**, 659 (C ; N)

CAMP, J. D. and GIANTURCO, C. A. (1933). 'A simplified technique for roentgenographic examination of the optic canals.' *Am. J. Roentg.*, **29**, 547 (A)

CAMP, J. D. and NASH, L. A. (1944). 'Developmental thinness of the parietal bones.' *Radiology*, **42**; 42 (D)

CAMP, J. S. and OCHSNER, H. C. (1931). 'The osseous changes in hyperparathroidism associated with parathyroid tumour: roentgenologic study.' *Radiology*, **17**, 63 (M)

CAMPBELL, D. (1930). 'Syphillis des Schädeldaches als Ursache von Kopfschmerzen.' *Röntgenpraxis*, **2**, 429 (I)

CAMPBELL, J. A. (1966). 'Roentgen aspects of cranial configurations.' *Radiol. Clin. N. Am.*, **4**, 11–31 (G)

CAPITANIO, M. A. and KIRKPATRICK, J. A. (1969). 'Widening of cranial sutures. A roentgen observation during periods of accelerated growth in patients treated for deprivation dwarfism.' *Radiology*, **92**, 53–59 (M)

CARR, G. L. (1917). 'Roentgen ray findings in the skull in cases of brain tumours.' *Am. J. Roentg.*, **4**, 405 (G)

CARTER, T. L., GABRIELSEN, T. O. and ABELL, M. R. (1968). 'Mechanism of split cranial sutures in metastatic neuroblastoma.' *Radiology*, **91**, 461–475 (M)

CASATI, A. (1926). 'Die senilen Schädelveränderungen im Röntgenbild.' *Fortschr. RöntgStrahl.*, **34**, 335 (G)

CASATI, A. (1954). 'Le alterazioni presenili del cranio nil radiogramma.' *Radiologia med.*, **40**, 872 (G)

CASTELLANO, Fr. and RUGGIERO, G. (1953). 'Meningiomas of the posterior fossa.' *Acta Radiol.*, Suppl. 104, 1 (N)

CASTRO, M. and LEPE, A. (1963). 'Cerebral tuberculosis.' *Acta Radiol.*, **1**: 821 (I)

CAUGHEY, J. E. (1951). 'Bone changes in the skull in dystrophia myotonica.' *J. Bone Jt Surg.*, **34B**, 343 (D)

CAWTHORNE, T. and GRIFFITHS, A. (1961). 'Primary cholesteatoma of the temporal bone.' *Archs Otolar.*, **73**, 252 (E ; N)

CHAMBERLAIN, W. E. (1939). 'Basilar impression (platybasia): a bizarre developmental anomaly on the occipital bone and upper cervical spine with striking and misleading neurologic manifestations.' *Yale J. Biol. Med.*, **11**, 487 (D)

CHAMBERLAIN, W. E., WAYSON, N. E. and GARLAND, L. H. (1931). 'The bone and joint changes of leprosy: a roentgenologic study.' *Radiology*, **17**, 930 (I)

CHASLER, C. N. (1967). 'The newborn skull: the diagnosis of fracture.' *Am. J. Roentg.*, **100**, 92–99 (T)

CHEMKE, J. and ROBINSON, A. (1969). 'The third fontanelle.' *J. Pediat.*, **75**, 617–622 (A)

CHILDE, A. E. (1941). 'Calcification of the choroid plexus and its displacement by expanding intracranial lesions.' *Am. J. Roentg.*, **45**, 523 (C ; N)

CHONG-WAH, A. and MASEL, J. P. (1972). 'Cerebral calcification following pseudomonas meningitis in an infant.' *Australas. Radiol.*, **16**, 56–58 (I ; C)

CHONT, L. K. (1941). 'Osteogenesis imperfecta. Report of 12 cases.' *Am. J. Roentg.*, **45**, 850 (D)

CHOROBSKI, J. and DAVIS, L. (1934). 'Cyst formation of the skull.' *Surg. Gynec. Obstet.*, **58**, 12 (G)

CHOROBSKI, J., JARZYMSKI, J. and FERENS, E. (1939). 'Intracranial solitary chondroma.' *Surg. Gynec. Obstet.*, **68**, 677–686 (N)

CHUANG, V. P. and VINES, F. S. (1973). 'Roentgenology of the posterior superior alveolar foramina and canals.' *Am. J. Roentg.*, **118**, 426–430 (A)

CHYNN, K. Y. (1966). 'Neuroradiologic exploration in intra- and parasellar conditions.' *Radiol. Clin. N. Am.*, **4**, 93–115 (P)

CLARKE, E. (1954). 'Cranial and intracranial myelomas.' *Brain*, **77**, 61 (N)

CLEMENS, F. and SANDSTRÖM, J. (1975). 'Double-barrelled hypoplastic internal auditory canal in unilateral deafness.' *Acta Radiol.*, **16**, 342–346 (D)

COCKAYNE, E. A. (1936). 'Dwarfism with retinal atrophy and deafness.' *Archs Dis. Child.*, **11**, 1–8 (D)

COCKSHOTT, W. P., CLARK, B. M. and MARTINSON, F. D. (1968). 'Upper respiratory infection due to *Entomophthora coronata*.' *Radiology*, **90**, 1016–1019 (I)

COFFIN, G. S., SIRIS, E. and WEGIENKA, L. C. (1966). 'Mental retardation with osteocartilaginous anomalies.' *Am. J. Dis. Child.*, **112**, 205–213 (D)

COHEN, J. (1951). 'Osteoporosis. Case report, autopsy findings and pathological interpretation: failure of treatment with vitamin A.' *J. Bone Jt Surg.*, **33A**, 923 (M)

COHEN, M. E., ROSENTHAL, A. D. and MATSON, D. D. (1976). 'Neurological abnormalities in achondroplastic children.' *J. Pediat.*, **71**, 367–376 (D)

COLE, M. and DAVIES, H. (1964). 'Carotid siphon calcification.' *Br. J. Radiol.*, **35**, 289 (C)

COLEMAN, E. N. and FOOTE, J. B. (1954). 'Craniostenosis with familial vitamin D-resistant rickets.' *Br. med. J.*, **1**, 561 (M ; D)

COLEY, B. L. (1949) (also 2nd ed. 1960). *Neoplasms of Bone and Related Conditions: Etiology Pathogenesis, Diagnosis and Treatment.* New York; Hoeber (G ; N)

COMINGS, D. E., PAPAZIAN, C. and SCHOENE, H. R. (1968). 'Conradi's disease. Chondrodystrophia calcificans congenita, congenital stippled epiphyses.' *J. Pediat.*, **72**, 63–69 (D)

COONEY, J. P. and CROSBY, E. H. (1944). 'Absorptive bone changes in leprosy.' *Radiology*, **42**, 14 (I)

COOPER, R. (1953). 'Acrocephalosyndactyly with report of a case.' *Br. J. Radiol.*, **26**, 533 (D)

CORNELIUS, E. A. and McCLENDON, J. L. (1969). 'Cherubism—hereditary fibrous dysplasia of the jaws. Roentgenographic features.' *Am. J. Roentg.*, **106**, 136–143 (D)

COURVILLE, C. B., MARSH, C. and DEEB, P. (1952). 'Massive deforming meningiomatous hyperostosis. Report of a case long considered to be a cranial osteogenic sarcoma.' *Bull. Los Ang. neurol. Soc.*, **17**, 177 (N)

CRAIG, J. O. (1961). 'Enlargement of the sphenoidal fissure by rhinitis caseosa.' *Br. J. Radiol.*, **37**, 784 (I)

CRAWFORD, T., DENT, C. E., LUCAS, P., MARTIN, N. H. and NASSIM, J. R. (1954). 'Osteosclerosis associated with chronic renal failure.' *Lancet*, **2**, 981 (M)

CRITCHLEY, M. and MEADOWS, S. P. (1933). 'Calcified subdural haematoma.' *Proc. R. Soc. Med.*, **26**, 306 (C ; T)

CRONQVIST, S. (1961). 'Renal osteonephropathy.' *Acta Radiol.*, **55**, 17 (M)

CRONQVIST, S. (1968). 'Roentgenologic evaluation of cranial size in children. A new index.' *Acta Radiol.*, **7**, 97–111 (A)

CRONQVIST, S. and FÜRST, E. (1964). 'Pre- and post-therapeutical radiological changes in chromophobe adenoma of pituitary. A survey in connection with a clinical examination of 121 cases.' *Radiology*, **4**, 182–189 (P)

CROUZON, O. (1912). 'La dysostose cranio-faciale héréditaire.' *Presse méd.*, **20**, 737–739 (D)

CURRARINO, G., NEUHAUSER, E. B. D., REYERBACH, G. C. and SOBEL, E. H. (1957). 'Hypophosphatasia.' *Am. J. Roentg.*, **78**, 392–419 (M)

CUSHING, H. (1922). 'The cranial hyperostoses produced by meningeal endotheliomas.' *Archs Neurol. Psychiat., Chicago*, **8**, 139 (N)

CUSHING, H. and EISENHARDT, L. (1929). 'Meningiomas arising from the tuberculum sellae with the syndrome of primary optic atrophy and bitemporal field defects combined with a normal sella turcica in a middle-aged person.' *Archs Ophthal., Chicago*, **1**, 168 (P ; N)

CUSHING, H. and EISENHARDT, L. (1938). *Meningiomas, their Classification, Regional Behaviour, Life History, and Surgical Results.* Springfield, Ill.; Thomas (N)

CUSMANO, J., BAKER, D. H. and FINBY, N. (1956). 'Pseudohypoparathyroidism.' *Radiology*, **67**, 845 (M)

DAHLHAUS, Kh. (1939). *Über Turmschädel.* Müchen; Diss (D)

DAHLMANN, J. (1951). 'Osteoblastiches Meningeom im Orbitaldach.' *Fortschr. Röntgenstr.*, **74**, 306 (N)

DALE, T. (1934). 'Intracranial calcifications.' *Acta Radiol.*, **15**, 628 (C)

DALY, J. G. (1973). 'Osteoid osteoma of the skull. Case report.' *Br. J. Radiol.*, **46**, 392–393 (N)

DARLING, D. B. and LaCASSE, B. G. (1967). 'A radiographic base line for demonstrating sinuses and facial bones in pediatric radiography.' *Radiology*, **89**, 509–512 (A)

DARLING, D. B., FEINGOLD, M. and BERKMAN, M. (1968). 'The roentgenological aspects of Goldenhar's syndrome (oculoauriculovertebral dysplasia).' *Radiology*, **91**, 254–260 (D)

DAURELLE, G., SMITH, G. F. and REIMER, W. (1958). 'Periventricular calcification and cytomegalic inclusion disease in newborn infants.' *J. Am. med. Ass.*, **167**, 989 (C ; I)

DAVID, M. and STUHL, L. (1933). 'Les meningiomes de la petite aile du sphénoide étude radiologique.' *J. Radiol. Électrol.*, **17**, 193 (N)

DAVIDOFF, L. M. (1936). 'Convolutional digitations seen in the roentgenograms of immature human skulls.' *Bull. Neurol. Inst., N.Y.,* **5,** 61 (A)

DAVIDOFF, L. M. and DYKE, C. G. (1938). 'Relapsing juvenile chronic subdural haematoma: clinical and roentgenographic study.' *Bull. neurol. Inst., N.Y.,* **7,** 95 (T ; D)

DAVIDOFF, L. M. and GASS, H. (1949). 'Convolutional markings in the skull – roentgenograms of patients with headache.' *Am. J. Roentg.,* **61,** 317 (R)

DAVIDSON, K. C. (1966). 'Cranial and intracranial lesions in neurofibromatosis.' *Am. J. Roentg.,* **98,** 550–556 (W ; K)

DAVIS, H. W. (1967). 'Radiological changes associated with Arnold–Chiari malformation.' *Br. J. Radiol.,* **40,** 262–269 (D)

DAVIS, J. G. (1955). 'The osseous radiographic findings of chronic renal insuffiency.' *Radiology,* **60,** 406 (M)

DAVIS, L. (1933). 'Intracranial tumours roentgenographically considered.' *Ann. Roentg.,* **14,** 000 (N)

DAVIS, L. A. and DIAMOND, I. (1957). 'Metastic retino-blastomas as a cause of diffuse intracranial calcification.' *Am. J. Roentg.,* **78,** 437 (M)

DEAK, K. and FRIED, L. (1960). 'Über die einzelnen Formen der endostalen Hyperostosen.' *Radiol. Diag., Berlin,* **1,** 73 (G)

DECKER, K. (1960). *Klinische Neuroradiologie.* Stuttgart; Thieme (G)

DECKER, K. and HIPP, E. (1955). 'Spätveränderungen nach kindlichen Subduralblutungen.' *Fortschr. Röntg.,* **82,** 375 (T ; D)

DeMYER, W. (1967). 'The median cleft face syndrome: Differential diagnosis of cranium bifidum occultum, hypertelorism, and median cleft nose, lip and palate.' *Neurology,* **17,** 961–971 (D)

DENT, C. E. and HODSON, C. J. (1954). 'Generalized softening of bone due to metabolic causes. II: radiological changes associated with certain metabolic bone diseases.' *Br. J. Radiol.,* **27,** 605 (M)

DERRY, E. M. (1929). 'Note on calcification in pituitary adenomas.' *Endocrinology,* **13,** 455 (C ; P)

DESAI, M. G. and PATEL, C. C. (1961). 'Heredo-familial carotid body tumours.' *Clin. Radiol.,* **12,** 214–218 (N)

di CHIRO, G. (1953). 'Cordoma intracranici: studio radiografico.' *Radiologia, Roma,* **9,** 29 (N)

di CHIRO, G. (1960). 'The width (3rd dimension) of the sella turcica.' *Am. J. Roentg.,* **84,** 26 (A)

di CHIRO, G. and LINDGREN, E. (1951). 'Radiographic finding in 14 cases of Sturge–Weber syndrome.' *Acta Radiol.,* **35,** 387 (D)

di CHIRO, G. and LINDGREN, E. (1952). 'Bone changes in cases of suprasellar meningioma.' *Acta Radiol.,* **38,** 133 (N)

di CHIRO, G. and NELSON, K. B. (1962). 'The volume of the sella turcica.' *Am. J. Roentg.,* **87,** 989 (A)

di CHIRO, G., SALDINO, R., McGUFFIN, W. L., SACHSON, R. A., GORDEN, P. and BARTTER, F. C. (1975). 'Pituitary stones.' *Ann. intern. Med.,* **83,** 66–69 (P ; C)

DICKINSON, W. W. (1945). 'Characteristic roentgenographic changes associated with tuberose sclerosis.' *Archs Neurol. Psychiat.,* **53,** 199 (W)

DIETRICH, J. (1959). *Neuro-Röntgendiagnostik des Schädels.* Jena; Fisher (G)

DIXON, H. B. F. and HARGREAVES, W. H. (1944). 'Cysticercosis (*Taenia solium*): a further ten years clinical study covering 284 cases.' *Q. Jl Med.,* **13,** 107 (I)

DODGE, H. W., WOOD, M. W. and KENNEDY, R. L. J. (1959). 'Craniofacial dysostosis: Crouzon's disease.' *Pediatrics,* **23,** 98–106 (D)

DOEL, G. (1963). 'Bone involvement in Weber–Christian disease.' *Br. J. Radiol.,* **36,** 140 (D)

DORFSMAN, J. (1963). 'The radiologic aspects of cerebral cysticercosis.' *Acta Radiol.,* **1,** 836 (I)

DORST, J. P. (1964). 'Functional craniology: an aid in interpreting roentgenograms of the skull.' *Radiol. Clin. N. Am.,* **2,** 347–366 (G)

DRESSLER, W. and ALBRECHT, K. (1949). 'Über endokrane Kalkablagerungen und ihre Darstellung im Röntgenbild.' *Beitr. klin. Chir.,* **178,** 103 (C)

DUBLIN, A. B. and POIRIER, V. C. (1976). 'Fracture of the sella turcica.' *Am. J. Roentg.,* **127,** 969–972 (T ; P)

du BOULAY, G. (1956). 'The significance of digital impressions in children's skulls.' *Acta Radiol.,* **46,** 112 (R)

du BOULAY, G. (1957). 'The radiological evidence of raised intracranial pressure in children.' *Br. J. Radiol.,* **30,** 375 (R)

du BOULAY, G. (1964). 'Radiological examination of two pairs of craniopagus twins.' *Br. med. J.* **1,** 1337 (D)

du BOULAY, G. and BOSTICK, T. (1969). 'Linear tomography in congenital abnormalities of the ear.' *Br. J. Radiol.,* **42,** 161–183 (E)

du BOULAY, G. and EL GAMMAL, T. (1966). 'The classification, clinical value and mechanism of sella turcica changes in raised intracranial pressure.' *Br. J. Radiol.* **39,** 422–442 (G)

du BOULAY, G. and TRICKEY, S. E. (1962). 'Calcification in chromophobe adenoma.' *Br. J. Radiol.,* **35,** 793 (P ; C)

du BOULAY, G. and TRICKEY, S. E. (1967). 'The choice of radiological investigations in the management of tumours around the sella.' *Clin. Radiol.,* **18,** 349–365 (P)

DÜBEN, W. (1949). 'Epidermoide des Schadelknochens und Wirbelkanals und besonderer Berücksichtigung der Röntgenbefunde.' *Fortschr. Röntg.,* **72,** 484

DUGGAN, C. A., KEENER, E. B. and GAY, B. B. (1970). 'Secondary craniosynostosis.' *Am. J. Roentg.,* **109,** 277–293 (R ; D ; M)

DUNN, F. H. (1960). 'Non-familial and non-hereditary craniofacial dysostosis: a varient of Crouzon's disease.' *Am. J. Roentg.,* **84,** 472 (D)

DYKE, C. G. (1930). 'Indirect sign of brain tumour as noted in routine roentgen examinations. Displacement of the pineal shadow (a survey of 3,000 consecutive skull examinations).' *Am. J. Roentg.,* **23,** 598 and 628 (N ; C)

DYKE, C. G. (1941). 'The roentgen-ray diagnosis of diseases of the skull and intracranial contents.' In *Diagnostic Roentgenology,* Vol. 1, Ed. by R. Golden. New York; Nelson (G)

DYKE, C. G. WOLF, A., COWAN, D., PAIGE, B. H. and CAFFEY, J. (1942). 'Toxoplasmic encephalitis VIII: significance of roentgenographic findings in diagnosis of infantile or congenital toxoplasmosis.' *Am. J. Roentg.,* **47,** 830 (I)

EATON, L. M. and HAINES, S. F. (1939). 'Symmetrical cerebral calcification associated with parathyroid insufficiency: preliminary report.' *Proc. Mayo Clin.,* **14,** 48 (M ; C)

EATON, L. M., CAMP, J. D. and LOVE, J. G. (1939). 'Symmetrical cerebral calcification, particularly of the basal ganglia, demonstrable roentgenographically. Calcification of the finer cerebral blood vessels.' *Archs Neurol. Psychiat., Chicago,* **41,** 921 (C)

ECKER, A. (1950). 'Hyperostosing meningioma of pterion: clay model as an aid in surgical excision without bone flap.' *J. Neurosurg.,* **7,** 174 (N)

EINHORN, N. H., MOORE, J. R., OSTRUM, H. W. and ROWNTREE, L. G. (1941). 'Osteochondrodystrophia deformans (Morquio's disease).' *Am. J. Dis. Child.,* **61,** 776 (D)

ELKINGTON, J. St. C. (1932). 'Calcified pineal tumour.' *Proc. R. Soc. Med.,* **25,** 1533 (N ; C)

ELLEGAST, H. (1961). 'Zur Roentgensymptomatologie der Osteomalazie.' *Radio. Austy.,* **11,** 85 (M)

ELLEGAST, H. and JESSERER, H. (1958). 'Der roentgenologische Aspekt der renalen Osteopathie.' *Fortschr. Röntg.,* **89,** 450 (M)

ELLIS, K. and HOCHSTIM, R. J. (1960). 'The skull in hyperparathyroid bone disease.' *Am. J. Roentg.,* **83,** 732 (M)

ELLIS, R. W. B. and van CREVELD, S. A. (1940). 'A syndrome characterized by ectodermal dysplasia, polydactyly, chondrodysplasia and congenital morbus cordis. Report of 3 cases.' *Archs Dis. Child.,* **15,** 65 (D)

ELMORE, S. M. (1967). 'Pycnodysostosis; a review.' *J. Bone Jt Surg.,* **49A,** 153–162 (D)

ELSBERG, C. A. and SCHWARTZ, C. W. (1924). 'Increased cranial vascularity in its relation to intracranial disease. *Archs Neurol. Psychiat., Chicago*, **11**, 293

ENGELS, E. P. (1958). 'The roentgen appearances of the carotid sulcus of the sphenoid bone.' *Acta Radiol.*, **49**, 113 (A)

ENGELS, E. P. (1958). 'Roentgenographic demonstration of a hypophysial subarachnoid space.' *Am. J. Roentg.*, **80**, 1010 (A)

ENGESET, A. (1946). 'On roentgen examination in head trauma.' *Acta Radiol.*, **27**, 481 (T)

ENGESET, A. and TORKILDSEN, A. (1948). 'On changes of the optic canal in cases of intracranial tumour.' *Acta Radiol.*, **29**, 57–64 (N ; O)

EPINEY, J. (1949). 'L'Osteoporose circonscrite du crane.' *Rev. Rhum.*, **16**, 560 (K)

EPPLE, C. and RUCKENSTEINER, E. (1946). 'Die Röntgendiagnose des Clivuschordoms.' *Schweiz. med. Wschr.* **76**, 764 (N)

EPSTEIN, B. S. (1951). 'Shortening of the posterior wall of the sella turcica caused by dilatation of the 3rd ventricle or certain suprasellar tumours.' *Am. J. Roentg.*, **65**, 49 (P ; R)

EPSTEIN, B. S. (1953). 'The concurrence of parietal thinness with postmenopausal, senile, or idiopathic osteoporosis.' *Radiology*, **60**, 29 (M)

EPSTEIN, B. S. and DAVIDOFF, L. M. (1951). 'Advanced atrophy and enlargement of the sella turcica with destruction of the sphenoid.' *Am. J. Roentg.*, **66**, 884 (P)

EPSTEIN, B. S. and DAVIDOFF, L. M. (1953). *An Atlas of Skull Roentgenograms.* London; Kimpton, and Philadelphia; Fiebiger (G)

ERASMIE, U. and RINGERTZ, H. (1976). 'Normal width of cranial sutures in the neonate and infant.' *Acta Radiol.*, **17**, 565–572 (A)

ERDELYI, J. (1928). 'Über die Beschatung des Sinus sphenoidalis bei Hypophysen tumoren.' *Fortschr. Röntg.*, **37**, 674 (P)

ERDELYI, J. (1928). 'Diagnostische Verwertung der mit Hypophysen-geschwülsten-zusammenhängenden Röntgenveränderungen.' *Fortschr. Röntg.*, **38**, 280 (P ; D)

ERDELYI, J. (1930). 'Schädelveränderungen bei gesteigertem Hirndruck.' *Fortschr. Röntg.*, **42**, 153 (R ; P)

ERDELYI, J. (1935). 'Die Röntgendiagnostik der Hypophysengeschwulste.' *Fortschr. Röntg.*, **51**, 125 (N ; P)

EUNG, Ho Kim and YONG, Whee Bahk (1964). 'Intracranial calcification in cerebral paragonimiasis.' *Br. J. Radiol.*, **37**, 670 (I ; C)

EVANS, P. S. (1971). 'Sotos' syndrome (cerebral gigantism) with peripheral dysostosis.' *Archs Dis. Child.*, **46**, 199–202 (D)

FAGET, G. H. and MAYORAL, A. (1944). 'Bone changes in leprosy: a clinical and roentgenologic study of 505 cases.' *Radiology*, **42**, 1 (I)

FAIRBANK, H. A. T. (1949). 'Chondro-osteo-dystrophy: Marquio-Brailsford type.' *J. Bone Jt Surg.*, **31B**, 291 (D)

FAIRBANK, H. A. T. (1951). *An Atlas of General Affections of the Skeleton.* Edinburgh; Livingstone (G)

FAIRMAN, D. and HORRAX, C. (1949). 'Classification of craniostenosis.' *J. Neurosurg.*, **6**, 307 (D)

FALCK, I. (1954). 'Intrazerebrale Verkalkungen nach Brucellosen-Meningozephalitis.' *Fortschr. Röntg.*, **81**, 91 (I ; C)

FALCONER, M. A., BAILEY, I. C. and DUCHE, L. W. (1968). 'Surgical treatment of chordoma and chondroma of the skull base.' *J. Neurosurg.*, **29**, 261–275 (N)

FALK, B, (1951). 'Calcifications in the track of the needle following ventricular puncture.' *Acta Radiol.*, **35**, 304 (C)

FANCONI, G. (1952). 'Chronische Hypercalcämie Kombiniert mit Osteoskleros, Hyperazotämie Minderwuchs und Kongenitalen Missbildungen.' *Helv. paediat. Acta*, **7**, 314 (M)

FARBEROW, B. J. (1924). 'Röntgendiagnostik der Tumoren der Gegen der sella turcica.' *Fortschr. Röntg.*, **50**, 445 (P ; N)

FARRELL, V. J. and HAWKINS, T. D. (1967). 'Glomus jugulare tumours with special reference to the radiological features.' *Br. J. Surg.*, **54**, 789–795 (N)

FASSBENDER, C. W. and HÄUSSLER, G. (1959). 'Über multiple Hämangiome des Schädeldaches.' *Fortschr. Röntg.*, **91**, 137 (N)

FASSBENDER, C. W., HÄUSSLER, G. and STÖSSEL, H. G. (1961). 'Schädelbasis-Chondrome mit intrakraniller Ausdehnung.' *Fortschr. Röntg.*, **94**, 718 (N)

FAURE, C. and GRUSEN, B. (1959). 'L'exploration radiologique des craniopharyngiomes de l'enfant (as propos de 17 observations).' *Ann. Radiol., Paris*, **2**, 197 (N)

FAURE, C., BONAMY, P. and RAMBERT-MISSET, C. (1967). 'Les craniosténoses par fusion prématurée unilatérate de la suture coronale. *Ann. Radiol.*, Paris, **10**, 32–42 (D)

FEINGOLD, M., O'CONNOR, J. F., BERKMAN, M. and DARLING, D. B. (1969). 'Kleeblattschädel syndrome.' *Am. J. Dis. Child.*, **118**, 589–594 (D)

FERNER, H. (1960). 'Die Hypophysenzisterne des Menschen und ihr Beziehungs zum Entstehungsmechanismus der sekundären Sellaerweiterung.' *Z. Anat. Entwickl. Gesch.*, **121**, 407 (P ; R)

FISCHGOLD, H., DAVID, M. and BREGEAT, D. (1952). *La tomographie de la base du crane en neuro-chirurgie et neuroophthalmologie.* Paris; Masson (G ; D)

FISCHGOLD, H., METZGER, J. and JUSTER, M. (1956). 'Radiographic segmentaire du conduit auditif interne dans les neurinomes de la 8ième paire.' *Acta Radiol.*, **46**, 130 (N)

FISHER, C. M., GORE, I., OKABE, N. and WHITE, P. D. (1965). 'Calcification of the carotid siphon.' *Circulation*, **32**, 538–548 (C)

FISHMAN, M. A., HOGAN, G. R. and DODGE, R. R. (1971). 'The concurrence of hydrocephalus and craniosynostosis.' *J. Neurosurg.*, **34**, 621–629 (R)

FITCH, N., PINSKY, L. and LACHANCE, R. C. (1970). 'A form of bird-headed dwarfism with features of premature senility.' *Am. J. Dis. Child.*, **120**, 260–264 (D)

FITZ, C. R., HARWOOD-NASH, D. C. F. and THOMPSON, J. R. (1974). 'Neuroradiology of tuberous sclerosis in children.' *Radiology*, **110**, 635–642 (W)

FOLEY, J. (1951). 'Calcification of the corpus striatum and dentate nuclei occurring in a family.' *J. Neurol., Neurosurg. Psychiat.*, **14**, 253 (C ; D)

FORSYTHE, R. W., BAKER, G. S., DOCKERTY, M. S. and CAMP, J. D. (1947). 'Intracranial osteochondroma.' *Proc. Staff Meet. Mayo Clin.*, **22**, 350–356 (N)

FOSMOE, R. J., HOLM, R. S. and HILDRETH, R. C. (1968). 'Van Buchem's disease (hyperostosis corticalis generalisata familaris).' *Radiology*, **90**, 771–774 (D)

FOURNIER, A. M. and DENIZET, D. (1965). 'La sella Turcique en oméga. *Marseille Med.*, **102**, 260–264 (P)

FRANCESCHINI, P., GRASSI, E. and MARCHESE, G. S. (1971). 'Main radiological signs of the 4P-syndrome.' *Ann. Radiol.*, **14**, 335–340 (D)

FRANCIS, C. C. (1948). 'Growth of the human pituitary fossa.' *Hum. Biol.*, **20**, 1 (A)

FRANCONI, J. (1958). 'A new syndrome: dyscephalia with bird face and dental anomalies, nanism, hypotrichosis, cutaneous atrophy, microphthalmia and congenital cataract.' *Archs Ophthal., N.Y.*, **60**, 842–862 (D)

FRANKEN, E. A. (1969). 'The midline occipital fissure: diagnosis of fracture versus anatomic variants.' *Radiology*, **93**, 1043–1046 (T)

FRANKLIN, E. L. and MATHESON, I. (1942). 'Melorheostosis; report on a case with a review of the literature.' *Br. J. Radiol.*, **15**, 185 (D)

FRASER, D. (1957). 'Hypophosphatasia.' *Am. J. Med.*, **22**, 730–746 (M)

FRAY, W. W. (1936). 'A study of the effect of skull rotation on roentgenological measurements of the pineal gland.' *Radiology*, **27**, 433 (C)

FRAY, W. W. (1939). 'Methods for determining pineal position with analysis of their errors.' *Am. J. Roentg.*, **42**, 490 (C)

FREIMANIS, A. K. (1966). 'Fractures of the facial bones.' *Radiol. Clin. N. Am.*, **4**, 341–363 (T)

FREY, K. W. (1964). 'Die Tomographie zur Diagnostik er Gehörknöchlen.' *Röntgen-Blatter*, **17**, 527 (E)

FREY, K. W. (1965). 'Die Tomographie zur Diagnostik der "kleinen" Ohrmissbildungen.' *Röntgen-Blatter*, **18**, 1 (E)

FREY, K. W. (1965). 'Die Tomographie der Labyrinthmissbildungen.' *Fortschr. Röntg.*, **102**, 1–13 (E)

FRIEDENBERG, R. M. and SAYEGH, V. (1960). 'Advanced skeletal changes in hyperparathyroidism.' *Am. J. Roentg.*, **83**, 753 (M)

FRIES, J. W. (1957). 'The roentgen features of fibrous dysplasia of the skull and facial bones: a critical analysis of thirty-nine pathologically proved cases.' *Am. J. Roentg.*, **77**, 71 (D ; K)

FRY, I. K. and du BOULAY, G. (1965). 'Some observations on the sella in old age and arterial hypertension.' *Br. J. Radiol.*, **38**, 16 (G)

GABRIELE, O. F. (1960). 'Mucormycosis.' *Am. J. Roentg.*, **83**, 227–235 (I)

GASSMAN, W. (1960). 'Senile grubige Atrophie des Schäldedaches.' *Radiol austriaca*, **10**, 177 (A ; G)

GERSHON-COHEN, J., SCHRAER, H. and BLUMBERG, N. (1953). 'Hyperostosis frontalis interna among the aged.' *Am. J. Roentg.*, **73**, 396 (G)

GESCHICKTER, C. F. and COPELAND, M. M. (1949). *Tumours of Bone*, 3rd ed. Philadelphia; Lippinott (N)

GEYLIN, H. R. and PENFIELD, W. (1929). 'Cerebral calcification in epilepsy.' *Archs Neurol. Psychiat., Chicago*, **21**, 1020 (C)

GIFFORD, R. D., GOREE, J. A. and JIMENEZ, J. P. (1971). 'Tumour bulge into the sphenoid sinus. A roentgen sign of parasellar meningioma.' *Am. J. Roentg.*, **112**, 324–328 (N)

GLANCY, J. J. (1967). 'Some radiological aspects of acromegaly.' *Australas. Radiol.*, **11**, 226–233 (M)

GLEESON, J. A., SWANN, J. C., HUGHES, D. T. D. and LEE, F. I. (1967). 'Dystrophia myotonica—a radiological survey.' *Br. J. Radiol.*, **40**, 96–100 (D)

GLEN, J. A., GALINDO, J. and LAWRENCE, C. E. (1960). 'Chronic radium poisoning in a dial painter: case report.' *Am. J. Roentg.*, **83**, 465 (M)

GOALWIN, H. A. (1925). 'The precise roentgenography and measurement of the optic canal.' *Am. J. Roentg.*, **13**, 480 (A ; O)

GOALWIN, H. A. (1927). 'One thousand optic canals: a clinical anatomic and roentgenographic study.' *J. Am. med. Ass.*, **89**, 1745 (A ; O)

GOETSCH, E. (1955). 'Schädelveränderungen bei Neurofibromatose Recklinghausen.' *Fortschr. Röntg.*, **33**, 894 (W ; K)

GOLD, L. H., KIEFFER, S. A. and PETERSON, H. O. (1969). 'Intracranial meningiomas. A retrospective analysis of the diagnostic value of plain skull films.' *Neurology*, **19**, 873–878 (N)

GOLDHAMER, K. and SCHÜLLER' A. (1925). 'Die varietäten der Sella turcica.' *Fortschr. Röntg.*, **33**, 984 (A ; P)

GORDON, I. R. S. (1970). 'Microcephaly and craniostenosis.' *Clin. Radiol.*, **21**, 19–31 (D)

GORDON, M. B. and BELL, A. L. L. (1922). 'A Roentgenographic study of the sella turcica in normal children. *N.Y. Med.*, **22**, 54 (A ; P)

GORDON, M. B. and BELL, A. L. L. (1936). 'Further roentgenographic studies of the sella in abnormal children.' *J. Pediat.*, **9**, 781 (P)

GORLIN, R. J. and PSAUME, J. (1962). 'Orodigitofacial dysostosis – a new syndrome. A study of 22 cases.' *J. Pediat.*, **61**, 520–530 (D)

GORLIN, R. J., KOSZALKA, M. F. and SPRANGER, J. (1970). 'Pyle's disease (familial metaphyseal dysplasia). A presentation of two cases and argument for its separation from craniometaphyseal dysplasia.' *J. Bone Jt Surg.*, **52**, 347–354 (D)

GORLIN, R. J., MESKIN, L. H. and ST. GEME, J. W. (1963). 'Oculodentodigital dysplasia.' *J. Pediat.*, **63**, 69–75 (D)

GORLIN, R. J., JUE, K. L., JACOBSEN, U. and GOLDSCHMIDT, E. (1963). 'Oculo-auriculovertebral dysplasia.' *J. Pediat.*, **63**, 991–999 (D)

GRANTHAM, E. G. and SMOLIK, E. A., (1942). 'Calcified intracerebral haematoma.' *Ann. Surg.*, **115**, 465 (C)

GRASHEY, R. (1935). 'Variationen der Schädeldaches.' *Fortschr. Röntg.*, **52**, 22 (G)

GREIG, D. M. (1924). 'Hypertelorism.' *Edinb. med. J.* **31**, 560 (D)

GREITZER, L. J., JONES, K. L., SCHNALL, B. S. and SMITH, D. W. (1974). Craniosynostosis – radial aplasia syndrome.' *J. Pediat.*, **84**, 723–724 (D)

GRIFFITHS, T. (1957). 'Observations on cranial radiography in a series of intracranial tumours.' *Br. J. Radiol.*, **30**, 57 (N)

GRISCOM, N. T. and OH, K. S. (1970). 'The contracting skull: Inward growth of the inner table as a physiologic response to intracranial contact in children.' *Am. J. Roentg.*, **110**, 106–110 (D)

GROS, C. M. and WACKENHEIM, A. (1964). 'Critique radiologique de l.impression basilaire.' *J. Radiol.*, **45**, 781–788 (D)

GROS, J. (1956). 'Über die grubige Atrophie des Scheitelbeings.' *Fortschr. Röntg.*, **85**, 154 000

GROSS, H. (1956). 'Der Hypertelorismus.' *Ophthalmologica*, **131**, 137–156 (D)

GROSSMAN, C. B. and POTTS, D. G. (1974). 'Arachnoid granulations: radiology and anatomy.' *Radiology*, **113**, 95–100 (D)

GROSSMAN, H., WINCHESTER, P.H., DECK, M. and GUISTRA, P. (1971). 'Brain tumors in children with normal skull roentgenograms.' *Am. J. Roentg.*, **112**, 329–331 (N)

GRUNDY, L., GOREE, J. A. and JIMENEZ, J. P. (1970). 'Oxycephaly in the adult simulating pituitary tumour.' *Am. J. Roentg.*, **108**, 762–766 (D)

HASS, L. (1937). 'Über die Enstehung der Sella vergrösserungen extrasellaren Ursprungs.' *Fortschr. Röntg.*, **55**, 458 (P)

HAHN, E. V. (1928). 'Sinus pericranii (reducible blood tumor of cranium); its relation to hemangioma and abnormal arteriovenous communication: report of case.' *Archs Surg., Chicago*, **16**, 31 (D)

HALLIDAY, J. (1949). 'A rare case of bone dystrophy.' *Br. J. Surg.*, **37**, 52–63 (D)

HANSMAN, C. F. (1966). 'Growth of interorbital distance and skull thickness as observed in roentgenographic measurement.' *Radiology*, **86**, 87–96 (A)

HARBISON, J. B. and NICE, C. M. (1971). 'Familial pachydermoperiostosis presenting as an acromegaly-like syndrome.' *Am. J. Roentg.*, **112**, 532–536 (D)

HARDING, W. G. J. and COURVILLE, C. B. (1934). 'Bone formation with metastases of osteogenic sarcoma: report of a case with metastases to the brain.' *Am. J. Cancer*, **21**, 787 (N)

HARRISON, M. W. (1954). 'Osteomyelitis of the frontal bone.' *J. Laryng.*, **68**, 282 (I)

HARTLEY, J. B. (1943). 'Radiological diagnosis of craniolacuna.' *Br. J. Radiol.*, **16**, 99 (R ; M)

HARTLEY, J. B. and BURNETT, C. W. F. (1944). 'Enquiry into the causation and characteristics of cephalohaematoma.' *Br. J. Radiol.*, **17**, 33 (T)

HARTMANN, E. and GILES, E. (1959). *Roentgenologic diagnosis in Ophthalmology*. Philadelphia; Lippincott (O)

HARWOOD-NASH, D. C. (1970). 'Fractures of the petrous and tympanic parts of the temporal bone in children: a tomographic study of 35 cases.' *Am. J. Roentg.*, **110**, 598–607 (T)

HARWOOD-NASH, D. C. (1970). 'Axial tomography of the optic canals in children.' *Radiology*, **96**, 367–374 (D)

HARWOOD-NASH, D. C. (1972). 'Optic gliomas and pediatric neuroradiology.' *Radiol. Clin. N. Am.*, **10**, 83–100 (O ; N)

HARWOOD-NASH, D. C., HENDRICK, E. B. and HUDSON, A. R. (1971). 'The significance of skull fractures in children. A study of 1,187 patients.' *Radiology*, **101**, 151–156 (T)

HARWOOD-NASH, D. C., REILLY, B. J. and TURNBULL, I. (1970). 'Massive calcification of the brain in a newborn infant.' *Am. J. Roentg.*, **108**, 528–532 (C)

HASTINGS-JAMES, R. (1970). 'Lenticulodentate calcification.' *Radiology*, **101**, 571–576 (C)

HAYMAKER, W., GIRDANY, B. R., STEPHENS, J., LILLIE, R. D. and FETTERMAN, G. H. (1954). 'Cerebral involvement with advanced periventricular calcification in generalized cytomegalic inclusion disease in the newborn: a clinico-pathological report of a case diagnosed during life.' *J. Neuropath. exp. Neurol.*, **13**, 562 (I ; C)

HEMMINGSSON A. and LINDGREN, P. G. (1974). 'The cochlear aqueduct.' *Acta Radiol.*, **15**, 612–618 (A ; E)

HENSCHEN, F. (1911). 'Die Akustikastumoren, eine neue Gruppe radiographisch datstellbarer Hirntumoren.' *Fortschr. Röntg.*, **18**, 207 (N)

HERSCHBERG, A. D. and CREFF, A. (1956). 'Modifications radiologiques de la sella turcique au cours du syndrome hyperhormonal de la menopause et de la castration.' *Sem. Hôp., Paris*, **32**, 499 (M ; P)

HERTZ, H. (1949). 'Haemangioma of the skull.' *Acta med. scand.*, Suppl. 234, 158 (N)

HERTZ, H. and ROSENDAL, Th. (1956). 'Roentgen changes in the cranium in 153 intracranial tumours in children aged 0–15 years.' *Acta Radiol.*, Suppl. 141 (N)

HODES, P. J. and DENNIS, J. M. (1951). 'Cerebello-pontine angle tumors: their roentgenologic manifestations.' *Radiology*, **57**, 395 (N)

HODES, P. J., PENDERGRASS, E. P. and YOUNG, B.R. (1949). 'Eighth nerve tumors.' *Radiology*, **53**, 633 (N)

HODGES, F. J. and JOHNSON, V. C. (1935). 'Reliability of brain tumour localization by roentgen methods.' *Am. J. Roentg.*, **33**, 744 (N)

HOEFNAGEL, D. and BENIRSCHKE, K. (1965). 'Dyscephalia mandibulo-oculo-facialis (Hallerman-Streiff syndrome).' *Archs Dis. Child.*, **40**, 57–61 (D)

HOLDEN, W. S. and WHITEHEAD, A. S. (1951). 'The radiological appearances in congenital toxoplasmosis.' *Br. J. Radiol.*, **24**, 38 (I)

HOLMAN, C. B. (1952). 'Roentgenologic manifestations of vitamin D intoxication.' *Radiology*, **59**, 805 (M)

HOLMAN, C. B. (1959). 'Roentgenologic manifestations of glioma of the optic nerve and chiasm.' *Am. J. Roentg.*, **82**, 462 (O ; N)

HOLMGREN, B. S. (1947). 'Radiographic changes produced by intracranial arteriovenous aneurysms.' *Acta psychiat. scand.*, Suppl. 46, 145 (D)

HOLT, J. F. and WRIGHT, E. M. (1948). 'The radiologic features of neurofibromatosis.' *Radiology*, **51**, 647 (W ; K)

HOPE, J. W., SPITZ, E. B. and SLADE, H. W. (1955). 'The early recognition of premature cranial synostosis.' *Radiology*, **65**, 183 (D)

HORRIGAN, W. D. and BAKER, D. H. (1961). 'Gargoylism: review of the roentgen skull changes with a description of a new finding.' *Am. J. Roentg.*, **86**, 473 (D)

HOUSTON, C. S. (1967). 'Roentgen findings in the XXXXY chromosome anomaly.' *J. Can. Ass. Radiol.*, **18**, 258–267 (D)

HOUSTON, C. S., ZALESKI, W. A. and ZALESKI, L. A. (1974). 'Cranial growth retardation from maternal phenylketonuria.' *Am. J. Roentg.*, **122**, 33–37 (M)

HOWLAND, W. J., PUGH, D. G. and SPRAGUE, R. C. (1958). 'Roentgenologic changes of the skeletal system in Cushing's syndrome.' *Radiology*, **71**, 69 (M)

HÜNERMANN, C. (1933). 'Die diagnostiche Bedeutung der Impressiones digitatae under der Schädelnahtdehiszenzen im Röntgenbilde des kindlichen Schädels.' *Mschr. Kinderheilk*, **58**, 415 (R)

HURWITZ, L. J. and SHEPHERD, W. H. T. (1966). 'Basilar impression and disordered metabolism of bone.' *Brain*, **89**, (Pt. II), 223–234 (M)

LANNACCONE, G. and GERLINI, G. (1974). 'The so-called 'cloverleaf skull syndrome': a report of three cases with a discussion of its relationship with thanatophoric dwarfism and the craniostenoses.' *Pediat. Radiol.*, **2**, 175–183 (D)

IRVINE, E. D. and TAYLOR, F. W. (1936). 'Hereditary and congenital large parietal foramina.' *Br. J. Radiol.*, **9**, 456 (D)

ISAMAT, F., MIRANDA, A. M. and RIPOLL, M. (1968). 'Parajugular foramen chondroma. Case report.' *J. Neurosurg.*, **28**, 490–494 (N)

ISHERWOOD, I. and MAWDSLEY, C. (1963). 'Familial aspects of radiological changes in dystrophia myotonica.' *Acta Radiol.*, **1**, 110 (D)

ISRAEL, H. (1967). 'Loss of bone and remodeling-redistribution in the craniofacial skeleton with age.' *Fed. Proc.*, **26**, 1723–1728 (A)

ISRAEL, H. (1968). 'Continuing growth in the human cranial skeleton.' *Archs oral Biol.*, **13**, 133–138 (A)

ISRAEL, H. (1970). 'Continuing growth in sella turcica with age.' *Am. J. Roentg.*, **108**, 516–527 (A ; P)

JAMES, A. E., ATKINS, L., FEINGOLD, M. and JANOWER, M. L. (1969). 'The Cri du Chat syndrome.' *Radiology*, **92**, 50–52 (D)

JAMES, A. E., BELCOURT, C. L., ATKINS, L. and JANOWER, M. L. (1969). 'Trisomy 18.' *Radiology*, **92**, 37–43 (D)

JAMES, A. E., BELCOURT, C. L., ATKINS, L. and JANOWER, M. L. (1969). 'Trisomy 13–15.' *Radiology*, **92**, 44–49 (D)

JAMES, W. and MOULE, B. (1966). Hypophosphatasia.' *Clin. Radiol.*, **17**, 368–376 (D)

JEFERSON, G. (1936). 'Radiography of the optic canals.' *Proc. R. Soc. Med.*, **29**, 1169 (O ; A)

JENSEN, J. and ROVSING, H. (1968). 'Tomography in congenital malformations of the middle ear.' *Radiology*, **90**, 268–275 (E)

JENSEN, J., ROVSING, H. and BRÜNNER, S. (1966). 'Tomography of the inner ear in otosclerosis.' *Br. J. Radiol.*, **39**, 669–672 (E)

JOHNSON, R. T. and DUTT, P. (1947). 'Dural lacerations over paranasal and petrous air sinuses.' *Br. J. Surg.*, War Suppl. **1**, 141 (T)

JOHNSON, V. C. and HODGES, F. J. (1943). 'Reliability of brain tumour localization by roentgen methods.' *Radiology*, **41**, 117 (N)

JUHL, J. S., WESENBERG, R. L. and GWINN, J. L. (1967). 'Roentgenographic features in Fanconi's anemia.' *Radiology*, **89**, 646–653 (M)

JUPE, M. (1938). 'The reaction of the bones of the skull to intracranial lesions.' *Br. J. Radiol.*, **11**, 146 (G)

KADRUKA, S. and MERDGO, A. (1938). 'Apropos des manifestations osseous de la lepre.' *Radiol. Rdsch.*, **7**, 269 (I)

KAHN, E. A. and LUROS, J. T. (1952). 'Hydrocephalus from overproduction of cerebrospinal fluid (and experiences with other papillomas of the choroid plexus).' *J. Neurosurg.*, **9**, 59–67 (R ; N)

KALAN, C. and BURROWS, E. H. (1962). 'Calcification in intracranial gliomata.' *Br. J. Radiol.*, **35**, 589 (C ; N)

KASABACH, H. H. and DYKE, C. G. (1932). 'Osteoporosis circumscripta of the skull as a form of osteitis deformans.' *Am. J. Roentg.*, **28**, 192 (K)

KASEFF, L. G. (1969). 'Tomographic evaluation of trauma to the temporal bone.' *Radiology*, **93**, 321–327 (T)

KATTAN, K. R. (1970). 'Calvarial thickening after Dilantin medication.' *Am. J. Radiol.*, **110**, 102–105 (M)

KAUFMAN, B. (1968). 'The 'empty' sella turcica – a manifestation of the intrasellar subarachnoid space.' *Radiology*, **90**, 931–941 (P)

KAUFMAN, B., SANDSTROM, P. H. and YOUNG, H. F. (1970). 'Alteration in size and configuration of the sella turcica as the result of prolonged cerebrospinal fluid shunting.' *Radiology*, **97**, 537–542 (R ; P)

KEATS, T. E. (1966). 'Diffuse thickening of calvarium in osteogenesis imperfecta: further observations.' *Radiology*, **86**, 97–99 (D)

KEATS, T. E. (1970). 'Ocular hypertelorism (Greig's syndrome) associated with Sprengel's deformity.' *Am. J. Roentg.*, **110**, 102–105 (D)

KEATS, T. E. and SMITH, T. H. (1972). 'Excessive development of the frontal bone and frontal sinuses secondary to overlying soft tissue angioma.' *Am. J. Roentg.*, **115**, 592–594 (D)

KEATS, T. E., RIDDERVOLD, H. O. and MICHAELIS, L. L. (1970). 'Thanatophoric dwarfism.' *Am. J. Roentg.,* **108,** 573–480 (D)

KEATS, T. E., SMITH, T. H. and SWEET, D. E. (1975). 'Craniofacial dysostosis with fibrous metaphyseal defects.' *Am. J. Roentg.,* **124,** 271–275 (D)

KIEFFER, S. A. and GOLD, L. H. A. (1974). 'Intracranial physiologic calcifications.' *Semin. Roentg.,* **9,** 151–162 (C)

KIENBÖCK, R. and ROESLER, H. (1932). 'Neurofibromatose.' *Fortschr. Röntgenstr.,* **42,**   (W ; K)

KIER, E. L. (1966). 'Embryology of the normal optic canal and its anomalies. An anatomic and roentgenographic study.' *Invest. Radiol.,* **1,** 346–362 (A ; O)

KIER, E. L. (1967). ' "J" and "omega" shape of sella turcica.' *Acta Radiol.,* **9,** 91–94 (P)

KING, A. B. and GOULD, D. M. (1952). 'Symmetrical calcification in the cerebellum. A report of two cases.' *Am. J. Roentg.,* **67,** 562 (C)

KING, L. S. and BUTCHER, J. (1944). 'Osteochondroma of base of skull.' *Archs Path.,* **37,** 282–285 (N)

KISTLER, M. and PRIBRAM, H. W. (1975). 'Metastatic disease of the sella turcica.' *Am. J. Roentg.,* **123,** 13–21 (P ; N)

KLAUS, E. and FISHER, Z. (1960). 'Haemangioma des knochernen Schädels.' *Radiol. Diag., Berlin,* **1,** 435 (N)

KÖHLER, A. and ZIMMER, E. A. (1953). 'Grenzen des Normalen und Anfänge des Pathologischen.' im *Röntgenbilde des Skelets.* 9 Aufl. Stuttgart; Thieme (G)

KÖHLER, B. (1939). 'dysostosis cleido-cranialis beim Neugeborenen.' *Z. Kinderheilk,* **6,** 536 (D)

KOLODNY, A. (1929). 'Schädelveränderungen beim Meningeom, dem duralen Endotheliom.' *Fortschr. Röntgenstr.,* **40,** 343 (N)

KOPYLOV, M. B. (1936). 'Roentgen signs in hydrocephalus and their diagnostic value.' *Am. J. Roentg.,* **56,** 569 (R)

KORNBLUM, K. (1932). 'Alterations in the structure of the sella turcica as revealed by the roentgen ray.' *Archs Neurol. Psychiat., Chicago,* **27,** 305 (P)

KORNBLUM, K. (1934). 'Deformation of the sella turcica in tumors of the middle cranial fossa.' *Am. J. Roentg.,* **31,** 23 (P ; N)

KORNBLUM, K. and OSMUND, L. H. (1935). 'Deformation of the sella turcica by tumors in the pituitary fossa.' *Ann. Surg.,* **101,** 201 (P ; N)

KORNBLUM, K. and OSMUND, L. H. (1935). 'Effects of intracranial tumours on the sella turcica; an analysis of 446 cases of verified intracranial tumors.' *Archs Neurol. Psychiat., Chicago,* **34,** 111 (P ; N)

KOSOWICZ, J. and RZMISKI, K. (1975). 'Radiological features of the skull in Klinefelter's syndrome and male hypogonadism.' *Clin. Radiol.,* **26,** 371–378 (M ; D)

KRAUS, B. S. and DECKER, J. D. (1960). 'The prenatal interrelationships of the maxilla and premaxilla in the facial development of man.' *Acta anat., Basel,* **40,** 278 (A)

KRAYENBÜHL, H. (1937). 'Hilfsmethoden der Diagnostik raumsbeschrankender intrakranieller Erkrankungen.' *Schweiz. med. Wschr.,* **67,** 89 (N)

KRUSE, R. (1968). 'Osteopathien bei antiepileptischer Langzeittherapie (Vorläufige Mitteilung).' *Mschr. Kinderheilk,* **116,** 378–381 (M)

KRUYFF, E. (1965). 'Occipital dysplasia in infancy.' *Radiology,* **85,** 501–507 (D)

KRUYFF, E. (1967). 'Transverse cleft in the basi-occiput.' *Acta Radiol.,* **6,** 41–48 (D)

KRUYFF, E. and JEFFS, R. (1966). 'Skull abnormalities associated with the Arnold–Chiari malformations.' *Acta Radiol.,* **5,** Pt I, 9–24 (D)

KURLANDER, C. J., DeMYER, W. and CAMPBELL, J. A. (1967). 'Roentgenology of the median cleft face syndrome.' *Radiology,* **88,** 473–478 and 483 (D)

KURLANDER, G. J., DeMEYER, W., CAMPBELL, J. A. and TAYBI, H. (1966). 'Roentgenology of holoprosencephaly (arrhinencephaly).' *Acta Radiol.,* **5,** Pt. I, 25–40 (D)

LABRUNE, M., LEFEBVRE, J., LAFOURCADE, J. and LEJEUNE, J. (1967). 'Ètude des signes radiologiques de la maladie du cri du chat.' *Annls radiol.,* **10,** 303–310 (D)

LACEY, S. H., EYRING, E. J. and SHAFFER, T. E. (1970). 'Pycnodysostosis: a case report of a child with associated trisomy X.' *J. Pediat.,* **77,** 1033–1038 (D)

LAGOS, J. C., HOLMAN, C. B. and GOMEZ, M. R. (1968). 'Tuberous sclerosis: neuro-roentgenological observations.' *Am. J. Roentg.,* **104,** 171–176 (W)

LAGUNDOYE, S. B., MARTINSON, F. D. and FAJEMISIN, A. A. (1975). 'Tomography of the petrous bones in keratosis obturans.' *Br. J. Radiol.,* **48,** 170–175 (E)

LAITINEN, L. (1951). 'Craniosynostosis – premature fusion of the cranial sutures.' *Ann. Paediat. Fenn.* **2,** Suppl. 6, 1 (D ; M)

LAND, V. J. and NOGRADY, M. B. (1969). 'Cockayne's syndrome.' *J. Can. Ass Radiol.,* **20,** 194–203 (D)

LANG, E. K. and BESSLER, W. T. (1961). 'The roentgenologic features of acromegaly.' *Am. J. Roentg.,* **86,** 321 (M)

LANGER, L. O. (1967). 'The roentgenographic features of the oto-palato-digital (OPD) syndrome.' *Am. J. Roentg.,* **100,** 63–70 (D)

LANGER, L. O., BAUMAN, P. A. and GORLIN, R. J. (1968). 'Achondroplasia.' *Am. J. Roentg.,* **100,** 12–26 (D)

LANGER, L. O., BAUMAN, P. A. and GORLIN, R. J. (1968) 'Achondroplasia: clinical radiologic features with comment on genetic implications.' *Clin. Pediat.,* **7,** 474–485 (D)

LANGER, L. O., PETERSEN, D. and SPRANGER, J. (1970). 'An unusual bone dysplasia: parastremmatic dwarfism.' *Am. J. Roentg.,* **110,** 550–560 (D)

LANGER, L. O., SPRANGER, J. W., GREINACHER, I. and HERDMAN, R. C. (1969). 'Thanatophoric dwarfism.' *Radiology,* **92,** 285–294 and 303 (D)

LANGFELT, B. (1963). 'Tomography of the middle ear in sound transmission disturbances.' *Acta Radiol.,* **1,** 133 (E)

LANZKOWSKY, P. (1968). 'Radiological features of iron-deficiency anemia.' *Am. J. Dis. Child.,* **116,** 16–29 (M)

LARSEN, L. J., SCHOTTSTAEDT, E. R. and BOST, F. C. (1950). 'Multiple congenital dislocations associated with characteristic facial abnormality.' *J. Pediat.,* **37,** 574–581 (D)

LAWRENCE, D. A., NOGRADY, M. B. and CLOUTIER, A. M. (1970). 'Cherubism, a case report.' *Am. J. Roentg.,* **108,** 468–472 (M)

LEE, F. A. and KENNY, F. M. (1967). 'Skeletal changes in the Cornelia de Lange syndrome.' *Am. J. Roentg.,* **100,** 27–39 (D)

LEE, K. F., HODES, P. J., GREENBERG, L. and SINOTTI, A. (1968). 'Three rare causes of unilateral exophthalmos.' *Am. J. Dis. Child.,* **116,** 16–29 (O)

LEE, K. F., LIN, S–R. and HODES, P. J. (1972). 'New roentgenologic findings in myotonic dystrophy.' *Am. J. Roentg.,* **115,** 179–185 (D)

LEE, W. M. and ADAMS, J. E. (1968). 'The empty sella syndrome.' *J. Neurosurg.,* **28,** 351–356 (P)

LEEDS, N. and SEAMAN, W. B. (1962). 'Fibrous dysplasia of skull and its differential diagnosis: a clinical and roentgenographic study of 46 cases.' *Radiology,* **78,** 570 (D ; K)

LEGER, L. and WITZIG, E. (1950). 'Essai de classification et de diagnostic des lacunes craniennes.' *Helv. chir. Acta,* **17,** 109 (G)

LEHMANN, W. and KIRCHHOFF, H. W. (1954). 'Die Bedeutung der Schädeldiagnostik dür die Beurteilung Kindlicher Wuchsund Reifestörungen.' *Homo,* **5,** 93 (M)

LEHRER, H. Z. and FAMILANT, J. W. (1969). 'A concordant craniofacial dysostosis with enlarged parietal foramina in twins.' *Radiology,* **92,** 127–129 and 114 (D)

LEIGHT, T. F., FINCHER, E. F. and HALL, M. F. (1956). 'Evaluation of routine skull films in intracranial meningiomas.' *Radiology,* **66,** 509 (N)

LEROY, J. G. and CROCKER, A. C. (1966). 'Clinical definition of the Hurler–Hunter phenotypes. A review of 50 patients.' *Am. J. Dis. Child.,* **112,** 518–530 (D)

LEUPOLD, E. and MAYER, E. G. (1933). 'Verknöcherung der Falx cerebri.' *Röntgenpraxis*, **5**, 309 and 476 (C)

LEVIN, E. J. (1956). 'Congenital biliary atresia with emphasis on the skeletal abnormalities.' *Radiology*, **67**, 714 (K)

LEVINSON, A. and HARTENSTEIN, H. (1951). 'Intracranial calcification following pneumococcal meningitis.' *J. Pediat.*, **38**, 624 (C ; I)

LICHENSTEIN, L. and JAFFE, H. L. (1942). 'Fibrous dysplasia of bone: a condition affecting one, several or many bones the graver cases of which may present abnormal pigmentation of skin, premature sexual development, hyperthyroidism, or still other extra-skeletal abnormalities.' *Arch. Path.*, **33**, 777 (D)

LIEVRE, J. A., FISCHGOLD, H., CLEMENT, J. C. and ECOIFFER, J. (1952). 'Opacification des cavites diploiques du crane dans le maladie de Paget.' *Bull. Mém. Soc. Méd., Paris*, **68**, 306 (K)

LIGHTWOOD, R. (1955). 'Discussion about eosinophilic granuloma. Letterer–Siwe disease, Hand–Schüller–Christian disease.' *Proc. R. Soc. Med.*, **48**, 711 (K ; M)

LILJA, B. (1934). 'On the localization of calcified pineal bodies under normal and pathological conditions.' *Acta Radiol.*, **15**, 659 (C)

LILJA, B. (1939). 'Displacement of the calcified pineal body in roentgen pictures as an aid in diagnosing intracranial tumours.' *Acta Radiol.*, Suppl. 37 (C)

LILJA, B. (1948). 'The tentorial pressure cone, its significance and its diagnosis through dislocation of the calcified pineal body.' *Acta Radiol.*, **30**, 129 (C)

LILIEQUIST, B. (1966). 'Tomography with the mimer in otosclerosis of the temporal bone.' *Acta Radiol.*, **4**, 639–644 (E)

LILIEQUIST, B. (1968). 'Roentgenologic changes in otosclerosis.' *Acta Radiol.*, **7**, 129–139 (E)

LIM, G. H. K. (1975). 'Clivus chordoma with unusual bone sclerosis and brainstem invasion: A case report with review of the radiology of cranial chordomas.' *Australas. Radiol.*, **19**, 242–250 (N)

LIN, S–R., LEVY, W., GO, E. B., LEE, I. and WONG, W. K. (1973). 'Unusual osteosclerotic changes in sarcoidosis, simulating osteoblastic metastases.' *Radiology*, **106**, 311–312 (I)

LINDBLOM, K. (1936). 'A roentgenographic study of the vascular channels of the skull.' *Acta Radiol.*, Suppl. 30 (A)

LINDGREN, E. (1939). 'Über corticale Verkalkungen im Gehirn.' *Nervenarzt.*, **12**, 138 (C)

LINDGREN, E. (1941). 'Roentgenological views on basilar impression.' *Acta Radiol.*, **22**, 297 (D)

LINGREN, E. (1942). 'Zur Röentgendiagnose Subduralhämatoms.' *Acta Radiol.*, **23**, 268 (T)

LINDGREN, E. and di CHIRO, G. (1951). 'Suprasellar tumours with calcification.' *Acta Radiol.*, **36**, 173 (P ; C)

LINDGREN, E., OLIVECRONA, H. and TONNIS, W. (1954). 'Handbuch der Neurochirurgie.' Bd. II *Roentgenologie: einschilliesslich Kontraztmethoden*. Berlin; Springer (G)

LIST, C. F., HOLT, Y. G. and EVERETT, M. (1946). 'Lipoma of the corpus callosum: a clinico-pathologic study.' *Am. J. Roentg.*, **55**, 125 (N)

LLOYD, G. A. S. (1966). 'Orbital emphysema.' *Br. J. Radiol.*, **39**, 933–938 (O)

LLOYD, G. A. S., (1973). 'Radiographic measurement in the diagnosis of orbital space-occupying lesions.' *Trans. Ophthal. Soc. U.K.*, **93**, 301–310 (O)

LOEPP, W. (1937). 'Der Wert der einfachen Kraniographic für die Erkenning endokranieller Druckstelgerungen.' *Arch. Psychiat. Nervenkr.*, **106**, 410 (R)

LOEPP, W. and LORENZ, R. (1954). *Röntgendiagnostik der Schädels*. Stuttgart; Thieme

LOESCHCKE, H. and WEINNOLDT, H. (1922). 'Über den Einflus von Struck und Eutspannung auf das Knockenwachstrum des Hirnschädels.' *Beitr. path. Anat.* **70**, 406 (A)

LOFSTROM, J. E. (1966). 'Injuries of the cranial vault and brain.' *Radiol. Clin. N. Am.*, **4**, 323–340 (T)

LOMBARDI, G. (1956). 'L'ematoma subdurale calcificato.' *Nunt. radiol., Roma*, **22**, 727 (T ; C)

LOMBARDI, G. (1961). 'The occipital vertebra.' *Am. J. Roentg.*, **86**, 260 (D)

LOMBARDI, G. (1961). 'Les Malformations osseuses de la charnière occipito-cervicale et leurs retentissements neurologiques.' Proc. V. Congres des Medecine R. et E. de Culture latine. Paris, July (D)

LOMBARDI, G. (1967). *Radiology in Neuro-Ophthalmology*, pp 111–147 and 207–230. Baltimore; Williams and Wilkins (O)

LOMBARDI, G., PASSERINI, A. and CECCHINI, A. (1968). 'Pneumosinus dilatans.' *Acta Radiol.*, **7**, 535–542 (S)

LOOP, J. W. and FOLTZ, E. L. (1972). 'Craniostenosis and diploic lamination following operation for hydrocephalus.' *Acta Radiol.*, **13**, 8–13 (R)

LORBER, J. (1958). 'Intracranial calcifications following tuberculous meningitis in children.' *Acta Radiol.*, **50**, 204 (I)

LORENZ, R. (1949/50). 'Das Verhalten der Sella Turcica bei Pathologischen endokraniellen Prozessen.' *Fortschr. Röntgenstr.*, **72**, 10 (P)

LOVE, J. G. and MARSHALL, T. M. (1949). 'Craniopharyngioma (intracranial adamantinomas).' IV International Congr. Neurol. Vol. 2, Communications, p. 138. Paris; Masson (P ; N)

LÖW-BEER, A. (1931). 'Über die in Röntgenbild sichtbaren Tumoren der Sellagegand.' *Endokrinologie*, **9**, 268 (P ; N)

LÖW-BEER, A. (1932). 'Intrakranielle Verkalkungen in Röntgenbilde.' *Fortschr. Röntgenstr.*, **45**, 420 (C)

LOWMAN, R. M., ROBINSON, F. and McALLISTER, W. B. (1966). 'The craniopharyngeal canal.' *Acta Radiol.*, **5**, Pt. I, 41–54 (A)

LUCK, J. V. (1950). *Bone and Joint Diseases*, 1st ed., p. 468. Springfield, Ill. Thomas (G)

LÜDIN, M. (1935). 'Veränderungen der Sella Turcica bei sellafernen intracraniellen Tumoren.' *Acta Radiol.*, **16**, 48 (P ; N)

LYSHOLM, E. (1931). 'Apparatus and technique for roentgen examination of the skull.' *Acta Radiol.*, Suppl. 12, 1 (G)

LYSHOLM, E. (1934). 'About axial projections of the cranial vertex.' *Acta Radiol.*, **15**, 683 (G)

LYSHOLM, E. (1951). 'Röntgenologische Diagnostik in der Chirurgie der Gehirnkrankheiten.' In *Neue deutsche Chirurgie*, 50 (bd. 3). Stuttgart; Ferdinand (G)

LYSHOLM, E. and OLIVECRONA, H. (1932). 'On changes of optic canals in cases of intracranial tumour.' *Acta chir. scand.*, **72**, 197–209 (O)

MACAULEY, D. (1951). 'Digital markings in the radiographs of the skull in children.' *Br. J. Radiol.*, **24**, 647 (R)

MACPHERSON, R. I., (1974). 'Craniodiaphyseal dysplasia, a disease or group of diseases?' *J. Can. Ass. Radiol.*, **25**, 22–23 (D)

MACPHERSON, R. I. and DUNBAR, J. S. (1965). 'The radiology of mastoid disease in infants and children.' *J. Can. Ass. Radiol.*, **2**, 35 (E)

MAHMOUD, M.El-S. (1958). 'The sella in health and disease: the value of radiographic study of the sella turcica in the morbid anatomical and topographic diagnosis of intracranial tumours.' *Br. J. Radiol.*, Suppl. 8, 1-100 (P)

MALONEY, A. F. J. (1954). 'Two cases of congenital atresia of the foramina of Magendie and Luschka.' *J. Neurol., Neurosurg. Psychiat.*, **17**, 134 (N)

MAROTEAUX, P. and LAMY, M. (1962). 'La pycnodysostose.' *Présse med.*, **70**, 999-1002 (D)

MAROTEAUX, P. and LAMY, M. (1962). 'Deux observations d'une affection osseuse condensante la pycnodysostose.' *Arch. franc. pediat.*, **19**, 267–274 (D)

MAROTEAUX, P. and LAMY, M. (1965). 'The malady of Toulouse-Lautrec.' *J. Am. med. Ass.*, **191**, 715–7171 (D)

MAROTEAUX, P. and LAMY, M. (1968). 'Le diagnostic des nanismes chondrodystrophiques chez les nouveau-nes.' *Arch. franc. pediat.*, **25**, 241–262 (D)

MAROTEAUX, P., LAMY, M. and ROBERT, J. M. (1967). 'Le nanisme thanatophore.' *Présse med.*, **75**, 2519–2524 (D)

MARSHALL, R. E. and SMITH, D. W. (1970). 'Frontodigital syndrome: a dominantly inherited disorder with normal intelligence.' *J. Pediat.*, 77, 129–133 (D)

MARTIN, J. P. (1937). 'Calcified intracranial tuberculomata.' *Br. J. Radiol.*, 10, 5 (I; C)

MARTINEZ-FARINAS, L. O. (1967). 'The sellar-cranial index.' *Radiology*, 88, 264–267 and 286 (P)

MASCHERPA, F. and VALENTINO, V. (1959). *Intracranial Calcification*. Springfield, Ill.; Thomas (C)

MASON, R. C. and KOZLOWSKI, K. (1973). 'Chondrodysplasia punctata.' *Radiology*, 109, 245–250 (D)

MASSLER, M. and SCHOUR, I. (1951). 'The growth pattern of the cranial vault in the albino rat as measured by vital staining with alizarine red "S".' *Anat. Rec.*, 110, 83 (A)

MASSON, C. B. (1930). 'The occurrence of calcification in gliomas.' *Bull. neurol. Inst., N.Y.*, 1, 31 (C; N)

MAY, E., DEBRAY, C., GAUTHIER-VILLARS, P. and GUJAR (1942). 'Kyste épidermoid du crâne simulant une maladie de Schüller-Christian.' *Bull. Soc. méd. Hôp., Paris*, 58, 279 (N)

MAYER, E. G. (1930). *Otologische Röntgendiagnostik*. Ed. by G. Holzknecht. Berlin; Springer (E)

MAYER, E. G. (1932). 'Über die röntgenologische Diagnose der Hypophysen-tumoren.' *Fortschr. R¼*

MAYER, E. G. (1932). 'Über die röntgenologische Diagnose der Hypophysen-tumoren.' *Fortschr. Röntgenstr.*, 46, 497 (P; N)

MAYER, E. G. (1932). 'Die Röntgendiagnose den Erkrankanger der Schädelbasis.' *Wien. med. Wschr.*, 1932b, 1510 (G)

MAYER, E. G. (1935). 'Richtlinien für die Röntgenuntersuchung des Schädels bei endokraniellen Affektionen.' *Röntgenpraxis*, 7, 223 (G)

MAYER, E. G. (1939). 'Die ersten Kennzeichen endokranieller Erkrankungen Röntgenbilde ohne Kontrastimitalwendung.' *Radiol. clin., Basel*, 8, 41 (G)

MAYER, E. G. (1950). 'Über "Sella Diagnostik".' *Radiol. Aust.*, 3, 77 (P)

MAYER, E. G. (1954). 'Über den Gesamteindruck des Röntgenbildes des Schädels.' *Radiol. Aust.*, 8, 57 (G)

MAYER, E. G. (1955). 'Der diagnostische Wert des einfachen Röntgenbildes des Schädels.' *Acta neurochir., Wien*, Suppl. 3, 41 (G)

MAYER, E. G. (1955). 'Über Röntgenbefunde bei Kopfschmerz.' *Wien. med. Wschr.*, 105, ii, 925 (G)

MAYER, E. G. (1955). 'Die Zeichen endokranieller Drucksteigerung im nativen Röntgenbild.' *Woen. Z. Nervenheilk*, 10, 378 (R)

MAYER, E. G. (1959). *Diagnose und Differentialdiagnose in der Schädelronntgenologie*. Berlin; Springer (G)

McAFEE, J. G. (1958). 'The roentgen signs of systemic disease in the skull.' *Am. J. med. Sci.*, 236, 634 (G)

McGREGOR, M. (1948). 'The significance of certain measurements of the skull in diagnosis of basilar impression.' *Br. J. Radiol.*, 21, 171 (A)

McKENZIE, K. G. and SOSMAN, M. C. (1924). 'The Roentgenological diagnosis of craniopharyngeal pouch tumours.' *Am. J. Roentg.*, 11, 171 (N)

McKUSIK, U. A. (1909). 'The nosology of the mucopolysaccharidoses.' *Am. J. Med.*, 47, 730–747 (D)

McLACHLAN, M. F., WRIGHT, A. D. and DOYLE, F. H. (1970). 'Plain film and tomographic assessment of the pituitary fossa in 140 acromegalic patients.' *Br. J. Radiol.*, 43, 360–369 (P; M)

McRAE, D. L. (1953). 'Bony abnormalities in the region of the foramen magnum: correlation of the anatomic and neurologic findings.' *Acta Radiol.*, 40, 335 (D)

McRAE, D. L. (1966). 'Observations on craniolacuna.' *Acta Radiol.*, 5, (Pt. I). 55–64 (R; M)

McRAE, D. L. and ELLIOTT, A. W. (1958). 'Radiological aspects of cerebellar astrocytomas and medulloblastomas.' *Acta Radiol.*, 50, 52 (N)

MEADOR, C. K. and WORRELL, J. L. (1966). 'The sella turcica in postpartum pituitary necrosis (Sheehan's syndrome).' *Ann. intern. Med.*, 65, 259–264 (P)

MEDILL, E. V. (1951). 'Bilateral symmetrical calcification of the basal ganglia associated with parathyroid insufficiency.' *Br. J. Radiol.*, 24, 685 (M; C)

MEINARDUS, K. (1958). 'Über Schädelveränderungen bei der Neurofibromatosis Recklinghausen.' *Radiol. clin., Basel*, 27, 357 (P; K; W)

MELHEM, R., DORST, J. P., SCOTT, C. I. and McKusick, V. A. (1973). 'Roentgen findings in mucolipidoses III (pseudo-Hurler polydystrophy).' *Radiology*, 106, 153–160 (D)

MELLINGER, W. J. (1940). 'The venous circulation as a factor in osteomyelitis of the skull.' *Ann. Otol. St. Louis*, 49, 438 (I)

MENG, C. M. and Wu, Y-K. (1942). 'Tuberculosis of flat bones of vault of skull. Study of 40 cases.' *J. Bone Jt Surg.*, 24, 341–353 (I)

MENNE, F. R. and FRANK, W. W. (1937). 'So-called primary chondroma of ethmoid.' *Archs Otolaryng.*, 26, 170–178 (S; N)

MEREDITH, H. V. (1953). 'Growth in head width during the first twelve years of life.' *Pediatrics*, 12, 411 (A)

MEREDITH, J. M. and SAHYOUN, P. F. (1951). 'Ependymoblastoma grossly eroding and involving overlying dura and skull.' *J. Neurosurg.*, 8, 214 (N)

MESCHAN, I. (1974). 'The normal adult cranial vault.' *Sem. Roentg.*, 9, 125–136 (A)

METZGER, J. (1951). 'Description et Classification des calcifications intracraniennes chez l'enfant.' *These, Paris* (C)

MIDDLEMISS, I. B. D. (1959). 'Bone changes in adult cretins.' *Br. J. Radiol.*, 32, 685 (M)

MIFKA, P. and SWOBODA, W. (1951). 'Zur Röntgendiagnostik der Toxoplasmose.' *Ost. Z. Kinderheilk*, 6, 78 (I)

MILLER, F. (1953). 'Die Knochenveranderungen bei der Neurofibromatosis Recklinghausen.' *Fortschr. Röntgenstr.*, 78, 669 (K; W)

MILLS, J. and FOULKES, J. (1967). 'Gorlin's syndrome. A radiological and cytogenetic study of nine cases.' *Br. J. Radiol.*, 40, 366–371 (D)

MINAGI, H. and STEINBACH, H. L. (1968). 'Röntgen aspects of pituitary tumours manifested after bilateral adrenalectomy for Cushing's syndrome.' *Radiology*, 90, 276–280 (P; N)

MOEHLIG, R. C. (1949). 'Arachnodactyly (Marfan's syndrome): 2 cases reported with etiological implication.' *Am. J. Roentg.*, 61, 797 (D)

MOLLER, P. F. (1939). 'Chronic fluorine poisoning, seen from roentgenological standpoint.' *Br. J. Radiol.*, 12, 20 (M)

MOLLER, P. F. and GUDJONSSON, K. V. (1932). 'Massive fluorosis of bones and ligaments.' *Acta Radiol.*, 13, 269 (M)

MOLLOY, P. and LOWMAN, R. M. (1965). 'The lack of specificity of neonatal intracranial paraventricular calcification.' *Radiology*, 80, 98–102 (C)

MOMOSE, K. J. (1971). 'Developmental approach in the analysis of roentgenograms of the pediatric skull.' *Radiol. Clin. N. Am.*, 9, 99–116 (D)

MOODY, D. M., GHATAK, N. R. and KELLY, D. C. (1976). 'Extensive calcification in a tumour of the glomus jugulare.' *Neuroradiology*, 12, 131–136 (C; N)

MOORE, S. (1936). 'Metabolic craniopathy.' *Am. J. Roentg.*, 35, 30 (M)

MOORE, S. (1952). 'Acromegaly and contrasting conditions. Notes on roentgenology of the skull.' *Am. J. Roentg.*, 68, 565 (M)

MOORE, S. (1953). 'The Troell-Junet syndrome.' *Acta Radiol.*, 39, 485 (D)

MOSELEY, J. E., RABINOWITZ, J. G. and DZIADIW, R. (1966). 'hyperostosis cranii *ex vacuo*.' *Radiology*, 87, 1105–1107 and 1115 (M)

MUDD, R. J., STRAIN, R. E. and PERLMUTTER, I. (1955). 'Calcified intracranial tuberculoma.' *Am. J. Roentg.*, 73, 19 (I; C)

MUENTER, M. D. and WHISNANT, J. P. (1968). 'Basal ganglia calcification, hypoparathyroidism and extrapyramidal motor manifestations.' *Neurology*, 18, 1075–1083 (C; M)

MULLER, C. J. B. (1964). 'Gardner's syndrome.' *Sth Afr. J. Radiol.*, **2**, 35 (D)

MÜLLER, E. (1966). 'Narben und Defektbildung im Mittelohr und begeitende chronische Entzündungen.' In J. Berendes, R. Link and F. Zöllner, *Hals-Nasen-Phren-Heilkunde in Praxis und Klinik.* Vol. III, Pt. 2. Stuttgart; Thieme (E)

MURASE, Y., TANAKA, S., FUTAMURA, A., ITO, T., IMAMURA, K. and SAKATA, K. (1970). 'A new simple measurement of pineal calcification in the lateral craniogram.' *Am. J. Roentg.*, **110**, 92–95 (C)

MURDOCK, J. R. and HUTLER, H. J. (1932). 'Leprosy: a roentgenological survey.' *Am. J. Roentg.*, **28**, 598 (I)

MURPHY, J. and GOODING, C. A. (1970). 'Evolution of persistently enlarged parietal foramina.' *Radiology*, **97**, 391–392 (D)

MURRAY, R. O. (1960). 'Radiological bone changes in Cushing's syndrome and steroid therapy.' *Br. J. Radiol.*, **33**, 1 (M)

MURRAY, R. S. (1949). 'Orbital emphysema following fracture of the nasal sinus.' *J. Fac. Radiol., Lond.*, **1**, 121 (O ; T ; S)

MÜSSBICHLER, H. (1968). 'Radiologic study of intracranial calcifications in congenital toxoplasmosis.' *Acta Radiol.*, **7**, 369–379 (I ; C)

MUSUMECI, V. (1942). 'Contributo allo studio radiologico della cisticercosi.' *Quad. Clin. ostet. Ginec.*, **7**, 34 (I)

MUTHUKRISHNAN, N. and SHETTY, M. V. K. (1972). 'Pycnodysostosis. A report of a case.' *Am. J. Roentg.*, **114**, 247–252 (D)

NAKAYAMA, T. and MATSUKADO, Y. (1975). 'Sinus pericranii with aneurysmal malformation of the internal cerebral vein.' *Surg. Neurol.*, **3**, 133–137 (D)

NATTZIGER, H. C. (1925). 'Method for the localization of brain tumours: the pineal shift.' *Surg. Gynec. Obstet.*, **40**, 481 (C)

NEGRE, A. and FONTAN, R. (1955). 'Aspects radiologiques des lésions osseuses de la lèpre.' *J. Radiol. Électrol.*, **36**, 141 (I)

NELSON, J. D. (1958). 'The Marfan syndrome with special reference to congenital enlargement of spinal canal.' *Br. J. Radiol.*, **31**, 561 (D)

NEMANSKY, J. and HAGEMAN, M. J. (1975). 'Tomographic findings of the inner ears of 24 patients with Waardenburg's syndrome.' *Am. J. Roentg.*, **124**, 250–255 (E)

NESBIT, M. E., WOLFSON, J. J., KIEFFER, S. A. and PETERSON, H. O. (1970). 'Orbital sclerosis in histiocytosis X.' *Am. J. Roentg.*, **110**, 123–128 (O ; K)

NEUHAUSER, E. B. D. (1970). 'Infantile cortical hyperostosis and skull defects.' *Postgrad. Med.*, **48**, 57–59 (D ; T)

NEUHAUSER, E. B. D. and TUCKER, A. (1948). 'The roentgen changes produced by diffuse torulosis in the newborn.' *Am. J. Roentg.*, **59**, 805

NEW, P. F. J. (1966). 'Sella turcica as mirror of disease.' *Radiol. Clin. N. Am.*, **4**, 75–92 (P)

NEW, P. F. J. and WEINER, M. A. (1971). 'The radiological investigation of hydrocephalus.' *Radiol. Clin. N. Am.*, **9**, 117–140 (R)

NEWTON, T. H. and POTTS, D. G. (1971). *Radiology of the Skull and Brain*, Vol. 1. St. Louis; Mosby (G)

NICHOLSON, J. T. and SHERK, H. H. (1968). 'Anomalies of the occipitocervical articulation.' *J. Bone Jt Surg.*, **50–A**, 295–304 (R)

NIXON, G. W. and RAVIN, C. E. (1974). 'Malposition of the attached portion of the falx cerebri and the superior sagittal sinus: an indicator of severe cerebral maldevelopment.' *Am. J. Roent.*, **122**, 44–51 (D)

NOONAN, J. A. (1968). 'Hypertelorism with Turner phenotype. A new syndrome with associated congenital heart disease.' *Am. J. Dis. Child.*, **116**, 373–380 (D)

NORDMARK, B. (1949). 'Pressure changes in the sella turcica in the presence of glioma in the cerebral hemispheres.' *Acta Radiol.*, **32**, 461 (R)

NORRELL, H. and HOWIESON, J. (1970). 'Gas-containing brain abscesses.' *Am. J. Roentg.*, **109**, 273–276 (I)

NUMAGUCHI, Y., HOFFMAN, J. C. and SONES, P. J. (1975). 'Basal ganglia calcification as a late radiation effect.' *Am. J. Roentg.*, **123**, 27–30 (C)

OBRADOR, S. (1959). 'Intracranial tuberculomas: a review of 47 cases.' *Neurochirurgia*, **1**, 150 (I)

OGAWA, T. K., BERGERON, R. T., WHITAKER, C. W., MILES, J. W. and RUMBAUGH, C. L. (1976). 'Air-fluid levels in the sphenoid sinus in epistaxis and nasal packing.' *Radiology*, **118**, 351–354 (S)

OH, S. J. (1968). 'Roentgen findings in cerebral paragonimiasis.' *Radiology*, **90**, 292–299 (I)

OHTA, T., WAGA, S., HANDA, H., NISHIMURA, S. and MITANI, T. (1975). 'Sinus pericranii.' *J. Neurosurg.*, **42**, 704–701 (D)

OLIVERCRONA, H. (1935). 'Bedeutung des Röntgenbildes fur die Anzeigestellung und Behandlung der Gehirntumoren.' *Fortschr. Röntgenstr.*, **52**, 355 (N)

OON, C. L. (1963). 'The size of the pituitary fossa in adults.' *Br. J. Radiol.*, **36**, 294–299 (P ; A)

OON, C. L., LAVENDER, J. P. and JOPLIN, G. F. (1962). 'The width of the normal pituitary gland. A comparison of two radiological methods of measurement.' *Br. J. Radiol.*, **35**, 418 (A ; P)

ORLEY, A. (1949). *Neuroradiology.* Springfield, I11.; Thomas (G)

OSTERTAG, B. and SCHIFFER, K. H. (1949). 'Der Gerichtete Schädelbinnendruck und seine röntgenologische Erfassung.' *Dt. med. Wschr.*, **74**, 1116 (R)

O'SULLIVAN, J. (1925). 'Some rarer intracranial calcifications.' *Br. J. Radiol.*, **30**, 295 (C)

OTT, A. (1955). 'Die Kleine Sella Turcica.' *Wien, klin. Wschr.*, **67**, 778 (P)

OVERZIER, C. (1943). 'Das Randwachstum der Schädelknochen bei Hyperämie der Nähte.' *Virchows Arch. path. Anat. Physiol.*, **311**, 544 (D)

PACIFICO, A. (1939). 'Nuovi orientamenti sulla genesi della "Inpronte digitate" del cranio.' *Studi sassaresi*, **17**, 153 (R)

PALACIOS, E., (1970). 'Intracranial solitary chondroma of dural origin.' *Am. J. Roentg.*, **110**, 67–70 (N)

PALACIOS, E., (1970). 'Chemodectomas of the head and neck.' *Am. J. Roentg.*, **110**, 129–140 (N)

PALACIOS, E. and MacGEE, E. E. (1972). 'The radiographic diagnosis of trigeminal neurinomas.' *J. Neurosurg.*, **36**, 153–156 (N)

PALACIOS, E. and SCHIMKE, R. N. (1969). 'Craniosynostosis-syndactylism.' *Am. J. Roentg.*, **106**, 133–155 (D)

PANCOAST, H. K. (1932). 'The interpretation of roentgenograms of pituitary tumors.' *Am. J. Roentg.*, **27**, 697 (P ; N)

PARADIS, R. W. and SAX, D. S. (1972). 'Familial basilar impression.' *Neurology*, **22**, 554–560 (D)

PARK, E. A. and POWERS, G. F. (1920). 'Acrocephaly and scaphocephaly with symmetrically distributed malformation of the extremities. A study of the so-called acrocephalo-syndactylism.' *Am. J. Dis. Child.*, **20**, 235 (D)

PARNITZKE, K. H. (1961). *Endokranielle Verkalkungen im Röntgenbilde.* Leipzig; Thieme (C)

PARSONS, F. G. and BOX, C. R. (1905). 'The relation of the cranial suture to age.' *J. R. anthrop. Inst.*, **35**, 30 (A)

PATERSON, D. E. (1955). 'Radiological bone changes and angiographic findings in leprosy with special reference to the pathogenesis of "atrophic" conditions of the digits.' *J. Fac. Radiol., Lond*, **7**, 35 (I)

PEARSON, K. D., STEINBACH, H. L. and BIER, D. M. (1971). 'Roentgenographic manifestations of the Prader-Willi syndrome.' *Radiology*, **100**, 369–377 (D)

PEIMER, R. (1954). 'Benign giant-cell tumors of skull and nasal sinuses.' *Archs Otolaryng., Chicago*, **60**, 186 (S ; N)

PENDERGRASS, E. P. and de LORIMIER, A. A. (1936). 'Osteolytic lesions involving the calvarium.' *Am. J. Roentg.*, **35**, 9 (G)

PENDERGRASS, E. P. and HOPE, J. W. (1953). 'An extracranial meningioma with no apparent intracranial source. Report of a case.' *Am. J. Roentg.*, **70**, 967 (G)

PENDERGRASS, E. P. and PEPPER, O. H. P. (1939). 'Observations on the process of ossification in the formation of persistent enlarged parietal foramina.' *Am. J. Roentg.*, **41**, 343 (D)

PENDERGRASS, E. P. and PERRYMAN, C. R. (1949). 'The roentgen diagnosis of meningiomas of the sphenoidal ridge.' *Radiology*, **53**, 675 (N)

PENDERGRASS, E. P., SCHAEFFER, P. J. P., and HODES, P. J. (1956). *The Head and Neck in Roentgen Diagnosis*, 2nd ed. Oxford; Blackwell (G)

PENFIELD, W. (1923). 'Cranial and intracranial endotheliomata – hemicraniosis.' *Surg. Gynec. Obstet.*, **36**, 657–674 (N)

PENFIELD, W. (1952). 'Cranial clues to intracranial abnormality.' Caldwell Lecture 1951. *Am. J. Roentg.*, **67**, 535 (G)

PENFOLD, J. L. and SIMPSON, D. A. (1975). 'Premature craniosynostosis – a complication of thyroid replacement therapy.' *J. Pediat.*, **86**, 360–363 (M; D)

PERLBERG, H. J. and KRUGER, A. L. (1939). 'Osteoma of the skull.' *Am. J. Roentg.*, **41**, 587 (N)

PETASNICK, J. P. (1969). 'Tomography of the temporal bone in Paget's disease.' *Am. J. Roentg.*, **105**, 838–843 (E; K)

PETERSON, H. O. and KIEFFER, S. A. (1972). *Introduction to Neuroradiology*. New York; Harper and Row (G)

PFEIFFER, K. (1958). 'Ungewöhnlicher Schädeldachbedfund bei tertiarer Knochenlues unter der Behandlung.' *Fortschr. Röntgenstr.* **88**, 574 (I)

PFEIFFER, R. A. (1964). 'Akrocephalosyndaktylie.' *Z. Kinderheilk*, **90**, 301–320 (D)

PHILIP, A. G. S. (1975). 'Fontanelle size and epiphyseal calcification in neonatal twins discordant by weight.' *N. Pediat.*, **86**, 417–419 (D)

PORKORNA, L. (1949). 'Das Röntgenbild der Osteoporose im Konzentrationslager Theresienstadt.' *Radiol. clin. Basel*, **18**, 360 (M)

POMERANZ, M. M. (1948). 'Werner's syndrome.' *Radiology*, **51**, 521 (D)

POSCHL, M. (1956). 'Skelettveränderungen am Schädel bei kavernösen Gefässgeschwülsten.' *Fortschr. Röntgenstr.*, **84**, 209 (D)

POTTER, G. D. (1970). 'Sclerosis of the base of the skull as a manifestation of nasopharyngeal carcinoma.' *Radiology*, **100**, 35–38 (N)

POWELL, J. W., WEENS, H. S. and WENGER, N. K. (1965). 'The skull roentgenogram in iron deficiency anemia and in secondary polycythemia.' *Am. J. Roentg.*, **95**, 143–147 (M)

POZNANSKI, A. K. and STEPHENSON, J. M. (1967). 'Radiographic findings in hypothalamic acceleration of growth associated with cerebral atrophy and mental retardation (cerebral gigantism).' *Radiology*, **88**, 446–456 (D)

POZNANSKI, A. K., NOSANCHUK, J. S., BAUBLIS, J. and HOLT, J. F. (1970). 'The cerebro-hepato-renal syndrome (CHRS) (Zellweger's syndrome).' *Am. J. Roentg.*, **109**, 313–322 (D)

PRIBRAM, H. W. and du BOULAY, G. H. (1971). 'The sella turcica.' In *Radiology of the Skull and Brain*, Vol I pp357–405. ed. by T. H. Newton and D. G. Potts. St. Louis; Mosby

PRIBRAM, H. W. and SWANN, G. F. (1960). 'The radiological changes and clinical incidence of endocrine effects in sellar and parasellar tumours.' *Radiology*, **75**, 877–884 (P)

PRITCHARD, J. J., SCOTT, J. H. and GIRGIS, F. G. (1956). 'The structure and development of cranial and facial sutures.' *J. Anat., Lond.*, **90**, 73 (A)

PSENNER, L. (1941). 'Die Osteomyelitis der Schadelkapsel.' *Fortschr. Röntgenstr.*, **63**, 141 (I)

PSENNER, L. (1951). 'Die anatomischen Varianten des Hirnschädels.' *Fortschr. Röntgenstr.*, **75**, 197 (A)

PSENNER, L. (1952). 'Ein Beitrag zur Diagnose und Differentialdiagnose der Meningeome.' *Fortschr. Röntgenstr.*, **76**, 567 (N)

PSENNER, L. (1954). 'Ein weiterer Bericht über ein rein intraossares meningeom.' *Radiol. Austraca*, **7**, 91 (N)

PUGH, D. G. (1945). 'Fibrous dysplasia of the skull. A probable explanation for leontiasis ossea.' *Radiology*, **44**, 548 (D)

PUGH, D. G. (1951). *The Roentgenologic Diagnosis of Diseases of Bones*. Baltimore; Williams and Wilkins (G)

PUGH, D. G. (1952). 'The roentgenologic diagnosis of hyperparathyroidism.' *Surg. Clin. N. Am.* **32**, 1017 (M)

PYLE, E. (1931). 'A case of unusual bone development.' *J. Bone Jt Surg.*, **13**, 874–876 (D)

RÄDBERG, C. E. (1963). 'Some aspects of the asymmetric enlargement of the sella turcica.' *Acta Radiol.*, **1**, 152 (P)

RÄDBERG, C. E. and THIBAUT, A. (1971). *Supine Skull Radiography with Orbix*. Solna, Sweden; Elema Schönander

RAND, C. W. and REEVES, D. L. (1943). 'Dermoid and epidermoid tumors (cholesteatomas) of the central nervous system: report of 23 cases.' *Archs Surg., Chicago*, **46**, 350 (N)

RAO, B. N. B. (1945). 'Intradiploic epidermoid of the skull.' *Indian med. Gaz.*, **80**, 125 (N)

RATHBUN, J. C. (1948). ' "Hypophosphatasia", a new developmental anomaly.' *Am. J. Dis. Child.*, **75**, 822–831 (D; M)

RAUSCH, F. (1953). 'Die röntgenologische Bedeutung von Schadelverkalkungen fur die Differentialdiagnose der Hirntumoren Bericht 35 Tag.' *Dtsch. Röntgen-Gesell.*, *S.* 47 (C; N)

RAUSCH, F. (1954). 'Die Bedeutung von Verkalkungen fur die Artdiagnose intracranieller, raumbeengender Prosesse.' *Fortschr. Röntgenstr.*, **81**, 768 (C; N)

RAVELLI, A. (1956). 'Luetischer Herd im Schadeldach.' *Radiol. Clin. Basel*, **25**, 51 (I)

RECKLINGHAUSEN, F. von (1891). 'Die fibrose oder derfomierende Ostitis die Osteomalacie und die osteoplastische Carcinose.' In Virchow, R. *Festschrift*. Berlin; Reimer (N)

REINERT, H. (1927). 'Beitrag zur röntgenologischen Selladiagnostik.' *Fortschr. Röntgenstr.*, **35**, 553 (P)

REISNER, K. (1969). 'Tomography in inner and middle ear malformations.' *Radiology*, **92**, 11–20 (E)

REYNOLDS, J. (1965). *The Roentgenological Features of Sickle Cell Disease and Related Haemoglobinopathies*. Springfield, Ill.; Thomas (D)

RHOTON, A. L., PULEC, J. L., HALL, G. M. and BOYD, A. G. (1968). 'Absence of bone over the geniculate ganglion.' *J. Neurosurg.*, **28**, 48–53 (A; E)

RIACH, I. C. F. (1966). 'The sellar-index-relationship between the area of the sella turcica and the lateral area of the skull.' *Br. J. Radiol.*, **39**, 824–826 (A)

RIGGS, W. (1970). 'Roentgen findings in Noonan's syndrome.' *Radiology*, **96**, 393–395 (D)

RIGGS, W. and SEIBERT, J. (1972). 'Cockayne's syndrome.' *Am. J. Roentg.*, **116**, 623–633 (D)

RIGGS, W., WILROY, R. S. and ETTELDORF, J. N. (1972). 'Neonatal hyperthyroidism with accelerated skeletal maturation, craniosynostosis and brachydactyly.' *Radiology*, **105**, 621–625 (M)

RITVO, M. (1949). 'Roentgen diagnosis of diseases of the skull.' *Ann. Roentgenol.*, **19**, (G)

ROBERTS, F. and SHOPFNER, C. E. (1972). 'Plain skull roentgenograms in children with head trauma.' *Am. J. Roentg.*, **114**, 230–240 (T)

ROBERTSON, G. E. (1946). 'The roentgenographic appearance of the falx cerebri.' *Am. J. Roentg.*, **56**, 230 (A)

ROBIN, P. (1934). 'Glossoptosis due to atresia and hypertrophy of the mandible.' *Am. J. Dis. Child.*, **48**, 541–547 (D)

ROBINSON, A. E., MEARES, B. M. and GOREE, J. A. (1967). 'Traumatic sphenoid sinus effusion. An analysis of 50 cases.' *Am. J. Roentg.*, **101**, 795–801 (T; S)

RODRIGUEZ, M. F., de la Higuera Rojas, J. and Ortiz de Landazuri, E. (1952). 'Estudio de la superficie de la silla turca en la radiografia lateral del craneo para la interpretacion de los proceros endocrinos.' *Rev. Clin. Esp.*, **46**, 291 (P)

ROSEN, I. W. and NADEL, H. I. (1969). 'Button sequestrum of the skull.' *Radiology*, **92**, 969–971 (I)

ROSENBLUTH, P. R., LEUDERS, H. W. and MOYER, J. L. (1954). 'Traumatic diploic hematomas of skull.' *U. S. arm. Forces med. J.*, **5**, 378 (T)

ROSENCRANTZ, M. (1969). 'Widened vascular grooves in fibrous dysplasia of the skull.' *Acta Radiol.*, **9**, 95–100 (D)

ROSENOER, V. M. and MITCHELL, R. C. (1959). 'Skeletal changes in Wilson's disease.' *Br. J. Radiol.*, **32**, 805 (W;K)

ROSS, R. J. and GREITZ, T. B. V. (1966). 'Changes of the sella turcica in chromophobic adenomas and eosinophilic adenomas.' *Radiology*, **86**, 892–899 (P;N)

ROTH, I. and LEMKE, R. (1932). 'Das Röntgenbilde des Schädelse bei gesteigetern Hirndruck (DruckSchädel).' *Klin. Wschr.*, **11**, 949 (R)

ROTMAN, M. Z. and SIEGELMAN, S. S. (1967). 'Emphysematous encephalopathy. Report of a case with abnormal skull roentgenograms.' *Radiology*, **89**, 486–487 (R)

ROUKKULA, M. (1964). 'Roentgenologic findings in chondromas.' *Acta Radiol.*, **2**, 120 (N)

ROVIT, R. L., SCHECHTER, M. M. and CHODROFF, P. (1970). 'Choroid plexus papilloma: observations on radiographic diagnosis.' *Am. J. Roentg.*, **110**, 608–617 (N)

ROVSING, H. (1970). 'Otosclerosis: a tomographic-clinical study.' *Acta Radiol.*, Suppl. 296 (E)

ROVSING, H. and JENSEN, J. (1968). 'Tomographic visualization of labyrinthine fistula: complication of chronic otitis.' *Radiology*, **90**, 261–267 (E)

ROWBOTHAM, G. F. (1938/39). 'The hyperostoses in relation with the meningiomas.' *Br. J. Surg.*, **26**, 593 (N)

ROWEN, M., SINGER, M. I. and MORAN, E. T. (1972). 'Intracranial calcification in the congenital rubella syndrome.' *Am. J. Roentg.*, **115**, 86–91 (C)

RUBERTI, R., GALLIGIONI, F. and CARTERI, A. (1966). 'Considerations radiologiques dans les neurinomes du ganglion de Gasser.' *Acta Radiol.*, **5**, 465–469 (N)

RUBIN, P. (1965). *Dynamic Classification of Bone Dysplasias.* Chicago; Year Book Publishers (P)

RUBINSTEIN, J. H. and TAYBI, H. (1963). 'Broad thumbs and toes and facial abnormalities: a possible mental retardation syndrome.' *Am. J. Dis. Child.*, **105**, 588–608 (D)

RUCKENSTEINER, E. (1950). 'Zur Differentialdiagnose der meningeomatösen Schädelverändenrungen.' *Fortschr. Röntgenstr.*, **72**, 698 (N)

RUMBAUGH, C. L. and DAVIS, D. O. (1974). 'The normal skull: techniques and indications.' *Sem. Roentg.*, **9**, 91–100 (A)

RUMBAUGH, C. L. and POTTS, D. G. (1966). 'Skull changes associated with intracranial arteriovenous malformations.' *Am. J. Roentg.*, **98**, 525–534 (D)

RUSSELL, W. J., BIZZOZERO, O. J. and OMOIR, Y. (1968). 'Idopathic osteosclerosis. A report of 6 related cases.' *Radiology*, **90**, 70–76 (E)

RYNA, M. S. (1957). 'Radiological manifestations of ectopic salivary adenoma showing the cylindroma pattern.' *Proc. R. Soc. Med.*, **50**, 96 (N)

RZYMSKI, K. and KOSOWICZ, J. (1975). 'The skull in gonadal dysgenesis: a roentgenometric study.' *Clin. Radiol.*, **26**, 379–384 (D;M)

RZYMSKI, K. and KOSOWICZ, J. (1976). 'Abnormal basal angle of the skull in sex chromosome aberrations.' *Acta Radiol.*, **17**, 669–675 (D)

SACKETT, G. L. and FORD, M. M. (1956). 'Cytomegalic inclusion disease with calcification outlining cerebral ventricles.' *Am. J. Roentg.*, **76**, 512–515 (I)

SAJID, M. H. and COPPLE, P. J. (1968). 'Familial aqueductal stenosis and basilar impression.' *Neurology*, **18**, 260–262 (D)

SAKATI, N., NYHAN, W. L. and TISDALE, W. K. (1971). 'A new syndrome with acrocephalosyndactyly, cardiac disease and distinctive defects of the ear, skin and lower limbs.' *J. Pediat.*, **79**, 104–109 (D)

SALDINO, R. M. (1971). 'Lethal short-limbed dwarfism: achondrogenesis and thanatophoric dwarfism.' *Am. J. Roentg.*, **112**, 185–197 (D)

SALDINO, R. M. and di CHIRO, G. (1974). 'Tentorial calcification.' *Radiology*, **111**, 207–210 (C;A)

SALDINO, R. M., STEINBACH, L. and EPSTEIN, C. J. (1972). 'Familial acrocephalosyndactyly (Pfeiffer syndrome).' *Am. J. Roentg.*, **116**, 609–622 (D)

SAMUEL, E. (1952). *Clinical Radiology of the Ear, Nose and Throat.* London; Lewis (E;S)

SANSTRÖM, B. and WILBRAND, H. F. (1971). 'Anatomic cause for intraossicular cavities in temporal bone tomography.' *Acta Radiol.*, **11**, 225–231 (A)

SARWAR, M., SWISCHUK, L. E. and SCHECHTER, M. M. (1976). 'Intracranial chondromas.' *Am. J. Roentg.*, **127**, 973–977 (N)

SASSIN, J. T. and CHUTORIAN, A. M. (1967). 'Intracranial chordoma in children.' *Archs Neurol.*, **17**, 89–93 (N)

SAUNDERS, W. W. (1943). 'Basilar impression; position of normal odontoid.' *Radiology*, **41**, 589 (D)

SAUVEGRAIN, J. and MARESCHAL, J. L. (1972). 'Craniocervical joint malformations in childhood.' *Ann Radiol.*, **15**, 263–277 (D)

SAVINO, A. M. (1945). 'Significando y valor de las impressiones digitiformes de la calota en el sindrome radiografico de la lipertension endocraneal.' *Rev. esp. Cir. Traum. Ortop.*, **2**, 89 (R)

SCHATZ, C. J. and VIGNAUD, J. (1976). 'The inclined lateral projection: A new view in temporal bone tomograph.' *Radiology*, **118**, 355–361 (E;A)

SCHECHTER, M. M. and CHUSID, J. G. (1966). 'Chemodectomas of the carotid bifurcation.' *Acta Radiol.*, **5**, 488–508 (N)

SCHECHTER, M. M. and ZINGESSER, L. H. (1967). 'The radiology of aqueductal stenosis.' *Radiology*, **88**, 905–916 and 929 (D)

SCHEUERMANN, H. (1932). 'The roentgenological picture of the normal and the pathologic sella turcica.' *Acta Radiol.*, **13**, 404 (P)

SCHEUERMANN, H. (1944). 'On the size and form of the sella turcica in the various pituitary adenomas.' *Acta Psychiat.*, **19**, 347 (P;N)

SCHEY, W. L. (1973). 'Plain film skull roentgenographic changes in hydrocephalus.' *Am. J. Roentg.*, **118**, 134–146 (R)

SCHIEFER, W. and MARGUTH, F. (1954/56). 'Intraselläre Aneurysmen.' *Acta neurochir.*, **4**, 344 (P)

SCHIFFER, K. H. and STRUBEL, H. (1960). 'Über Störungen der Entwickelungsmechanik des Gehirnschädels beim Mongolinsmus und anderen Konstitution-sanomalien.' *Nervenarzt*, **31**, 340 (G)

SCHINZ, H. R., BAENSCH, W. E., FRIEDL, E. and UEHLINGER, E. (1952). *Roentgen Diagnostics*, Vol. 2. London; Heinemann (G)

SCHMIDT, H. and HOLTHUSEN, W. (1972). 'Die Schädelform Frühgeborener Kinder.' *Acta Radiol.*, **13**, 14–24 (A)

SCHOEPS, J. (1949/50). 'Die Röntgendiagnose der toxoplasmorgenen Defekterkrankungen.' *Fortschr. Röntgenstr.*, **72**, 577 (I)

SCHOTT, H. (1953). 'Bedeutung von Schädelgrösse und sekundürer Sellaerweiterung fur die Diagnostik raumfordernder intracranieller Prozess.' im *Wachtstumsalter.* Köln; Diss (G)

SCHREIBER, R. (1930). 'Intracranial pressure. The correlation of choked disc and roentgenologic pressure signs.' *Am. J. Roentg.*, **23**, 607 (R)

SCHÜLLER, A. (1905). *Die Schädelbasis im Röntgenbilde.* Hamburg; Gräfe & Sillem (G)

SCHÜLLER, A. (1907). 'Über Halisterese der Schädelknochen bei intrakranieller Drucksteigerung.' *Fortschr. Röntgenstr.*, **11**, 217 (R)

SCHÜLLER, A. (1908). 'Über Schädelröntgenogramme mit positiven Befunde im Sinne von Folgeerscheinungen längerbestehender Drucksteigerung.' *Fortschr. Röntgenstr.*, **12**, 354 (R)

SCHÜLLER, A. (1908). 'Die röntgenographische Darstellung der diploetischen Venenkanäle des Schädels.' *Fortschr. Röntgenstr.,* **12,** 232 (G)

SCHÜLLER, A. (1909). 'Die Röntgendiagnostik der Erkrankungen des Schädels und Gehirnes.' *Grenzgeb. med. und. Chir.,* **12,** Nr. 22 (G)

SCHÜLLER, A. (1910). 'Röntgendiastnostik der Hirntumoren.' *Fortschr. Röntgenstr.,* **15,** 45 (N)

SCHÜLLER, A. (1912). 'Röntgendiagnostik der Erkrankungen des Kopfes.' In *Spezielle Pathologie v Therapie,* ed. by. H. Nothnagel. Wien; Holder (G)

SCHÜLLER, A. (1918). *Roentgen Diagnosis of Diseases of the Head.* St. Louis; Mosby (G)

SCHÜLLER, A. (1926). 'The sella turcica.' *Am. J. Roentg.,* **16,** 336 (P)

SCHÜLLER, A. (1928). 'Röntgendiagnose der Akustikustumoren.' *Ergeb. med. Strahlenforsch.,* **3,** 89 (N)

SCHÜLLER, A. (1929). 'Craniostenosis.' *Radiology,* **13,** 377 (D ; M ; R)

SCHÜLLER, A. (1930). 'Kurze Darstellung der Röntgendiagnostic kraniozerebraler Affektionen.' *Röntgenpraxis,* **2,** 625 (G)

SCHÜLLER, A. (1933). 'Zyste de Cisterne chiasmati.' *Fortschr. Röntgenstr.,* **48,** 717 (D)

SCHÜLLER, A. (1935). 'Welche Bedeutung haben verstärkte Impressiones digitatae auf Schädel röntgenological von Kindern und Erwachsenen.' *Röntgenpraxis,* **7,** 68 (R ; A)

SCHÜLLER, S. (1935). 'Über supraselläre Tumoren.' *Wien. klin. Wschr.* **48,** 1007 (P ; N)

SCHÜLLER, A. (1936). 'Röntgenologie und Hypophyse.' *Wien. klin. Wschr.,* **49,** 1259 (P)

SCHÜLLER, A. (1937). 'Die Regio orbito-temporalise.' *Fortschr. Röntgenstr.,* **55,** 62 (G)

SCHÜLLER, A. (1940). 'The diagnosis of basilar impression.' *Radiology,* **34,** 214 (D)

SCHÜLLER, A. (1941). 'X-ray symptoms of intracranial hypertension.' *Confin. neurol., Basel,* **3,** 253 (R)

SCHÜLLER, A. (1950). 'Short review of cranial hyperostosis.' *Acta Radiol.,* **34,** 361 (G)

SCHUMACHER, F. (1949). *Über die pathognomonische Bedeutung, besonders für intrakranielle Drucksteigerung, von vertstärkten Impressiones digitatae, lokalen Knochenusuren, Nahtdehiszenzen und Veränderungen der sella turcica.* Marbug; Diss (R)

SCHUMANN, E. (1961). 'Cysticercose in Röntgenild.' *Fortschr. Röntgenstr.,* **75,** 694 (I)

SCHUNK, H. and MARUYAMA, Y. (1960). 'Two vascular grooves of the external table of the skull with simulate fractures.' *Acta Radiol.,* **54,** 186 (A)

SCHUSTER, G. and WESTBERG, G. (1967). 'Gliomas of the optic nerve and chiasm.' *Acta Radiol.,* **6,** 221–232 (N)

SCHWARTZ, A. and LAVY, S. (1962). 'Evolution of roentgenographic skull changes with loss of brain substance in children.' *Neurology,* **12,** 133–139 (W)

SCHWARTZ, C. W. (1933). 'Some evidences of intracranial disease as revealed by the roentgen ray.' *Am. J. Roentg.,* **29,** 182 (G)

SCHWARTZ, C. W. (1936). 'The gliomas roentgenologically considered.' *Radiology,* **27,** 419 (N)

SCHWARTZ, C. W. (1938). 'The meningiomas from a roentgenological viewpoint.' *Am. J. Roentg.,* **36,** 698 (N)

SCHWARTZ, C. W. (1938). 'Tumours of the hypophysis cerebri from a roentgenologic viewpoint.' *Am. J. Roentg.,* **40,** 548 (P ; N)

SCHWARTZ, C. W. (1941). 'The cranial and intracranial epidermoidomas from a roentgenologic viewpoint.' *Am. J. Roentg.,* **45,** 18 (N)

SCHWARTZ, C. W. and COLLINS, L. C. (1951). *The Skull and Brain Roentgenologically Considered.* Springfield, I11.; Thomas (G)

SCHWARZ, E. (1960). 'Craniometaphyseal dysplasia.' *Am. J. Roentg.,* **84,** 461 (D)

SCHWARZ, E. and FISH, A. (1960). 'Roentgenographic features of new congenital dysplasia.' *Am. J. Roentg.,* **84,** 511 (D)

SEAR, H. R. (1953). 'The congenital bone dystrophies and their co-relation.' *J. Fac. Radiol., Lond.,* **4,** 221 (D)

SEAFERTH, J. (1961). *Die diagnostische Bedeutung der Impressiones digitatae (gyroum) im Wachstumalter.* Köln; Diss (R ; A)

SEEGER, J. F. and GRABRIELSEN, T. O. (1971). 'Premature closure of the fronto-sphenoidal suture in synostosis of the coronal suture.' *Radiology,* **98,** 305–309 (D ; M ; R)

SHACKELFORD, G. D., SHACKELFORD, P. G. SCHWET-SCHERNAN, P. R. and McALISTER, W. H. (1974). 'Congenital occipital dermal sinus.' *Radiology,* **111,** 161–166 (D)

SHAPIRO, C. E. and ROSSI, J. O. (1973). 'Roentgen evaluation of the paranasal sinuses in children.' *Am. J. Roentg.,* **118,** 176–186 (I)

SHAPIRO, R. (1972). 'Anomalous parietal sutures and the bipartite parietal bone.' *Am. J. Roentg.,* **115,** 569–577 (D)

SHAPIRO, R. (1972). 'Compartmentation of the jugular foramen.' *J. Neurosurg.,* **36,** 340–343 (A)

SHAPIRO, R. and JANZEN, A. H. (1970). 'Osteoblastic metastases to the floor of the skull simulating meningioma en plaque.' *Am. J. Roentg.,* **81,** 964–966 (N)

SHAPIRO, R. and ROBINSON, F. (1967). 'The foramina of the middle fossa: a phylogenetic, anatomic and pathologic study.' *Am. J. Roentg.,* **101,** 779–794 (A)

SHAW, R. C. (1951). 'Metastasizing goitre, "Hurthle cell" tumour of the thyroid and skull.' *Br. J. Surg.,* **39,** 25 (N)

SHILLITO, J. and MATSON, D. (1968). 'Craniosynostosis. A review of 519 surgical patients.' *Pediatrics,* **41,** 829–853 (D ; R)

SHIRA, R. B. (1953). 'Manifestations of systematic disorders in the facial bones.' *J. oral Surg.,* **11,** 286 (S)

SHOLKOFF, S. D. and MAINZER, F. (1971). 'Button sequestrum revisited.' *Radiology,* **100,** 6491652 (I)

SHOPFNER, C. E. and ROSSI, J. O. (1953). 'Roentgen evaluation of the paranasal sinuses in children.' *Am. J. Roentg.,* **118,** 176–186 (S)

SIGLIN, I. S., EATON, L. M. CAMP, J. D. and HAINES, S. F. (1947). 'Symmetric cerebral calcification which followed postoperative parathyroid insufficiency.' *J. clin. Endocrin.,* **7,** 433 (C ; M)

SILVERMAN, F. N. (1968). 'Differential diagnosis of achondroplasia.' *Radiol. Clin. N. Am.,* **6,** 223–237 (D)

SINGLETON, E. B. (1957). 'The radiographic features of severe idiopathic hypercalcaemia of infancy.' *Radiology,* **68,** 721 (D ; M)

SMITH, C. G. (1953). 'The x-ray appearance and incidence of calcified nodules on the habenular commissure.' *Radiology,* **60,** 647 (C)

SMITH, T. R. and KIER, E. L. (1971). 'The unfused planum sphenoidale. Differentation from fracture.' *Radiology,* **98,** 305–309 (A ; T)

SMITH-AGREDA, V. (1955). 'Über die Verteilung der Impressiones gyrorum an der Innenseite des Gehirnschädels des Menschen.' *Dt. Z. Nervenheilk,* **173,** 37 (R ; A)

SNAPPER, I. (1940). 'Tuberose sclerosis of the brain (Bourneville's disease).' *China med. J.,* **57,** 401 (W)

SONDHEIMER, R. K. (197?). 'Suture diastasis following rapid brain weight gain.' *Archs Neurol. Psychiat.,* **23,** 314–318 (M)

SOSMAN, M. C. (1927). 'Radiology as an aid in diagnosis of skull and intracranial lesions.' *Radiology,* **9,** 396 (G)

SOSMAN, M. C. (1930). 'Xanthomatosis.' *Am. J. Roentg.,* **23,** 581 (K)

SOSMAN, M. C. (1936). 'The reliability of the roentgenographic signs of intracranial tumour.' *Am. J. Roentg.,* **36,** 737 (G)

SOSMAN, M. C. (1949). 'Cushing's disease – pituitary basophilism.' *Am. J. Roentg.,* **62,** 1 (M ; P)

SOSMAN, M. C. and PUTNAM, T. J. (1925). 'Roentgenological aspects of brain tumors – meningiomas.' *Am. J. Roentg.,* **13,** 1 (N)

SPENCE, A. W. (1958). 'The radiology of endocrine disorders.' *Br. J. Radiol.,* **31**, 341 (M)

SPENCE, A. W., ASTLEY, R. and LAWS, J. W. (1958). (Symposium) *Br. J. Radiol.,* **31**, 341 (M)

SPITZER, R., RABINOWITCH, J. Y. and WYBAR, K. D. (1961). 'A study of abnormalities of skull, teeth, lenses in mongolism.' *Can. med. Ass. J.,* **84**, 567 (D)

SPRANGER, J. W. and LANGER, L. O. (1970). 'Spondyloepiphyseal dysplasia congenita.' *Radiology,* **94**, 313–322 (D)

SPRANGER, J. W., LANGER, L. O. and WIEDERMANN, H. R. (1974). *Bone Dysplasias, An Atlas of Disorders of Skeletal Development.* Philadelphia; Saunders (D)

STANTON, J. B. and WILKINSON, M. (1949). 'Familial calcification of the petrosphenoidal ligament.' *Lancet,* **2**, 736 (C)

STARGARDTER, F. and MARGOLIS, M. T. (1972). 'Sella turcica destruction with chromophobe adenomas.' *Am. J. Roentg.,* **115**, 774–776 (P ; N)

STAUFFER, H. M., SNOW, B. L. and ADAMS, A. B. (1953). 'Roentgenologic recognition of habenular calcification as distinct from calcification in the pineal body: its application in cerebral localization.' *Am. J. Roentg.,* **70**, 83 (C)

STEINBACH, H. L., FELDMAN, R. and GOLDBERG, M. B. (1959). 'Acromegaly.' *Radiology,* **72**, 535 (M)

STEINBACH, H. L., KOLB, F. O. and CRANE, J. T. (1959). 'Unusual roentgen manifestations of osteomalacia.' *Am. J. Roentg.,* **82**, 875 (K)

STEINBACH, H. L., GORDON, G. S. EISENBERG, E., CRANE, J. T., SILVERMAN, S. and GOLDMAN, L. (1961). 'Primary hyperparathyroidism: a correlation of roentgen, clinical and pathological features.' *Am. J. Roentg.,* **86**, 329 (M)

STENHOUSE, D. (1948). 'Plain radiography of the skull in the diagnosis of intracranial tumours.' *Br. J. Radiol.,* **21**, 287 (G)

STENVER, H. W. (1917). 'Roentgenology of the os petrosum.' *Arch. Radiol. Electrother.,* **22**, 97 (E)

STENVER, H. W. (1921/22). 'Roentgenology of the os petrosum.' *Acta Otolaryng., Stockh.,* **3**, 266 (E)

STENVER, H. W. (1928). *Röntgenologie des Felsenbeines und des bitemporalen Schädelbildes.* Berlin; Springer (G)

STENVER, H. W. (1932). 'Röntgendiagnose der Tumoren der hinteren Schädelgrube.' *Dt. Z. Nervenheilk.,* **124**, 11 (G)

STENVER, H. W. (1935). 'Über Drucksymptome am knochernen Schädel bei den Hirngeschwülsten.' *Fortshr. Röntgenstr.,* **52**, 341 (R ; N)

STEWART, D. M. (1938). 'Roentgenological manifestations in bone syphilis.' *Am. J. Roentg.,* **40**, 215 (I)

STEWART, W. H. (1925). *Skull Fracture Roentgenologically Considered.* New York; Hoeber (T)

STIEHM, W. D. (1972). 'Facial Duplication.' *Am. J. Roentg.,* **116**, 598–601 (D)

STOOL, S., LEEDS, N. E. and SHULMAN, K. (1967). 'The syndrome of congenital deafness and optic meningitis: diagnosis and management.' *J. Pediat.,* **71**, 547–552 (O)

STOVIN, J. J., LYON, J. A. and CLEMMENS, R. L. (1960). 'Mandibulofacial dysostosis.' *Radiology,* **74**, 225–231 (D)

STRAND, R. D. and GREEN, B. (1974). 'A "calcified suprasellar mass" in association with spondylometaphyseal dysplasia.' *Ann. Radiol.,* **17**, 369–374 (D)

STRAUS, P., COMPERE, R., LIVCHITZ, J., PROT, D. and KAPLAN, M. (1968). 'L'apport de la radio-pédiatrie an dépistage des enfants maltraités.' *Ann. de Radiol.,* **11**, 1591169 (G)

STRICKLAND, B. (1954). 'Cushing's syndrome.' *Proc. R. Soc. Med.,* **47**, 341 (M)

STRICKLER, J. M. (1966). 'New and simple techniques for demonstration of the jugular foramen.' *Am. J. Roentg.,* **97**, 601–606 (A)

STROBOS, R. J., de la TORRE, E. and MARTIN, J. F. (1957). 'Symmetrical calcification of the basal ganglia with familial ataxia and pigmentation macular degeneration.' *Brain,* **80**, 313 (C ; D)

STURGE, W. A. (1879). 'A case of partial epilepsy, apparently due to a lesion of one of the motor centres of the brain.' *Trans. clin. Soc., Lond.,* **12**, 162 (G ; W)

SUSSE, H. J. (1955). 'Angiographische Untersuchungen bei der Ostitis deformans Paget.' *Fortschr. Röntgenstr.,* **83**, 498 (K)

SUSSE, H. J. (1961). 'Nerven- und Gefässkanäle am Os Zygomaticum und am Sinus maxillaris.' *Fortschr. Röntgenstr.,* **95**, 505 (A ; S)

SUSSE, H. J. (1961). 'Gefässtrukturen im Dach der Orbita.' *Fortsch. Röntgenstr.,* **95**, 510 (A ; O)

SUSSE, H. J. (1962). 'Zur Problematik der Duploevenen.' *Fortschr. Röntgenstr.,* **97**, 17 (A)

SUSSMAN, M. L. and COPLEMAN, B. (1942). 'The roentgenographic appearance of the bone in Cushing's syndrome.' *Radiology,* **39**, 288 (M)

SUSSMAN, M. L. and POPPEL, M. H. (1942). 'Renal osteitis.' *Am. J. Roentg.,* **48**, 726 (M)

SUTTON, D. (1949). 'The radiological diagnosis of lipoma of the corpus callosum.' *Br. J. Radiol.,* **22**, 534 (N)

SUTTON, D. (1951). 'Intracranial calcification in toxoplasmosis.' *Br. J. Radiol.,* **24**, 31 (C ; I)

SUTTON, D. and LIVERSEDGE, L. A. (1951). 'Radiological and pathological aspects of tuberose sclerosis with special reference to hydrocephalus.' *J. Fac. Radiol., Lond.,* **2**, 224 (W ; R)

SUTTON, D., BRAIN, W. R. and STRAUSS, E. B. (1955). *Recent Advances in Neurology and Neuropsychiatry.* London; Churchill (G)

SWANSON, H. A. and du BOULAY, G. (1975). 'Borderline variants of the normal pituitary fossa.' *Br. J. Radiol.,* **48**, 366–369 (G)

SWISCHUK, L. E. (1974). 'The normal newborn skull.' *Sem. Roentg.,* **9**, 101–113 (G ; A)

SWISCHUK, L. E. (1974). 'The growing skull.' *Sem. Roentg.,* **9**, 115–124 (G ; A)

SWOBODA, W. (1959). 'Kraniostenose und "Druckschädel" bei Rachitis.' *Neue Öst. Z. Kinderheilk.,* **4**, 302 (R ; D ; M)

TÄNSZER, A. (1966). 'Die Veränderungen am Schädel bei der Neurofibromatosis Recklinghausen. Versuch einer Einteilung.' *Fortschr. Röntgenstr.,* **105**, 50–62 (W ; K)

TAVERAS, J. M. (1960). 'Die neuroradiologische Untersuchung im Kindersalter.' In *Klinische Neuroradiologie.* ed. by K. Decker. Stuttgart; Thieme (G)

TAVERAS, J. M. and RANSOHOFF, J. (1953). 'Leptomeningeal cysts of the brain following trauma with erosion of the skull: a study of 7 cases treated by surgery.' *J. Neurosurg.,* **10**, 233 (T)

TAVERAS, J. M. and WOOD, E. H. (1964). *Diagnostic Neuroradiology.* Baltimore; Williams and Wilkins (G)

TAYBI, H. and LINDER, D. (1967). 'Congenital familial dwarfism with cephalo-skeletal dysplasia.' *Radiology,* **89**, 275–281 (D)

TAYLOR, J. (1928). 'Invasion of the skull by dural tumours.' *Br. J. Surg.,* **16**, 6 (N)

TEMTAMY, S. A. (1966). 'Carpenter's syndrome: acrocephalopolysyndactyly, an autosomal recessive syndrome.' *J. Paediat.,* **69**, 111–120 (D)

TENG, C–T. and NATHAN, M. H. (1960). 'Primary Hyperparathyroidism.' *Am. J. Roentgenol.,* **83**, 716 (M)

TEYMOORIAN, G. A. and BAGHERI, F. (1976). 'Hydatid cyst of the skull, report of four cases.' *Radiology,* **118**, 97–100 (I)

THAM, K. T., WEN, H. L. and TEOH, T. B. (1969). 'Case of papillary adenocarcinoma of choroid plexus.' *J. Path.,* **99**, 321–324 (N)

THOMPSON, J. R., HARWOOD-NASH, D. C. and FITZ, C. R. (1973). 'The neuroradiology of childhood choroid plexus neoplasms.' *Am. J. Roentg.,* **118**, 116–113 (N)

THOMPSON, R. C., GAULL, G. E., HORWITZ, S. J. and SCHENK, R. K. (1969). 'Hereditary hyperphosphatasia; studies of three siblings.' *Am. J. Med.,* **47**, 209–219 (D ; M)

THOMSON, J. L. G. (1955). 'Enlargement of the sella turcica: a report on 27 cases.' *Br. J. Radiol.,* **28**, 454–461 (P)

THORNHILL, E. H. and ANDERSON, B. (1944). 'Extradural diploic epidermoids producing unilateral exophthalmos.' *Am. J. Ophthal.*, **27**, 477 (N ; O)

THOYER-ROZAT, P., KLEIN, M. R. and MAZARS, M. (1944/5). 'Un cas de kyste demoid intra-cranien.' *J. Radiol. Électrol.*, **26**, 89 (N)

TIRONA, J. P. (1954). 'The roentgenological and pathological aspects of tuberculosis of the skull.' *Am. J. Roentg.*, **72**, 762 (I)

TOD, P. A. (1966). 'Radiology in head injury.' *Australas. Radiol.*, **10**, 91–100 (T)

TONNIS, W. (1938). 'Die Enstehung der intrakraniellen Drucksteigerung bei Hirngeschwülsten.' *Arch. klin. Chir.*, **193**, 669 (R)

TONNIS, W. (1938). 'Über Hirngeschwülste.' *Z. ges. Neurol. Psychiat.*, **161**, 114 (N)

TONNIS, W. (1939). 'Zirkulationsstörung en bei kraukhaftem Schadelinnendruck.' *Z. ges. Neurol. Psychiat.*, **167**, 462 (R)

TONNIS, W. (1939). 'Hydrozephalus infolge Liquorzirkulationsstorung.' *Arch. Kinderheilk*, **118**, 65 (R)

TONNIS, W. (1958). '43 Verhalten der Schädelnähte bei kraniellen und intrakraniellen Prozessen.' *Arch. klin. Chir.*, **289**, 418 (G)

TONNIS, W. (1959). 'Pathophysiologie und Klinik der intrakraniellen Druckstegerung.' In *Handbuch der Neurochirurgie*, Bd. 1. Berlin- Göttingen-Heidelberg; Springer (R)

TONNIS, W. and FRIEDMANN, G. (1959). 'Zur Differential diagnose der pathologischen intrakraniellen Verkalkungen.' *Münch. med. Wschr.*, **101**, 1252 (C)

TONNIS, W. and KLEINSASSER, O. (1959). 'Über die roentgenologischen Zeichen enhohten Schädelinnendruckes im Kindes- und Jirgendalte.' *Z. Kinderheik*, **82**, 387 (R)

TONNIS, W. and SCHURMANN, K. (1951). 'Meningeome der Keilbeinflugal (Ein Bericht über 73 einige Fälle).' *Zbl. Neurochir.*, **11**, 1 (N)

TONNIS, W., FRIEDMANN, G. and ALBRECHT, H. (1957). 'Zur röntgenologischen. Differentialdiagnose der Hypophysenadenome.' *Fortschr. Röntgenstr.*, **87**, 677 (P ; N)

TONNIS, W., FRIEDMANN, G. and ALBRECHT, H. (1957). 'Veränderungen der Sella Turcica bei sellanahen Tumoren und Tumoren der Schädelbasis.' *Fortschr. Röntgenstr.* **87**, 686 (P ; N)

TONNIS, W., SCHIEFER, W. and RAUSCH, F. (1954). 'Sellaveränderung en bei gesteigerten Schädelinnendruck.' *Dt. Z. Nervenheilk*, **171**, 35 (N)

TOWNE, E. B. (1926). 'Erosion of the petrous bone by acoustic nerve tumours.' *Archs Otolaryng., Chicago*, **4**, 515 (N)

TRISTAN, T. A. and HODES, P. J. (1958). 'Meningiomas of the posterior cranial fossa.' *Radiology*, **70**, 1 (N)

TRUFANT, S. A. and SEAMAN, W. B. (1952). 'Unilateral calcification of the basal ganglia.' *Radiology*, **59**, 521 (C)

TSAI, F. Y., LISELLA, R. A., LEE, K. F. and ROACH, J. F. (1975). 'Osteoslerosis of base of skull as a manifestation of tumor invasion.' *Am. J. Roentg.*, **124**, 256–264 (N)

TUCKER, A. S. (1961). 'Intracranial calcification in infants: is it possible roentgenographically to distinguish between toxoplasmosis and cytomegalic inclusion disease?' *Am. J. Roentg.*, **86**, 458–461 (C ; I)

TUCKER, R. L., HOLMAN, C. B., MacCARTY, C. S. and DOCKERTY, M. B. (1959). 'The roentgenologic manifestations of meningiomas in the region of the tuberculum sellae.' *Radiology*, **72**, 348–355 (N)

TWINING, E. W. (1936). 'The value of radiology in neurosurgery.' *Proc. R. Soc. Med.*, **29**, 1155 (G)

UEHLINGER, E. (1941). 'Osteofibrosis deformans juvenilis.' *Fortschr. Röntgenstr.*, **64**, 41 (D)

UNGER, A. S. and POPPEL, M. H. (1939). 'Developmental skull anomalies.' *Am. J. Roentg.*, **41**, 347 (D)

UNGER, S. M. and ROSWIT, B. (1959). 'Restoration of the sella turcica after treatment of pituitary adenomas.' *Am. J. Roentg.*, **81**, 967 (P ; N)

VALVASSORI, G. E. (1964). 'Laminagraphy of the temporal bone.' Book II. In *Radiographic Atlas of the Temporal Bone*. American Academy of Ophthalmology and Otolaryngology (E)

VALVASSORI, G. E. (1965). 'Radiologic diagnosis of cochlear otosclerosis.' *Laryngoscope*, **75**, 1563–1571 (E)

VALVASSORI, G. E. (1966). 'The interpretation of the radiographic findings in cochlear otosclerosis.' *Ann. Otol.*, **75**, 172–178 (E)

VALVASSORI, G. E. (1966). 'The radiological diagnosis of acoustic neuromas.' *Archs Otolaryng., Chicago*, **83**, 582–587 (N)

VALVASSORI, G. E. (1969). 'The abnormal internal auditory canal: the diagnosis of acoustic neuromas.' *Radiology*, **92**, 449–459 (N)

van BUCHEM, F. S. P., HADDERS, H. N. and UBBENS, R. (1955). 'An uncommon familial systemic disease of the skeleton: hyperostosis corticalis generalisata familiaris.' *Acta Radiol.*, **44**, 109–120 (D)

van BUCHEM, F. S. P., HADDERS, H. N., HANSEN, J. F. and WOLDRING, M. G. (1962). 'Hyperostosis corticalis generalisata: a report of seven cases.' *Am. J. Med.*, **33**, 387–397 (D)

van der HOEVE, J. L. and de Kleyn, K. (1918). 'de Blaue Sclera Knochenbruchigkeit und Schwerhorigkeit.' *Archs Ophthal.*, **95**, 81 (D)

VANDOR, F. (1958). 'Über die Röntgendiagnostik des Foramen jugulare.' *Radiol. clin., Basel*, **27**, 114 (A ; G)

VARADARAJAN, M. G. and RAMAMURTHI, B. (1964). 'Assessment of normal physiological intracranial calcification occurring in Indian subjects.' *Mediscope*, **7**, 453–466 (C)

VASILIU, D. O. (1940). 'Sechs Fälle von symmetrischer intrazerebraler Kalkablagerung in der Stommganglien, verbunden mit epileptischen Anfällen und Geistesstörung disgnostiziert mid Hilfe der Kraniographie und Encephalographie.' *Wien. med. Wschr.*, **90**, 153 (C)

VASTINE, J. A. (1933). 'The pineal body: roentgenological considerations.' *Am. J. Roentg.*, **30**, 145 (C)

VASTINE, J. A. and KINNEY, K. K. (1927). 'The pineal shadow as an aid in the localization of brain tumors.' *Am. J. Roentg.*, **17**, 320 (C)

VERBRUGGHEN, A. and LEARMONTH, J. R. (1932). 'Chondroma of falx cerebri.' *J. nerv. ment. Dis.*, **76**, 463–466 (N)

VIGNAUD, J., JUSTER, M., LERICHE, H., LICHTENBERG, R. and KORACH, G. (1969). 'Radio-Anatomie de la cochlée.' *Acta Radiol.*, **9**, 117–123 (A ; E)

VOGT, A. (1949). 'Spörtschödigungen der Schädelkalotte nach Röntgenbehandlung intracerebraler Tumoren.' *Strahlentherapie*, **80**, 165 (N)

WALTON, J. N. and WARRICK, C. K. (1954). 'Osseous changes in myopathy.' *Br. J. Radiol.*, **27**, 1 (D)

WANG, C. C. and ROBBINS, L. L. (1956). 'Cushing's disease: its roentgenographic findings.' *Radiology*, **67**, 17 (M)

WARKANY, J., PASAARGE, E. and SMITH, L. B. (1966). 'Congenital malformations in autosomal trisomy syndromes.' *Am. J. Dis. Child.*, **112**, 502–517 (D)

WEAVER, D. D., GRAHAM, C. B., THOMAS, I. T. and SMITH, D. W. (1974). 'A new overgrowth syndrome with accelerated skeletal maturation, unusual facies and captodactyly.' *J. Pediat.*, **84**, 547–552 (D)

WEBER, F. P. (1929). 'A note on the association of extensive haemangiomatous naevus of skin with cerebral (meningeal) haemangiona, especially cases of facial vascular naevus with contralateral hemiplegia.' *Proc. R. Soc. Med.*, **22**, 25 (D)

WEICHERT, K. A., DINE, M. S., BENDON, T. and SILVERMAN, F. N. (1973). 'Macrocranium and neurofibromatosis.' *Radiology*, **107**, 163–166 (D ; W ; K)

WEIDNER, W., ROSEN, L. and HANAFEE, W. (1965). 'The neuroradiology of tumors of the pituitary gland.' *Am. J. Roentg.*, **95**, 884–889 (P ; N)

WEINSTEIN, M., TYRRELL, B. and NEWTON, T. H. (1976). 'The sella turcica in Nelson's syndrome.' *Radiology*, **118**, 363–365 (P ; N)

WELIN, S. (1941). 'Roentgendiagnostik dermotitis media acuta.' *Acta Radiol.*, Suppl. 42 (E)

WELLS, P. O. (1956). 'The button sequestrum of eosinophilic granuloma of the skull.' *Radiology*, 67, 746–747 (K)

WESENBERG, R. L., GWINN, J. C. and BARNES, G. R. (1969). 'Radiological findings in the kinky-hair syndrome.' *Radiology*, 92, 500–506 (D)

WEYAND, R. D. and CAMP, J. D. (1954). 'Roentgenographic examination in meningioma of the tuberculum sellae or olfactory groove.' *Am. J. Roentg.*, 71, 947–951 (N)

WHITAKER, P. H. (1959). 'Radiological manipulations in tuberose sclerosis.' *Br. J. Radiol.*, 32, 152 (W)

WICHTL, O. (1952). 'Zur Kenntnis der fibrösen Knochendyplasie.' *Radiol. Austr.*, 5, 61 (D)

WIEDEMANN, H. R. (1964). 'Complexe malformatif familial avec hernie ombilicale et macroglossie–au syndrome nouveau.' *J. Genet, Hum.*, 13, 223–232 (D)

WIEGAND, H. R. (1959). 'Die impressiones digitatae (gyrorum) und die endokranialen Impressionen überhaupt.' *Psychiat. Neurol., Basel*, 138, 272 (R)

WILBRAND, H. F., RASK-ANDERSEN, H. and GILSTRING, D. (1974). 'The vestibular aqueduct and the para-vestibular canal. An anatomic and roentgenologic investigation.' *Acta Radiol.*, 15, 337–355 (A)

WILLIAMS, E. R. (1957). 'The skull at birth.' *J. Fac. Radiol., Lond.*, 8, 290 (A)

WILLIAMS, H. J. (1971). 'Posterior choanal atresia.' *Am. J. Roentg.*, 112, 1–11 (S)

WILLIAMS, J., FOWLER, G. W., PRIBRAM, H. F., DELANEY, C. A. and FISH, C. H. (1972). 'Roentgenographic changes in headbangers.' *Acta Radiol.*, 13, 37–42 (T)

WILSON, A. K. (1944). 'Roentgenological findings in bilateral symmetrical thinness of the parietal bones (senile atrophy).' *Am. J. Roentg.*, 51, 685 (D)

WILSON, A. K. (1947). 'Thinness of the parietal bones.' *Am. J. Roentg.*, 58, 724 (D)

WINDHOLZ, F. (1947). 'Cranial manifestations of fibrous dysplasia of bones: their relation to leontiasis ossea and to simple bone cysts of the vault.' *Am. J. Roentg.*, 58, 51 (D)

WOOD, E. H. (1944). 'Some roentgenological and pathological aspects of calcification of the choroid plexus.' *Am. J. Roentg.*, 52, 388 (C)

WOOD, E. H. and HIMADI, G. M. (1950). 'Chordomas: a roentgenologic study of 16 cases previously unreported.' *Radiology*, 54, 706 (N)

WORLD FEDERATION OF NEUROLOGY (1962). 'Problem Commission of Neuroradiology.' *Br. J. Radiol.*, 35, 501 (G)

WORTH, H. M. and WOLLIN, D. G. (1966). 'Hyperostosis corticalis generalisata congenita.' *J. Can. Ass. Radiol.*, 17, 67–74 (D)

WYKE, B. D. (1949). 'Primary hemangioma of the skull. a rare cranial tumour. Review of the literature and reports of a case, with special reference to the roentgenographic appearance.' *Am. J. Roentg.*, 61, 302 (N)

YOUNG, B. R. (1948). *The Skull, Sinuses and Mastoids. A Handbook of Roentgen Diagnoses.* Chicago; Year Book Publishers (G)

YOUNG, B. R. (1949). 'Roentgen demonstration of displaced intracranial physiologic calcification and its significance in the diagnosis of brain tumor and other space-occupying diseases.' *Radiology*, 53, 625 (C)

YOUNG, R. S., POCHACZEVSKY, R., LEONIDAS, J. C., WEXLER, I. B. and RATNER, H. (1973). 'Thanatophoric dwarfism and cloverleaf skull (Kleeblattschädel).' *Radiology*, 106, 401–405 (D)

YU, H. C. and DECK, M. D. F. (1971). 'The clivus deformity of the Arnold–Chiari malformation.' *Radiology*, 101, 613–615 (D)

YUHL, E. T. and SCHMITZ, A. L. (1969). 'The occipital emissary channel and increased intracranial pressure.' *Acta Radiol.*, 9, 124–127 (R)

YUNE, H. Y., HOLDEN, R. W. and SMITH, J. A. (1975). 'Normal variations and lesions of the sphenoidal sinus.' *Am. J. Roentg.*, 124, 129–138 (S)

ZATZ, L. M. (1968). 'Atypical choroid plexus calcification associated with neurofibromatosis.' *Radiology.*, 91, 1135–1139 (C)

ZAUNBAUER, W. (1955). 'Über das Vorkommen von Verkalkungen bei Epidermoiden des Schädels.' *Forschr. Röntgenst.*, 82, 548 (C ; N)

ZDANSKY, E. (1936). 'Zwei seltene Fälle von Knochenhämangiom.' *Fortschr. Röntgenstr.*, 54, 263 (N)

ZIMMERMAN, R. and LEEDS, N. E. (1976). 'Calvarial and vertebral sarcoidosis. Case report and review of literature.' *Radiology*, 119, 384 (I)

ZIPPEL, H. and SCHÜLER, K-H. (1969). 'Dominant vertebral acrocephalosyndactyly.' *Fortschr. Röntgenstr.*, 110, 234–245 (D)

ZOEPRITZ, U. and SCHMIDT, H. (1961). 'Tuberöse Sklerose une röntgenologische Notfalldiagnostik.' *Fortschr. Röntgenstr.*, 94, 399 (W)

ZYLAK, C. J., CHILDE, A. E., ROSS, R. T. and PARKINSON, D. (0000). 'Lucent unilateral supratentorial dermoid cyst. Report of an unusual case.' *Am. J. Roentg.*, 106, 329–332 (N)

INDEX

Many diseases are mentioned again and again in different chapters, sometimes repetitively. The three about which information is most widely scattered are meningioma, malignant tumours in bone, and Paget's disease.

For the convenience of the reader who wishes to make a systematic study of these without frequent tiresome returns to the index, a separate cross-reference system has been included.

In this system, at the end of each relevant section, there is an instruction for finding the next section in order through the book, omitting only those paragraphs that are pure repetition.

The opening page numbers for these three conditions are:

Malignant disease in bone,	57
Meningioma,	36
Paget's disease.	49

(The page numbers of textual references are in arabic type; the page numbers of illustrations are in italics).